AI-Assisted Medical Diagnostics

A Clinical Guide to Next-Generation Diagnostics

By

Milan Toma, PhD, SMIEEE

2025

Published by: Dawning Research Press
Contact: admin@dawningresearch.org
Website: www.dawningresearch.org

ISBN Numbers

Paperback: 979-8-9998324-3-6
Hardcover: 979-8-9998324-4-3

All information has been carefully verified, and sources are cited throughout the text. The content reflects the author's commitment to evidence-based research and is intended for educational and informational purposes. The views expressed are those of the author and do not necessarily reflect those of any affiliated institutions. While every effort has been made to ensure the accuracy of the information presented, errors or omissions may still occur. If you spot a serious inaccuracy, we encourage you to contact us so that we can make corrections in the next edition. The author and publisher assume no responsibility for errors or omissions, or for damages resulting from the use of the information contained herein.

First Edition

Contents

Preface

Artificial intelligence is rapidly transforming healthcare, offering unprecedented opportunities to enhance patient care, streamline operations, and inform policy. Yet, the promise of artificial intelligence is matched by its complexity and the need for critical, evidence-based evaluation. This book is designed as a practical, clinician-oriented guide to understanding, appraising, and integrating artificial intelligence and machine learning in medical diagnostics and clinical workflows.

The chapters are structured to move from foundational context to hands-on application:

- Chapters 1–2 provide a comprehensive overview of the landscape, definitions, and real-world applications of artificial intelligence in healthcare, highlighting both opportunities and risks. These chapters also address the ethical, legal, and societal considerations that must guide responsible adoption.

- Chapter 3 introduces the core principles of machine learning evaluation, explaining why traditional metrics like accuracy can be misleading and emphasizing the importance of learning curves, class imbalance, fairness, and robust validation.

- Chapter 4 focuses on imaging classification, detailing the modalities, pitfalls, and hallmarks of high-quality studies, and offering practical guidance for selecting and evaluating machine learning models in cardiovascular imaging.

- Chapter 5 surveys core machine learning algorithms, outlining their concepts, strengths, limitations, and clinical examples to help readers understand which tools are best suited for specific diagnostic challenges.

- Chapter 6 presents a standardized validation framework, guiding readers through end-to-end model training and evaluation using clinically oriented composite metrics and emphasizing the necessity of external validation for real-world reliability.

- Chapter 7 explores the critical issues of data leakage and feature selection, demonstrating how superficially strong metrics can mask clinical failure and providing strategies to ensure true generalizability.

- Chapter 8 addresses the practical integration of artificial intelligence in clinical practice, equipping clinicians with key questions to ask, governance considerations, and operational insights for safe deployment.

- Chapter 9 offers actionable checklists and tools to operationalize the appraisal of clinical artificial intelligence, enabling clinicians and decision-makers to rapidly and carefully evaluate artificial intelligence solutions for their own practice.

Throughout, the book emphasizes the importance of interdisciplinary collaboration, transparent reporting, and continuous learning. By combining technical rigor with clinical relevance, it aims to empower healthcare professionals to critically assess artificial intelligence tools, avoid common pitfalls, and harness the full potential of next-generation diagnostics for improved patient outcomes.

Whether you are a clinician, researcher, educator, or policymaker, this guide is intended to support your journey from understanding the fundamentals of artificial intelligence in healthcare to confidently integrating and evaluating these technologies in real-world settings.

Chapter 1

AI in Healthcare

Artificial Intelligence (AI) is a rapidly evolving field in healthcare, with new publications emerging daily, each contributing new perspectives and outputs. AI has become increasingly important in healthcare, offering the potential to enhance patient outcomes, streamline hospital operations, and inform health policy. Its integration into clinical practice, hospital management, and health policy presents both opportunities and challenges that necessitate comprehensive understanding and responsible implementation. A systematic literature review was conducted to assess the implications of AI in healthcare. Peer-reviewed articles, with the focus on AI applications in clinical practice, hospital management, or health policy, published in English from January 2023 onwards were identified. The review revealed that AI significantly enhances clinical practice by improving diagnostic accuracy, offering personalized treatment recommendations, and aiding in patient monitoring. In hospital management, AI contributes to operational efficiency by automating administrative tasks, optimizing resource allocation, and supporting decision-making through predictive analytics. In terms of health policy, AI facilitates evidence-based policymaking, data-driven insights for governance, and has the potential to improve health equity by identifying and addressing healthcare disparities. Despite these benefits, several limitations were identified, including risks of false positives and negatives in clinical applications, model overfitting due to inadequate validation, ethical concerns related to data privacy and fairness, and challenges in regulatory compliance. AI holds substantial promise for advancing healthcare across multiple domains. Realizing its full potential requires addressing ethical considerations, ensuring robust model validation, and fostering collaboration between healthcare professionals and AI experts. Establishing appropriate regulatory frameworks and integrating AI education into medical training are crucial steps toward responsible and effective AI integration in healthcare.

1.1   Introduction

A report by the National Academy of Medicine highlighted three potential advantages of AI in healthcare: enhancing outcomes for patients and clinical teams, reducing healthcare costs, and promoting better population health [1]. Hence, in the complex world of healthcare, AI serves as a pivotal hub, extending its influence into three vital areas (Figure 1.1): Clinical Practice, Hospital Management, and Health Policy. The Clinical Practice branch elucidates the multifaceted role of AI in patient care. It commences with diagnosis, where AI is instrumental in imaging and pathology, providing accurate and timely results. The journey continues to treatment, where AI's capabilities in personalized medicine come to the forefront, tailoring treatments to individual patient needs. The branch culminates with patient monitoring, underscoring AI's integration in wearable technology that enables real-time tracking of patient health metrics. The Hospital Management branch portrays AI's significant contribution to efficient hospital operations. It initiates with resource allocation, where AI's predictive capabilities are leveraged to anticipate patient flow, ensuring optimal utilization of resources. The path proceeds to staff scheduling, where AI optimizes shifts, contributing to improved staff productivity and patient care. The branch concludes with patient data management, emphasizing AI's role in managing electronic health records, ensuring secure and efficient handling of patient data. Lastly, the Health Policy branch demonstrates AI's profound influence on policy-making and regulation. It begins with policy-making, where AI's predictive modeling is utilized for anticipating policy outcomes, aiding in the formulation of effective health policies. The journey continues to regulation, where AI's monitoring capabilities ensure compliance with health regulations. The branch wraps up with public health, where AI's role in tracking disease outbreaks is highlighted, contributing to timely and effective public health responses.

   The integration of AI into healthcare is not just a technological shift but also a significant change in how clinical practices are conducted and

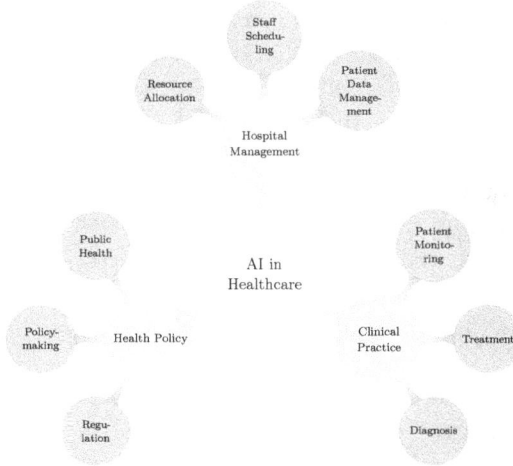

Figure 1.1: Encapsulation of the multifaceted role of AI in the healthcare sector. At the center of the map is the concept of 'AI', which branches out into three key areas 'Clinical Practice', 'Hospital Management', and 'Health Policy'.

how health policies are formulated. AI can enhance diagnostic accuracy, streamline hospital management, and improve patient outcomes. However, it also raises ethical concerns and challenges regarding data privacy, implementation barriers, and the need for regulatory frameworks to ensure safe and effective use.

AI's role in healthcare has been extensively discussed in recent literature. For instance, a study by Bagabir et al. discusses the integration of AI in clinical settings, focusing on its applications in genome sequencing, drug development, and vaccine discovery, particularly in the context of COVID-19 [2]. A review by Giordao et al. highlights various roles AI plays in healthcare, including its impact on patient management and clinical decision-making [3, 4]. A publication by Secinaro et al. examines how AI technologies are reshaping hospital operations and clinical practices, emphasizing efficiency and patient care improvements [5]. An article by Amini et al. reviews the ethical considerations and challenges faced in implementing AI in nursing and healthcare settings [6]. A qualitative interview study with healthcare leaders by Petersson et al. discusses the benefits and challenges of AI in healthcare, focusing on administrative and medical processes [7].

In light of these contributions, it is clear that AI, despite being a driving force for innovation in healthcare, also requires a balanced strategy for its ethical and responsible use. The ongoing discussions and research highlight the importance of continuous evaluation and adaptation in managing the complexities that artificial intelligence introduces into the healthcare field.

The literature search for this chapter was designed to capture the most relevant and recent publications on the implications of AI in healthcare, with a specific focus on hospital management and health policy. The inclusion criteria required that each publication have a Digital Object Identifier (DOI) to ensure traceability and credibility. Only articles published in the English language from January 2023 onwards were considered to ensure the timeliness and relevance of the information. The types of publications included were peer-reviewed research papers, reviews, and clinical studies that directly addressed the use of AI in the specified domains of healthcare.

The search was conducted across several academic databases known for their comprehensive coverage of scientific and medical literature, including PubMed/Medline, Scopus, EMBASE, Web of Science, Google Scholar, and ResearchGate. The search strategy employed a combination of keywords and phrases such as "artificial intelligence in healthcare," "AI in hospital management," and "AI implications for health policy" to filter and retrieve pertinent publications.

The recent literature underscores the transformative potential of AI in healthcare across clinical practice [8,9], hospital management [10], and health policy [5,11,12]. AI technologies have demonstrated the capacity to enhance diagnostic accuracy, personalize treatment, improve operational efficiency, and inform policymaking. However, realizing these benefits requires careful attention to ethical considerations, robust validation of AI models, and collaborative efforts among healthcare professionals, AI experts, and policymakers to ensure responsible and effective implementation.

1.1.1 Clinical Practice

In clinical practice, AI has demonstrated substantial potential in enhancing disease diagnosis, treatment recommendations, and patient monitoring. Studies have shown that AI applications, such as machine learning algorithms and neural networks, have improved diagnostic accuracy in areas like medical imaging, pathology, and chronic disease management [8, 9, 13, 14]. For instance, AI has been utilized in cancer screenings to produce faster and more accurate results [15,16], and in predicting declines in kidney function by analyzing total kidney volume [17]. Additionally, AI supports personalized medicine by optimizing medication dosages and tailoring treatment plans to individual patient profiles [8,11], leading to improved patient outcomes and reduced healthcare costs.

AI has also contributed to advancements in drug discovery and development. Through AI-driven autonomous experimentation systems and generative chemistry platforms, researchers have accelerated the identification of new drug candidates and materials [18–34]. Moreover, AI has enhanced patient safety by reducing the potential for human error and aiding in the management of chronic illnesses such as asthma, diabetes, and hypertension [35–38].

1.1.2 Hospital Management

AI has been instrumental in transforming hospital management by enhancing operational efficiency and resource allocation. The reviewed literature indicates that AI-driven systems automate routine administrative tasks such as scheduling, billing, and record-keeping, thereby reducing administrative burdens and minimizing errors [10,39–45]. AI tools analyze large datasets to provide evidence-based recommendations and predictive analytics, enabling hospital administrators to optimize resource allocation, forecast patient flow, and improve workforce management [5,8,11,13]. For example, AI applications in staff scheduling and capacity planning have contributed to improved productivity and patient care [46,47].

Furthermore, AI has been utilized to enhance patient data management, ensuring secure handling of electronic health records (EHRs) and compliance with regulations [42,43,48]. Predictive analytics help in identifying compliance risks and preventing costly mistakes [49–53]. Overall, AI integration in hospital management leads to streamlined processes, cost savings, and enhanced patient experiences [5,10,39].

1.1.3 Health Policy

In the context of health policy, AI offers new opportunities for evidence-based policymaking, data-driven insights, and promotion of health equity. The literature highlights that AI facilitates accurate data collection and analysis, supporting the formulation of effective health policies [5,11,12,54]. AI models assist policymakers in simulating potential policy outcomes and adjusting strategies in response to emerging health crises, such as pandemic preparedness and vaccine distribution [55, 56]. Additionally, AI helps identify healthcare disparities by analyzing patterns in health data, guiding interventions to address systemic inequities and improve access to healthcare services [6, 57–59].

Despite these benefits, ethical considerations related to data privacy, fairness, and regulatory compliance remain critical challenges that need to be addressed to ensure responsible AI integration in health policy [5, 6, 55]. The development of appropriate regulatory frameworks and global convergence on AI governance in healthcare are essential steps toward mitigating risks and leveraging AI's full potential [6, 60].

1.2   Clinical Practice

AI is making significant strides in clinical practice [9], offering enhanced diagnostic capabilities [61, 62], personalized treatment recommendations [63, 64], and improved patient safety [65, 66]. The articles reviewed demonstrate the diverse applications of AI [39], from drug discovery [19–22] and chronic disease management [67] to surgical assistance [68–71] and medical imaging. As AI technology continues to evolve, its integration into clinical practice promises to revolutionize patient care and health management [8, 9, 35].

AI is used in cancer screenings, such as mammograms [15] and lung cancer screenings [16], to produce faster results. In chronic kidney disease, AI helps predict the decline in kidney function by analyzing total kidney volume [17]. AI also identifies individuals at risk of left ventricular dysfunction [72], even without noticeable symptoms [73]. Additionally, AI assists in managing chronic illnesses like asthma [36], diabetes [37], and high blood pressure [38] by connecting patients with relevant screenings and therapies [35]. AI's role extends to predicting disease outbreaks [74] and aiding in communication [75] and decision-making [76] to prevent spread [77, 78]. It has also shown higher accuracy than traditional pathology methods in predicting survival rates for malignant mesothelioma [79] and improving colonoscopy accuracy [80] by identifying colon polyps [81].

AI, along with algorithm optimization and high-throughput experiments, has enabled rapid discovery of new chemicals [19,20,23–25] and materials [26]. Autonomous experimentation systems, powered by AI, enhance research and development by running numerous chemical experiments autonomously [27–29]. A notable breakthrough was the discovery of a protein kinase inhibitor, designed using AI, which entered clinical trials for its anti-tumor properties [30]. The study utilized AlphaFold [31], an AI program for protein structure prediction [32], integrated with a biocomputational engine and a generative chemistry platform to identify new drugs for hepatocellular carcinoma. AI-driven autonomous experimentation systems are expected to significantly impact biomedical research, particularly in drug discovery and molecular systems engineering [33, 34].

1.3 Hospital Management

The integration of AI-powered solutions in hospital management is significantly transforming operations [10, 46, 82, 83]. AI technologies automate repetitive tasks such as scheduling [40], billing [41], and record-keeping [42, 43], which helps to reduce administrative burdens [39] and minimize errors [44, 45]. AI tools are capable of analyzing large datasets quickly [84], providing evidence-based recommendations [85] and identifying patterns that may not be obvious to healthcare professionals [86]. Additionally, these tools assist in recognizing compliance risks [49] and anomalies in billing [87] and coding, ensuring that healthcare facilities remain compliant with regulations [48] and avoid costly mistakes [88]. By streamlining processes [89] and lessening manual workloads [90–92], AI enhances efficiency [93, 94] and can lead to substantial cost savings for hospitals [95]. Predictive analytics tools can identify areas of potential compliance [50, 51] and audit risk [52], enabling proactive measures to mitigate expensive errors [53, 96]. Overall, AI-driven systems significantly reduce the likelihood of human error [97], improve productivity, and free up staff to concentrate on more high-value responsibilities, including the detection and prevention of healthcare fraud [98].

AI systems have demonstrated their efficiency in reviewing EHRs [99] and updating treatment guidelines [100], significantly accelerating healthcare information processing [101]. Machine learning techniques are being leveraged to analyze unstructured data [102], enhancing decision-making [103] and operational efficiency in healthcare organizations [104]. AI's diverse applications extend to patient diagnosis [105, 106], medical document transcription [107], and drug development [18–34], with various AI types like neural networks [108, 109] and natural language processing [110, 111] playing a role in healthcare management [10, 13, 40, 42, 43, 65, 112]. Finally, AI-driven advancements promise to enhance healthcare with technologies like

whole-body MRI scans [113–115] for preventative screenings [116–118] and
the potential to significantly improve provider productivity while reducing
costs [119–121].

AI has also shown potential to aid in personalized patient flow optimization [122,123], predictive capacity planning [124], and advanced workforce
management tools [10]. AI scheduling algorithms are being leveraged to
customize individual patient pathways in real-time [125], considering specific
patient profiles and treatment timelines [126], which can decrease length of
stay and improved patient throughput [46]. Recent studies have highlighted
the potential of AI to predict and manage peak demand by integrating
hospital data with external factors such as social events [127], seasonal
patterns [128,129], and epidemiological trends, [130] allowing administrators
to deploy resources more effectively [82]. The integration of reinforcement
learning models for inventory and pharmaceutical supply chain management
is enabling hospitals to predict shortages and surpluses [131], maintaining
optimal stock levels without overburdening their storage systems [83]. Workforce allocation has also been improved, with AI identifying patterns of staff
burnout [92,132,133] and suggesting optimal rotation schedules to minimize
fatigue [13,47]. With the ability to constantly learn and adapt from evolving data, AI's role in hospital management is moving beyond basic task
automation to decision-making and strategic planning [39,134], ultimately
enhancing operational resilience and patient-centered care [135,136].

1.4   Health Policy

AI is changing healthcare policymaking by providing new opportunities to
address complex health challenges more effectively. For instance, integrating
AI into health policy has enabled more accurate data collection and analysis,
which directly supports the formulation of evidence-based policies [54]. By
automating the analysis of health data, AI reduces human error and provides
real-time insights that allow policymakers to adjust strategies swiftly, such
as in responding to emerging health crises [55]. This capability is particularly
crucial in addressing public health concerns like pandemic preparedness and
vaccine distribution [56], as AI models can optimize logistics and resource
allocation [137]. However, challenges such as data privacy and ethical
issues, including ensuring compliance with regulations like GDPR [138],
remain central to policy discussions, requiring well-structured AI governance
frameworks [6].

AI also contributes to more equitable health policies by uncovering healthcare disparities [57]. Machine learning algorithms can identify patterns in healthcare data, revealing gaps in service provision to underserved populations [58], which can then be addressed through targeted health interventions [59]. For example, AI's ability to analyze large datasets enables the identification of social determinants of health [139], guiding policymakers in formulating more inclusive policies that address systemic inequities [6]. Furthermore, AI-driven insights help develop proactive policies aimed at reducing healthcare inequalities across different demographic groups [58,140], ensuring that resources are allocated where they are most needed [141] based on emerging trends and outcomes [142].

Moreover, AI plays a pivotal role in evaluating the effectiveness of health policies. Through predictive modeling, AI allows policymakers to simulate the impact of potential policy changes before implementation [143], thereby optimizing decisions and minimizing risks [144]. This approach is particularly useful in assessing the long-term effects of policies related to chronic disease management [145] or public health initiatives [146,147]. AI also provides a mechanism for continuous feedback, enabling policies to be adjusted in real-time based on actual health outcomes [6]. However, the legal and ethical implications of AI in healthcare policy remain a concern, especially regarding accountability and transparency in decision-making processes, highlighting the need for comprehensive regulations to guide AI's role in policymaking [55].

1.5 Limitations

In the field of healthcare, the integration of reliable AI systems is essential, particularly in supporting clinical decision-making processes. These AI systems leverage patient data, including various forms of medical imaging, to aid healthcare professionals in diagnosing and treating diseases more effectively. However, the successful implementation of AI in clinical settings requires a collaborative approach between healthcare professionals and AI experts. Failing to establish this collaboration can lead to significant risks, including the potential for false positives and false negatives, which can have dire consequences for patient care.

1.5.1   False Positives/Negatives

When an AI system incorrectly identifies a disease that is not present, it can lead to unnecessary anxiety for patients, additional invasive testing, and potentially harmful treatments. For instance, if an AI model misclassifies a benign tumor as malignant, the patient may undergo unnecessary surgery or chemotherapy, exposing them to the risks and side effects of these interventions without any real benefit. This not only affects the patient's physical health but can also have profound psychological impacts, leading to stress and diminished quality of life.

Conversely, a false negative occurs when an AI system fails to detect a disease that is present. This can be particularly dangerous in cases of serious conditions such as cancer, where early detection is crucial for effective treatment. If a model overlooks a malignant tumor, the patient may miss the opportunity for timely intervention, leading to disease progression and potentially fatal outcomes. The implications of false negatives can be devastating, resulting in a loss of trust in medical professionals and the healthcare system as a whole.

To mitigate these risks, healthcare professionals must work closely with AI experts who understand the intricacies of machine learning algorithms and their limitations. AI systems are not infallible; they require careful tuning, validation, and continuous monitoring to ensure their accuracy and reliability. By collaborating with AI specialists, healthcare providers can better interpret AI-generated insights, understand the context of the data, and make informed decisions that prioritize patient safety.

Moreover, the integration of AI into clinical workflows should be accompanied by robust training programs for healthcare professionals. This training should focus on understanding how AI systems operate, their potential pitfalls, and the importance of human oversight in the decision-making process. By fostering a culture of collaboration and continuous learning, healthcare organizations can enhance the effectiveness of AI tools while minimizing the risks associated with their use.

1.5.2   Validation Issues

Many of the studies cited here report impressively high accuracy rates, often in the high 90s. However, without proper data splitting and validation, these results may be overoptimistic due to the risk of overfitting. Overfitting occurs when a model learns the training data too well–including the noise–and fails to perform adequately on new, unseen data.

It is common practice in many studies to split the dataset into 80% for training and 20% for testing, but there is often no mention of a separate validation set. Without a validation set, hyperparameters may have been tuned based on the test set, which should remain untouched until the final evaluation. This practice risks data leakage and overfitting, as it precludes the ability to detect overfitting during training and raises concerns about the optimization and tuning of the model [148].

Additionally, without testing on external data, the model's generalizability cannot be assessed. Patient data can vary significantly between individuals due to differences in physiology, device placements, geography, socioeconomics, noise characteristics, and many other factors. A model that generalizes well should perform consistently across diverse datasets. However, many studies do not include the use of an external testing set (or hold-out set) [149]. An external testing set–ideally sourced from a different dataset or collected under different conditions–is vital for assessing the model's generalizability. Without it, models may perform well on a specific dataset but fail to generalize to data from different patient populations or recording environments. Therefore, by not including an external testing set, it is difficult to ascertain how the proposed model would perform in real-world clinical settings.

1.6 Discussion

The integration of AI in healthcare goes beyond mere technology, encompassing significant moral and ethical considerations [150, 151]. To make AI more transparent, regulated, and usable, Explainable AI serves as a pivotal advancement in machine learning models, enhancing their clarity and applicability in various domains [152, 153]. In the current global regulatory landscape, most regulations governing AI primarily focus on Software as a Medical Device, which falls under the category of digital health products [60]. However, it is crucial to recognize that these existing regulations may be insufficient. AI technologies possess the ability to operate autonomously, adapt their algorithms, and enhance their performance over time based on new real-world data they encounter. To address these challenges, establishing a global regulatory convergence for AI in healthcare would be advantageous. This approach could mirror the voluntary AI code of conduct being developed by the US-EU Trade and Technology Council [154]. The use of AI for decision-making presents ethical challenges due to its complex characteristics, which can result in errors, a loss of human control, and difficulties in assigning responsibility, leading to a need for a careful evaluation of the costs and benefits in high-stakes situations [155]. The integration of AI in healthcare raises concerns about unfairly placing legal liability on clinicians for errors and adverse outcomes, as they may be held responsible for system malfunctions over which they have limited control [156]. To address the complexities of liability in AI-integrated healthcare systems, several potential solutions have been proposed. These include recognizing that liability should not rest solely on clinicians, as many individuals are involved in the AI's design, implementation, and operation. Risk pooling between clinicians and software development companies through insurance schemes has been suggested to cover AI-related damages [157]. Additionally, there is a call for a shift in how AI systems are treated legally, potentially viewing them as part of the clinical team rather than mere products [158], which could help clarify responsibility. However, current legal frameworks present significant challenges, making it difficult to establish clear liability for AI-related errors.

Fortunately, medical colleges are recognizing the importance of preparing future healthcare professionals for this new era. Many institutions are proactively integrating AI education into their curricula, ensuring that students are equipped with the knowledge and skills necessary to navigate the complexities of AI in clinical practice. By incorporating AI into medical education, students learn how these systems work, including the algorithms and data inputs that drive their functionality. This foundational knowledge is essential for interpreting AI-generated insights accurately and making informed clinical decisions. Education on AI also includes discussions about its limitations and potential biases. Understanding these factors helps future healthcare professionals critically evaluate AI recommendations and avoid over-reliance on technology, which can lead to errors in diagnosis and treatment. Training programs must emphasize the importance of human oversight in the decision-making process. Students learn that while AI can enhance diagnostic accuracy and efficiency, it should complement, not replace, the expertise and judgment of healthcare providers. By fostering a collaborative mindset, medical colleges prepare students to work alongside AI experts and data scientists [159]. This interdisciplinary approach is vital for optimizing the use of AI in clinical settings and ensuring that patient care remains the primary focus. The field of AI is rapidly evolving, and ongoing education is necessary to keep pace with new developments. Medical colleges traditionally instill a culture of continuous learning, encouraging future healthcare professionals to stay informed about advancements in healthcare technology and its applications in medicine.

Chapter 2

Definitions and Applications

Artificial intelligence (AI) has emerged as a crucial tool in healthcare with the primary aim of improving patient outcomes and optimizing healthcare delivery. By harnessing machine learning algorithms, natural language processing, and computer vision, AI enables the analysis of complex medical data. The integration of AI into healthcare systems aims to support clinicians, personalize patient care, and enhance population health, all while addressing the challenges posed by rising costs and limited resources. As a subdivision of computer science, AI focuses on the development of advanced algorithms capable of performing complex tasks that were once reliant on human intelligence. The ultimate goal is to achieve human-level performance with improved efficiency and accuracy in problem-solving and task execution, thereby reducing the need for human intervention. Various industries, including engineering, media/entertainment, finance, and education, have already reaped significant benefits by incorporating AI systems into their operations. Notably, the healthcare sector has witnessed rapid growth in the utilization of AI technology. Nevertheless, there remains untapped potential for AI to truly revolutionize the industry. It is important to note that despite concerns about job displacement, AI in healthcare should not be viewed as a threat to human workers. Instead, AI systems are designed to augment and support healthcare professionals, freeing up their time to focus on more complex and critical tasks. By automating routine and repetitive tasks, AI can alleviate the burden on healthcare professionals, allowing them to dedicate more attention to patient care and meaningful interactions. However, legal and ethical challenges must be addressed when embracing AI technology in medicine, alongside comprehensive public education to ensure widespread acceptance.

2.1   Introduction

The origins of AI can be traced back to more than 70 years ago, specifically during World War II. It was during this time that mathematician Alan Turing developed The Bombe, an electro-mechanical computer spanning almost 50 square feet in size. A remarkable feat at the time, The Bombe successfully broke the Enigma code, a task previously believed to be impossible even for the most brilliant human mathematicians [160]. This pivotal moment in history ignited further inquiry into the potential of creating machines capable of incorporating external data and processing it using algorithms to produce useful and efficient outcomes for various tasks. In 1950, Alan Turing examined the possibility of creating intelligent computational machines that could imitate human thought processes. He developed a method known as the Turing test to assess whether a machine's responses can be distinguished from those of a human [161]. If the machine's answers are indistinguishable from a human's, it is considered intelligent. Several years later in 1956, John McCarthy coined the term "Artificial Intelligence", describing it as the computational aspect of achieving goals and capable of being precisely defined for simulation by machines [162].

Despite the decades-long development of AI, as illustrated in Figure 2.1, public awareness of AI remained relatively limited until very recently. For much of its history, AI research and its applications advanced steadily but largely out of the public eye. Notable breakthroughs such as the invention of the perceptron in the 1950s, the introduction of backpropagation in the 1980s, and the rise of deep learning in the 2010s were milestones recognized primarily within academic and professional circles. It was not until the viral launch of large language models (LLMs), with ChatGPT's public release in late 2022 serving as a watershed moment, that AI moved into mainstream consciousness and everyday conversation. Prior to this popularization, AI had already been working "behind the scenes" in a range of domains, including medical diagnostics, where machine learning algorithms have supported tasks such as image analysis and disease detection for years. AI-based diagnostic systems, such as those used for radiology and pathology, have been researched and adopted since at least the early 2000s; e.g., [163]. The opportunity for the general public to directly interact with LLMs changed perceptions almost overnight, shifting AI from a background technology to a topic of widespread fascination and debate.

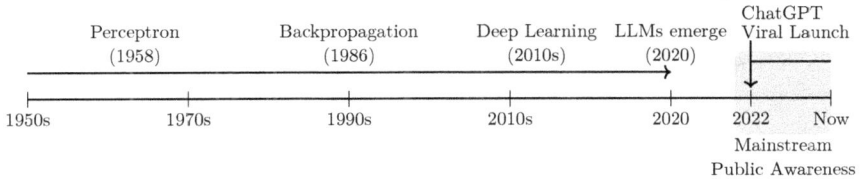

Figure 2.1: The timeline highlights key innovations in AI and machine learning, including the creation of the perceptron (1958), the development of backpropagation (1986), the advent of deep learning (2010s), and the emergence of large language models (2020). The shaded area marks the viral launch of ChatGPT in late 2022, which heralded the onset of mainstream public awareness. Prior to this, most AI advancements occurred without significant public attention, despite AI's integration into specialized domains such as healthcare and industry

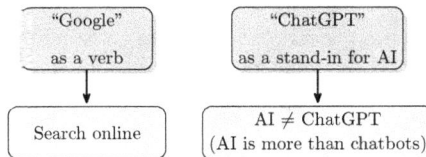

Figure 2.2: The rise of ChatGPT has led to its name becoming synonymous with AI in popular discourse, much like "Google" became shorthand for searching the web. However, just as searching predates Google and encompasses more than a single company, AI is a broad field with a rich history and diverse applications that extend far beyond any one system or interface.

While ChatGPT's explosive popularity dramatically elevated public awareness of AI, it also created a misconception: that ChatGPT is synonymous with AI itself. This phenomenon parallels how "Google" became a verb for online searching, despite being just one of many tools for that purpose, depicted in Figure 2.2. In reality, AI is a vast and multifaceted discipline that has existed for decades, encompassing a range of methods and applications; from early expert systems and symbolic reasoning to modern machine learning, robotics, and specialized diagnostic agents used in medicine, finance, and industry. The field includes numerous intelligent agents, each with their own strengths and specialties, many of which operate quietly behind the scenes without fanfare or public recognition. Conflating AI solely with ChatGPT or conversational agents overlooks the breadth and depth of AI's contributions and ongoing evolution. As the public conversation around AI continues, it is vital to recognize the distinction between the popular face of AI and the much larger, dynamic landscape it represents.

Since the inception of AI, this field has experienced rapid advancement. Following its successful demonstration in passing the Turing test, AI began to make significant contributions across various industries. One early adopter was the automotive industry, which witnessed an infusion of AI technology starting in the early 1960s. In particular, John Devol and Joseph Engelberger pioneered the development of Unimate, a groundbreaking industrial robot introduced in 1961. Originally designed for die-casting tasks, it later found application in workpiece handling and spot-welding processes involved in car body manufacturing [164]. Subsequently, advancements were made towards creating conversational systems using chatbots powered by AI algorithms. In 1966, Joseph Weizenbaum introduced Eliza, the first chatbot. Eliza could engage in conversations with humans by utilizing pattern matching to generate appropriate responses based on textual inputs [165]. During the same period, Charles A. Rosen created Shakey, a pioneering achievement that enabled an electronic entity capable of executing complex tasks and identifying errors for correction [166]. These significant milestones played a crucial role in shaping AI's impact across industries and its subsequent expansion into healthcare applications.

During the period from the 1970s to the 2000s, there was a decline in significant advancements in AI known as the "AI winter". However, this downturn resulted in increased utilization of AI in the medical field [167]. Ophthalmology emerged as one of the early adopters of incorporating AI technology. A notable example was the development of CASNET/glaucoma model in 1976, which utilized stored patient data to make informed decisions based on physiological parameter changes, clinical manifestations, and treatment outcomes [168]. This model showcased the potential of AI in ophthalmology and paved the way for further advancements in the field. A similar system known as the INTERNIST-1 was developed to assist physicians in accurately diagnosing complex internal medicine diseases [169]. In 1996, the ZEUS robotic surgery system was introduced as the first complete remote surgery system, designed to enhance laparoscopic procedures by eliminating motion scaling and tremors [170]. These early advancements in AI within the medical field have sparked renewed interest in AI applications throughout medicine in the 21st century. Figure 2.3 illustrates the significant surge in AI research over the past decade.

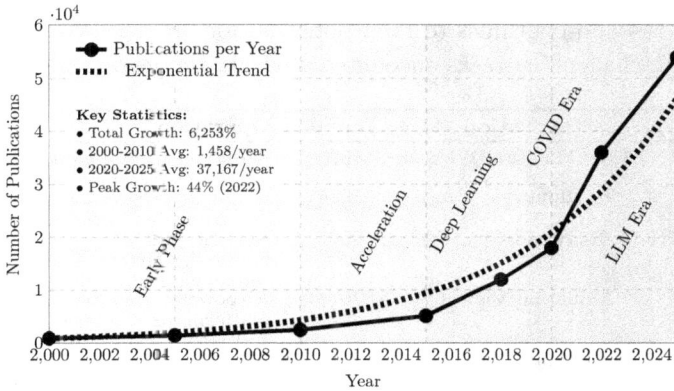

Figure 2.3: Exponential rise in AI in medicine/healthcare publications (2000-2025). PubMed-indexed publications per year showing growth from 850 (2000) to 54,000 (2025), a 6,253% increase across five developmental eras: Early Phase, Acceleration, Deep Learning, COVID Era, and LLM Era. The exponential trend line and phase-specific growth rates (10.7% to 38.5% annually) illustrate the dramatic acceleration of AI research in healthcare, particularly following major technological breakthroughs.

In recent years, there has been a significant surge of interest in integrating AI into the medical domain. Continuous advancements and enhancements of AI have paved the way for its application in complex medical cases. For instance, in 2017 AI technology was introduced to cardiology through CardioAI, an innovative clinical design that utilizes deep learning algorithms to analyze cardiac magnetic resonance images rapidly. This groundbreaking development enables the swift determination of essential information such as cardiac ejection fraction within seconds [171]. Subsequently, similar techniques were extended to lung imaging analysis and interpretation of musculoskeletal system X-ray images as well as head CT scans. A noteworthy step forward occurred in 2019, when AI was utilized collaboratively with endoscopies, demonstrating promising potential for future growth while remaining subject to ongoing refinement and improvement. The use of computer-aided diagnosis (CAD) has enabled accurate detection, differentiation, and characterization of both neoplastic and non-neoplastic colon polyps, with an average accuracy rate of 91.5% [171]. Moreover, the field of AI in healthcare has witnessed the emergence of several companies that contribute to various aspects of medicine; for examples, see Table 2.1. Such companies support robotic surgeries, data collection from patients, and prompt diagnosis and treatment through blood tests for early-stage cancers. This highlights how AI has evolved into an effective tool from its inception in the 1950s and continues to hold potential for further advancements in addressing challenging tasks encountered within the medical domain.

Name	Location	Founded	Operation
Accuray	Madison, WI	1990	AI-driven radiation oncology systems for cancer treatment
Intuitive	Sunnyvale, CA	1995	Robot-assisted minimally invasive surgeries (da Vinci Surgical System)
Auris Health	Redwood City, CA	2007	Robotic endoscopy systems for minimally invasive diagnostic and therapeutic procedures
Qventus	Mountain View, CA	2012	AI-powered hospital operations platform for real-time patient flow and resource optimization
H2O.ai	Mountain View, CA	2012	AI and machine learning platform for predictive analytics and clinical decision support in healthcare
Atomwise	San Francisco, CA	2012	AI-driven drug discovery and molecular analysis
Enlitic	Fort Collins, CO	2014	AI-powered medical imaging solutions for radiology workflow and diagnostic support
Freenome	Brisbane, CA	2014	AI-driven blood tests for early cancer detection using multi-omics data
Buoy Health	Boston, MA	2014	AI-powered digital health assistant for symptom assessment and care navigation
CloudMedx	Palo Alto, CA	2015	AI-driven clinical and operational analytics for population health and care management
Tempus AI	Chicago, IL	2015	AI-powered precision medicine platform for personalized cancer care
KenSci	Seattle, WA	2015	AI-based predictive analytics for risk and cost management in healthcare
PathAI	Boston, MA	2016	AI-powered pathology solutions for disease diagnosis from tissue samples

Table 2.1: *Examples of AI healthcare companies in the US.*

This chapter contributes to the book by: (a) providing readers with a clear and concise understanding of the topic through a detailed overview of AI, including its origins, evolution, and current state, with a particular focus on its uses within healthcare; (b) reviewing and analyzing varied applications of AI in healthcare, ranging from diagnostics and medical imaging to surgical assistance, patient prognosis, and treatment decision-making; (c) discussing AI's role and impact during pandemic scenarios, demonstrating its potential in disease identification, monitoring patients, determining mortality risk, managing data, and facilitating rapid response, accurate diagnosis, and efficient treatment; (d) highlighting the potential advantages and challenges associated with the integration of AI in healthcare, including ethical, legal, and social considerations, while raising awareness about the need for regulated and ethically guided use of AI in medicine; (e) detailing the role of AI in contemporary innovations such as remote monitoring, telehealth, drug discovery, vaccine development, and natural language processing; and (f) providing a thorough view of AI's transformative potential in various medical fields, such as rehabilitation, gastroenterology, nutritional assessment, and surgery.

This chapter is organized into several cohesive sections, each serving a specific purpose. (1) Introduction: introduces the topic at hand, establishes its relevance, and presents an overview of the current state of knowledge in the field. It also outlines the objectives of the paper. (2) Key principles of AI: describes the structured methodologies and advanced techniques used in AI, such as artificial neural networks and deep learning, and their successful applications in predictive modeling within the medical domain. (3) Key Applications of AI in Healthcare: explores the diverse applications of AI in health care, ranging from diagnostics and medical imaging to surgical assistance, patient prognosis, and treatment decision-making. (4) The Role of AI in Medicine: discusses the transformative potential of AI in various medical fields, touching upon areas such as rehabilitation, gastroenterology, nutritional assessment, and surgery, among others. (5) Considerations of AI Applications: tackles the crucial ethical, legal, and social considerations that arise from the integration of AI in healthcare, addressing issues related to accountability, liability, privacy protection, bias and discrimination, transparency, consent, and the balance between innovation and regulatory oversight. (6) Discussion: synthesizes the contents of the previous sections, contemplating the implications of the findings, examining potential challenges, and offering thoughts on future directions in the field of AI in healthcare. This structure ensures comprehensive coverage of the topic and aids readers in understanding the various aspects of the AI in healthcare.

2.2   Key Principles of AI

The field of AI utilizes a structured method to integrate external data, employing intricate algorithms that ultimately yield accurate predictions for specific scenarios [172]. This systematic process involves advanced techniques such as artificial neural networks and deep learning. By appropriately selecting and implementing the algorithm tailored to the technique being employed [173], AI has successfully found its applications in predictive modeling within the medical domain. Figure 2.4 depicts the use of neural networks for medical decision support. This process might encompass various steps such as collecting and preprocessing data, training the model, revising the model through cross-validation, choosing the best model, and integrating it with systems such as desktop applications or embedded devices and hardware.

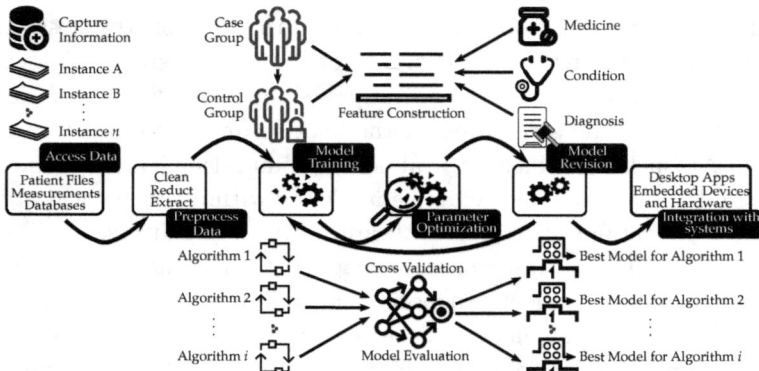

Figure 2.4: The use of neural networks for medical decision support. This procedure typically includes multiple stages such as gathering and preprocessing data, developing the model, refining the model via cross-validation, selecting the optimal model, and amalgamating it with systems like desktop software or embedded hardware and devices.

2.2.1 Artificial Neural Networks

Artificial Neural Networks (ANNs) have gained popularity in the medical domain due to their effectiveness in diagnostics and imaging detection. They are commonly used for clinical diagnosis, including histopathology evaluations and electrocardiograms (ECGs). In addition, ANNs have been integrated into surgical diagnostic procedures covering aspects such as abdominal pain assessment, appendicitis identification, detection of retained common bile duct stones, and evaluation of glaucomas [174]. These networks draw inspiration from the nervous system and employ a sophisticated methodology for gathering input data that ensures accurate results are obtained. In the medical field, accurate diagnosis is crucial for effective treatment and patient care.

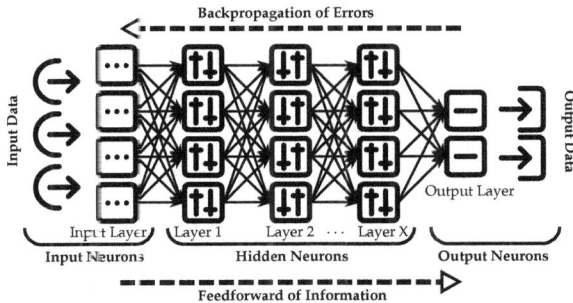

Figure 2.5: Neural elements of a multilayer feedforward backpropagation network.

As depicted in Figure 2.5, artificial neural networks comprise interconnected layers that guide input data towards the intended path in order to produce a reliable output. The input data are initially processed and gathered in the input layer, which captures general information. The data then traverse multiple subsequent layers (layer 1, layer 2, etc.), ensuring greater accuracy of the resulting output. Upon traversing these deeper layers, the data reach the final output layer, where an appropriate solution or answer is generated based on the provided input. ANNs effectively select optimal paths for data while minimizing inaccuracies by eliminating alternative pathways during processing. The application of ANNs in medical diagnosis is becoming increasingly prevalent, as they offer a promising solution for accurate and efficient diagnostics.

In the context of ANNs, "choosing the best path for the data" refers to the network's ability to evaluate input data and make informed decisions regarding which connections and pathways within the network should be activated. This process involves analyzing patterns and features in order to adjust connection strengths between neurons while giving priority to relevant information. By selecting an appropriate pathway through the network, the probability of producing accurate outputs is increased. To determine this optimal path, various factors are considered by the ANN, including the weights assigned to connections and the activation functions applied to the neurons. These considerations enable informed decision-making with the goal of minimizing errors or inaccuracies in the findings [175].

The "feed forward" model described here relies on a substantial amount of data to effectively determine the optimal pathway. Furthermore, this network commonly utilizes a backpropagation algorithm, in which information flows backwards from the deepest layer to match inputs and outputs by minimizing discrepancies between predicted values and known correct outputs [176]. In essence, the available data are meticulously analyzed to provide an accurate solution.

2.2.2 Deep Learning Networks

Deep Learning Networks (DLNs) are a subfield of AI with a broad scope, encompassing image diagnostics. DLNs are frequently combined with other networks in the same category, including Artificial Neural Networks and Convolutional Neural Networks (CNNs). CNNs specifically fall under the category of ANNs, and adopt a similar methodology. Inspired by the visual perception abilities of living organisms, CNNs consist of multiple layers and employ backpropagation algorithms to directly recognize visual patterns without extensive preprocessing [177]. DLNs share this cascading approach across several layers for information extraction; however, they incorporate additional learning modalities such as unsupervised pattern analysis and supervised classification into their framework as well. Supervised learning focuses on establishing a connection between input and desired output by utilizing the provided inputs and their corresponding correct outputs. The algorithm learns by comparing its actual output to the correct outputs, enabling it to identify errors and making it beneficial for tasks such as classification and prediction [178]. In contrast, unsupervised learning involves finding solutions to unlabeled information without any given guidance. The algorithm must explore the provided data in order to create a meaningful structure. This process relies on hierarchical representation, in which higher-level features are derived from lower-level ones, resulting in a hierarchy of concepts being formed [178]. Overall, deep neural networks play an integral role in incorporating neural networks alongside various learning modalities for efficient analysis of data and representation of images. Therefore, DLNs, particularly CNNs, are widely used in image diagnostics thanks to their ability to directly recognize visual patterns without extensive preprocessing.

2.2.3 Machine Learning

Machine Learning (ML) is an extensive branch of AI that encompasses various types of networks. It shares similarities with DLNs in terms of utilizing supervised and unsupervised learning techniques. Additionally, ML incorporates a third learning modality called semi-supervised learning, which combines aspects of both supervised and unsupervised approaches.

The primary objective of this approach is to leverage unlabeled data as a way to enhance model performance [179]. ML is a distinctive branch of AI that utilizes datasets to learn and draw correlations between variables [180]. Unlike traditional problem solving techniques, ML does not rely on predefined step-by-step processes. Instead, it leverages the power of data analysis to identify patterns and trends in specific characteristics for accomplishing complex tasks [181]. This integrative approach incorporating various subfields makes ML an invaluable tool applicable across diverse industries.

2.2.4 Key Principles of AI within the Context of Healthcare

To reiterate the above within the context of healthcare, the relationships between ANNs, DLNs, and ML are described below to provide a more comprehensive understanding of their interplay within the field of AI. ANNs play a fundamental role in AI for healthcare applications. ANNs are computational models inspired by the structure and functioning of biological neural networks. They have been extensively utilized in various healthcare applications, including disease diagnosis, prognosis, and treatment prediction. They consist of interconnected artificial neurons that process and transmit information in a manner similar to the human brain. ANNs have demonstrated remarkable capabilities in pattern recognition, feature extraction, and nonlinear mapping, making them highly effective in analyzing complex medical data. DLNs build upon the foundations of ANNs, and have revolutionized the field of AI in healthcare. DLNs are composed of multiple layers of artificial neurons, enabling the creation of deep neural networks capable of learning hierarchical representations of data. This depth allows DLNs to automatically extract complex and abstract features from medical images, signals, and textual data. Their ability to learn from large-scale datasets has facilitated significant advancements in medical imaging analysis, natural language processing, and clinical decision support systems.

The relationship between ANNs and DLNs is progressive, with DLNs representing a more advanced and complex form of neural network architecture. While ANNs laid the groundwork for neural network-based approaches, DLNs have extended these capabilities by introducing deeper architectures and more sophisticated learning algorithms. This progression has enabled the development of highly accurate and robust models in healthcare applications. ML encompasses a broader range of techniques including both ANNs and DLNs. It refers to the field of study that focuses on algorithms and models capable of automatically learning from data and making predictions or decisions without being explicitly programmed. ML techniques in healthcare leverage the power of ANN and DLN models, along with other approaches such as decision tree [182], support vector machine [183], and random forest [184]. These techniques enable the extraction of valuable insights from healthcare data, facilitating tasks such as patient risk stratification, treatment recommendation, and health outcome prediction. It is important to note that within the context of this manuscript ML refers to the specific range of techniques employed in the analysis of healthcare data, incorporating both ANN and DLN. This distinction is important to remember in order to avoid any potential confusion regarding the scope of ML in the context of this review.

Additionally, different ML algorithms are particularly suited to different applications. For example, certain models might perform better in image analysis for diagnosis, while others might be more effective in forecasting disease spread. Comparing the efficacy of different ML models using the same datasets is of paramount importance in the field of AI. Such comparisons allow researchers and practitioners to gain insights into the strengths and weaknesses of various models, enabling them to make informed decisions about which approach to adopt for a given task. By applying multiple models to the same dataset, it becomes possible to assess their performance, accuracy, and generalization capabilities, e.g., [81]. This process promotes a better understanding of the underlying algorithms and their suitability for specific problem domains, and can aid in identifying the most effective and efficient solution. Additionally, comparing different models on the same datasets fosters fair and unbiased evaluations, contributing to the advancement of machine learning techniques and driving innovation in the field.

2.3   Key Applications of AI in Healthcare

The various subfields and modalities of AI discussed earlier have the potential to greatly impact different industries, leading to overall improvements and growth. The recent COVID-19 pandemic has created a pressing need for digital solutions, particularly in the medical field. Machine learning has found applications in tasks such as medical imaging, disease diagnosis,

patient prognosis, and treatment decision-making [185–187]. Moreover, AI
has been successfully integrated into other important aspects of healthcare
such as virtual nursing assistants and reducing medication errors [188]. As
shown in Table 2.2, the majority of AI applications are within the medical
field due to several key factors that must be addressed for optimal patient
care outcomes. Notably, these advancements hold significant financial value,
with an estimated combined annual worth exceeding USD 100 billion over
the next three years.

Application	Value	Assists with...
Robot-assisted surgery	$40B	more types of surgery
Virtual nursing assistant	$20B	reduced labor shortage
Administrative workflow	$18B	writing, transcribing, infrastructure
Fraud detection	$17B	complex fraud attempts
Dosage error reduction	$16B	medical errors
Connected machines	$14B	proliferation of connected devices
Clinical trial participation	$13B	plethora of data
Preliminary diagnosis	$5B	increased diagnosis accuracy
Image diagnosis	$3B	storage capacity
Cybersecurity	$2B	protecting health data

Table 2.2: AI Applications in Healthcare: Estimated Annual Values and Primary
Functions (Source: Accenture; hbr.org).

The key applications of AI in healthcare include the following. In
medical imaging and radiology, AI is already reshaping diagnostics by
interpreting X-rays, CT scans, and MRIs with remarkable precision [189].
This technology is not limited to the radiology suite; it is equally valuable
in the realm of clinical trials and research, where it optimizes patient
selection, enhances monitoring, and streamlines data collection—ultimately
making research endeavors more efficient [190]. Managing electronic health
records (EHRs) remains a time-consuming task for many clinicians, but
AI is stepping in to simplify information capturing and facilitate nuanced
data analysis. Natural language processing is helping to extract meaningful
insights from clinical notes, improving workflow and supporting better
patient care [191]. Perhaps most compelling is AI's impact on diagnosis and
clinical decision-making. Sophisticated algorithms are assisting clinicians
in identifying complex diseases, including various cancers, with improved
accuracy, and are providing valuable support for critical decision points in
patient management [192, 193]. In the operating room, AI-powered robotic
systems such as the Da Vinci and Smart Tissue Autonomous Robot are

enhancing surgical precision, allowing for minimally invasive procedures and improved patient outcomes [194].

Personalized medicine is another area where AI is making significant inroads. By integrating individual genetic profiles and other patient-specific data, AI helps clinicians tailor therapies, which is especially promising in oncology, where it can improve treatment success rates [122, 195]. Risk assessment and prognostication are being revolutionized as well—AI can rapidly process vast amounts of historical and real-time data, flagging high-risk patients and predicting disease trajectories to inform clinical strategies [196–198]. The reach of AI extends beyond the hospital walls through telemedicine and virtual health assistants, offering assessments and healthcare recommendations that improve access and continuity of care, particularly for patients in remote or underserved areas [199, 200]. In the field of drug discovery and development, AI accelerates the identification of promising compounds and can suggest effective drug combinations for challenging diseases such as cancer [201]. Finally, AI plays a crucial role in patient monitoring and ongoing care. By tracking symptoms and physiological parameters in real time, AI supports clinicians in promptly detecting complications and responding to patient needs more effectively [202]. Collectively, these advances underscore how AI is enhancing efficiency, accuracy, and precision throughout every stage of healthcare delivery, from diagnosis through treatment and follow-up.

2.4   The Role of AI in Medicine

In order to fully comprehend the extent of AI's contribution to the healthcare industry, an examination of the existing state of medical care is necessary. This includes acknowledging any limitations that can potentially be addressed and resolved through the integration of AI. For example, when patients lack sufficient understanding of medical procedures it hinders their ability to provide informed consent. This inadequacy is mainly attributed to time constraints and a lack of personalization. To address this issue, the utilization of an AI-powered chatbot has been found to improve the informed consent process. In a study, patients were randomly assigned to either a conventional informed consent group or an AI-supported chatbot group [203]. The findings indicated that although satisfaction levels were comparable between the two groups, the AI group exhibited significantly higher levels of accurate comprehension regarding the procedure and its associated risks. The subsequent sections present a comprehensive outline of current challenges within healthcare that stand to benefit from advancements in AI technology.

2.4.1   Financial Burdens in Healthcare

Excessive spending poses a significant challenge to the US healthcare system. Previous research indicates that unnecessary costs in the range of USD 760 to 935 billion are incurred annually, which represents almost 25% of the country's total healthcare budget [204]. This substantial economic burden weighs heavily on the overall US economy and is predominantly due to inefficiencies within the current healthcare system. The integration of AI into this framework has emerged as a potential solution, with projected cost savings of nearly USD 150 billion anticipated by 2026 [167]. These extra funds generated through AI implementation could be directed towards addressing existing healthcare concerns, thereby enhancing patient care quality and improving outcomes for patients overall.

The integration of AI technologies in healthcare is offering significant opportunities to ease financial pressures in a variety of ways that go well beyond simply automating administrative tasks. One major benefit is in improving the accuracy and speed of both diagnosis and treatment. By supporting clinicians in making more precise decisions, AI reduces the likelihood of unnecessary tests and procedures, which in turn helps to lower overall healthcare costs. Predictive analytics powered by AI can also play a crucial role in preventing disease before it develops, minimizing the need for costly treatments and extended hospital stays.

AI is also enhancing the effectiveness of telemedicine platforms, enabling the remote diagnosis of patient symptoms. This not only helps reduce the expenses associated with in-person hospital visits but also makes healthcare more accessible and affordable for patients who may face barriers to reaching traditional facilities. In the realm of drug discovery, AI accelerates the identification of promising drug candidates by predicting interactions between drugs and the body. This can significantly shorten a process that is traditionally time-consuming and costly, leading to substantial savings in research and development. Personalized medicine is another area where AI demonstrates considerable value. By analyzing individual health and genetic data, AI can help clinicians tailor treatments to each patient's unique profile. This individualized approach can improve treatment efficacy while reducing the reliance on expensive trial-and-error prescribing.

Additionally, AI supports better resource allocation within hospitals and clinics by predicting patient inflow. This allows healthcare organizations to optimize the use of staff, equipment, and space, thereby minimizing wastage and avoiding cost overruns. AI also contributes to predictive maintenance of medical equipment. By forecasting when machines require servicing, healthcare facilities can prevent unexpected equipment failures and the associated costs, making it easier to plan for repairs or replacements within budget. Finally, AI is proving valuable in detecting insurance fraud. By identifying potentially false claims, AI helps generate significant cost savings for both healthcare providers and insurance companies, further alleviating financial strain across the healthcare system.

2.4.2   Redundant Administrative Tasks

The primary reason for excessive healthcare spending is due to significant allocations towards administrative expenses which encompass various redundant tasks such as reviewing patient records, documenting encounters, and managing medical files [205]. Administrative duties are indispensable in the healthcare system; however, they consume a substantial amount of time and effort that could otherwise be dedicated to providing direct patient care. On average, nurses in the United States spend 25% of their working hours on administrative tasks [206]. While it remains crucial for healthcare professionals to attend to these essential responsibilities, there exists an opportunity to enhance efficiency through the utilization of AI. AI has the potential to automate and streamline healthcare administrative systems, reducing the burden on healthcare providers and optimizing processes [207]. In the emerging era, AI has exhibited a remarkable ability to efficiently carry out administrative functions on par with human capabilities [208]. While it cannot completely supplant the indispensable role of humans in healthcare management, AI presents an opportunity to optimize and streamline these operations, thereby assisting providers in their day-to-day administrative responsibilities. By delegating repetitive organizational tasks to automated systems, valuable time can be liberated for meaningful patient-care interactions. Furthermore, AI can improve accuracy and reduce errors in administrative tasks such as reviewing patient records and managing medical files [209].

2.4.3   Provider Burnout

An increasingly prevalent issue in modern healthcare systems is the phenomenon of provider burnout. Studies have found that burnout is a prevalent issue among healthcare professionals, including physicians and other workers in the field [210]. This syndrome can have detrimental effects on mental well-being as well as on the quality and safety of patient care. To mitigate the effects of burnout and improve the overall well-being of healthcare providers, it is crucial to address the contributing factors that lead to burnout, such as excessive workload and burdensome administrative tasks. Provider burnout refers to a chronic stress reaction that arises from emotional exhaustion, mental health decline, and feelings of depersonalization experienced by healthcare professionals due to systemic and organizational factors [211]. According to recent research findings, approximately 25.6% of physicians reported experiencing symptoms associated with burnout [212]. Interestingly, it was discovered that EHR systems played a significant role in contributing to these symptoms, as indicated by 74.5% of survey respondents attributing EHR as the primary cause [212]. Recognizing the critical impact on patient well-being, it becomes essential to acknowledge the importance of maintaining good physical and mental health among healthcare providers who must perform at their utmost capacity to ensure high-quality care delivery. The issue of burnout among healthcare providers remains a persistent challenge for healthcare organizations globally. Efforts are currently underway to address this issue, including the introduction of natural language processing (NLP)-based AI systems [213]. These NLP analytics can generate insights and analyze patient data on a large scale, offering opportunities to optimize electronic health record systems cost-effectively and efficiently [214]. While integrating NLP in EHR requires continued effort and improvement, the potential benefits of increased efficiency and decreased provider burnout serve as strong motivation for further advancements in this area.

2.4.4   Diagnosis and Clinical Decision Making

The application of AI in the field of medical diagnosis and treatment is not a new concept. Researchers have been exploring whether AI can accurately suggest clinical diagnoses and recommend optimal treatment plans since the 1970s. The ability to improve the accuracy of clinical diagnoses is seen as an appealing aspect of AI in medicine, as early and precise detection of medical conditions may lead to better patient outcomes by reducing readmission rates, preventing progression to chronic conditions, and improving prognosis with a lower risk for complications. Currently, various subspecialties are showing growing interest in developing advanced AI tools that could assist with clinical problem-solving. These tools can analyze large amounts of medical data, including patient records [215], lab results, and imaging data, to identify patterns and correlations that might not be immediately apparent to human clinicians. Thus, the use of AI in clinical decision-making is based on its ability to analyze a vast amount of patient data and identify patterns that can accurately predict clinical outcomes and recommend appropriate treatments. AI algorithms are capable of examining various types of medical information, including radiographic images, laboratory results, and patient records, to assist healthcare professionals in recognizing abnormal patterns indicative of specific diagnoses. Machine learning, an integral component of AI, plays a crucial role in clinical decision-making by analyzing data to make informed decisions and predictions [216]. Deep learning (DL), a subfield within ML, has demonstrated considerable success in diagnosing heart failure (HF). In light of the significant global burden posed by HF, which affects approximately 26 million individuals worldwide, the achievements of DL hold great importance in the healthcare context [216, 217].

The integration of ML in the field of orthopedics has shown promising outcomes, as AI can provide valuable assistance to orthopedic surgeons by analyzing radiographic images, conducting preoperative risk assessments, and aiding in clinical decision-making [218]. Particularly for joint arthroplasty, which is a common elective procedure in orthopedics, AI offers significant advantages over traditional methods. By utilizing advanced vision models, sensors, and feedback mechanisms during robot-assisted arthroplasty surgery with augmented intelligence capabilities, AI technology demonstrates superior performance in achieving precise joint alignment and accurate implant placement tailored to individual patients' needs. This patient-centered approach sets AI-driven augmentation apart from conventional techniques and establishes it as the future direction for arthroplasty procedures [219].

An interdisciplinary application of ML lies in cancer diagnostics, risk stratification, and prognosis [220, 221]. These aspects play a crucial role in comprehending the progression of diseases and determining survival probabilities. In the past, medical professionals heavily relied on their expertise acquired through years of clinical practice to guide the diagnosis and treatment of cancer. However, traditional methods have shown limitations such as clinical errors and higher rates of misdiagnosis. By incorporating

ML algorithms into oncology practices, there is potential to mitigate these challenges, as AI algorithms have demonstrated superiority in early cancer detection compared to conventional approaches [222, 223]. Furthermore, the integration of AI in oncology has shown promising prospects for enhancing success rates in cancer treatments by tailoring therapies based on individual genetic information and patient-specific data [224].

AI algorithms have the ability to conduct clinical screenings for disease symptoms, allowing for an assessment of the probability prior to a diagnosis being made by a healthcare professional. One notable example of this is seen in the identification of Diabetic Retinopathy (DR), where several AI screening tools have been created and are now available for use in certain countries. In the past, identifying DR relied solely on human clinicians or graders [225]. However, deep learning screening tools can accurately classify individuals with DR at a statistically significant rate of 96.8% [226]. By making these automated screening tools accessible to the public, it becomes possible to initiate an appropriate follow-up plan with a clinician much more quickly, thereby reducing the chances of complications resulting from undiagnosed DR.

Numerous endeavors in the past and present have demonstrated AI's capacity to excel in clinical decision-making across various healthcare domains. In these instances, AI has successfully matched the vast knowledge and expertise of healthcare practitioners. However, it is crucial to recognize that the application of AI as both a diagnostic and treatment tool remains in its experimental stages and is not yet widely accessible for use within clinical settings. The widespread integration of AI into healthcare systems remains an additional hurdle on the path toward achieving full automation. The widespread integration of AI in clinical decision-making is expected to occur within the next 5–10 years. However, this timeline relies on obtaining approval from governing stakeholders, standardizing system operations, educating current professionals, and securing adequate funding [167]. It is important to note that AI currently does not pose an immediate threat to the job security of healthcare professionals, as their expertise remains crucial for providing the human touch in medicine [167]. The development of advanced clinical AI technology aims to enhance physicians' diagnostic abilities and offer optimal treatment plans rather than replace them entirely.

Physical disabilities are increasingly prevalent with advancing age, and rehabilitation plays a crucial role in restoring function and maintaining independence. However, the limited availability and accessibility of rehabilitation services have hindered their clinical impact. While AI has revolutionized several healthcare domains, its potential in rehabilitation remains uncertain. To address this gap, a systematic review of AI-supported physical rehabilitation technology in the clinical setting was conducted in [227]. The authors' objectives were to assess the availability of AI-supported physical rehabilitation technology, evaluate its clinical effects, and identify barriers and facilitators to implementation. They identified 28 projects encompassing five categories of AI solutions: app-based systems, robotic devices for function replacement or restoration, gaming systems, and wearables. Among these projects, they analyzed five randomized controlled trials that examined outcomes related to physical function, activity, pain, and health-related quality of life. The results revealed inconsistent clinical effects. Implementation barriers included technology literacy, reliability, and user fatigue, whereas enablers encompassed improved access to rehabilitation programs, remote monitoring of progress, reduced manpower requirements, and lower cost. Hence, while the application of AI in physical rehabilitation is a rapidly growing field, there is a need for more rigorous real-world clinical evaluations and post-implementation experiences in order to fully understand its potential and optimize its benefits. Developers and researchers must strive to conduct robust studies to unlock the true potential of AI in enhancing physical rehabilitation outcomes.

The global prevalence of irritable bowel syndrome (IBS) is approximately 4.1%, leading to decreased quality of life and increased healthcare costs. Current guidelines recommend using symptom-based criteria for diagnosing IBS; however, patients often undergo unnecessary medical interventions. To address this issue, the use of AI in medicine presents a promising solution. This paper aims to review the applications of AI in IBS. AI has proven useful in colonoscopy by detecting organic lesions, diagnosing them, and objectively evaluating the procedure's quality. Additionally, AI has been used to study biofilm characteristics in the large bowel and establish a potential correlation with IBS [228]. Furthermore, an AI algorithm has been developed to analyze specific bowel sounds associated with IBS. Smartphone applications based on AI have been created to aid in monitoring IBS symptoms. From a therapeutic perspective, an AI system has been designed to recommend personalized diets based on an individual's microbiota. In conclusion, the future of IBS diagnosis and treatment could greatly benefit from the integration of AI. The era of big data has necessitated the use of AI models to effectively handle the abundance of clinical data available. These data have become invaluable resources for machine learning, with DL models gaining prominence in analyzing unstructured data. However, traditional ML models continue to hold significant potential to enhance healthcare efficiency, especially for structured data. While ML models have been widely applied in predicting diagnoses and prognoses for various diseases, their adoption in gastroenterology has been relatively limited compared to traditional statistical models or DL approaches [229].

The prospect of patients reporting their symptoms to AI-powered NLP systems, followed by receiving diagnostic and treatment assistance from these AI systems, represents a promising avenue in healthcare. With the utilization of NLP, patients would have the capability to articulate their symptoms in a conversational manner, providing a comprehensive account of their medical condition. The AI systems would then employ advanced algorithms to process and interpret the information shared by the patients to integrate it with pertinent medical data. This amalgamation of patient-reported data and contextual knowledge would enable the AI systems to generate insightful analyses, potentially aiding physicians in arriving at accurate diagnoses and formulating tailored treatment plans. The integration of AI and NLP in this context has the potential to enhance patient outcomes by streamlining healthcare delivery and empowering healthcare providers with AI-facilitated decision support tools, thereby fostering more efficient and personalized medical care [230].

The application of AI in healthcare with potential benefits extending to the field of nutrition assessment has garnered significant attention in recent years. Nutrition assessment plays a pivotal role in healthcare, as it provides crucial insights into an individual's dietary intake, nutritional status, and overall health. Digital technologies such as mobile applications and wearable devices have emerged as valuable tools in facilitating the collection and analysis of dietary data. These technologies enable individuals to track their food consumption, monitor nutritional content, and receive personalized recommendations. AI algorithms enhance the capabilities of these digital tools by utilizing ML and data analytics techniques to process and interpret vast amounts of nutrition-related data. This allows for more accurate and timely assessment of nutritional status, identification of dietary patterns, and evaluation of health risks associated with inadequate or excessive nutrient intake [231].

2.4.5 AI in Surgical Procedures

The expanding application of AI in the healthcare field has brought about significant changes to surgical practices. Surgeons now have access to advanced robotic systems such as Da Vinci that enable less invasive and more independent procedures [232]. Robots are able to perform surgeries on previously inaccessible or delicate areas, such as neural structures, with improved dexterity, speed, and stability. As a result of these advancements, hospital stays have been shortened, recovery times have accelerated, and patient outcomes have been enhanced in terms of morbidity and mortality rates [233]. A recently developed semi-autonomous surgical robot called Smart Tissue Autonomous Robot (STAR) exhibits greater precision and accuracy than experienced surgeons when it comes to incising and suturing soft tissue [234]. Furthermore, studies have indicated that supervised autonomous robot surgery can outperform traditional manual surgery in complex intestinal anastomosis operations, which demand great skillfulness as well as delicacy from surgeons [232, 235].

One of the main challenges in traditional surgery is the lack of uniformity caused by variations in surgical experience, training, and skill levels among physicians. However, advancements such as the above-mentioned STAR have addressed this issue by demonstrating the ability to perform surgeries with greater precision and consistency. The STAR system utilizes three-dimensional techniques that result in more consistent suture spacing and improved resection margins compared to manual procedures. Consequently, this reduces the risk of post-surgical complications arising from variability between surgeons' performances [236]. Moreover, predicting surgical outcomes becomes challenging due to inconsistencies in patient anatomy. Nevertheless, STAR tackles this challenge effectively by adapting to inter-patient anatomical differences and tissue deformability during surgery through real-time data processing and regular updates to the surgical plan [236]. Advancements made on the development of STAR promise not only enhanced surgical outcomes but also increased predictability and standardization within surgeries.

Surgical procedures are widely acknowledged to pose significant risks to the well-being and safety of patients, primarily due to their unpredictable nature and the potential for human error. The integration of AI into surgical practices has been pursued as a means of addressing these concerns and ensuring enhanced levels of safety. Research indicates that robotic surgery boasts a notably lower mortality rate, with 0.097% compared to manual open surgery's rate of 0.92% per 10,000 surgeries [237]. Thus, by complementing physicians' expertise with precise robotic assistance, this technology improves surgical accuracy by approximately 6.4% while reducing surgeons' workload by up to 44% [238].

In addition to its applications in the operating room, AI technology has the potential to enhance healthcare outcomes by streamlining surgical decision-making and management both before and after surgery. As surgery is a significant and often anxiety-provoking event for patients, surgeons need to provide comprehensive support and counseling throughout the entire process. Conversely, surgical interventions necessitate extensive preparation that can be time-consuming; aside from performing procedures, surgeons must analyze various datasets such as patient scans and lab work to develop intricate surgical plans. Fortunately, AI offers a solution by efficiently processing large amounts of patient data within a short timeframe while generating optimal solutions. This allows surgeons more opportunity to engage in meaningful interactions with their patients [239].

A recent literature review analyzed 46 studies on the applications of AI and ML in spinal surgery [240]. The findings revealed that AI/ML models were accurate, with an average overall value of 74.9%. These models performed well in preoperative patient selection, cost prediction, length of stay, functional outcomes, and postoperative mortality prediction. Regression analysis was the most commonly used application, while deep learning/artificial neural networks had the highest sensitivity score of 81.5%. Despite AI/ML's relatively recent adoption, as shown by 77.5% of studies being published after 2018 (depicted in Figure 2.3), the results have been encouraging. The increasing prevalence of Big Data and National Registries suggests that the field of spine surgery will gradually adopt and integrate AI/ML into clinical practices, leading to significant improvements in patient care.

2.4.6   Medical Imaging

The introduction of X-ray imaging over 120 years ago revolutionized the way healthcare providers diagnose and treat patients [241]. Since then, advancements in imaging technologies have greatly enhanced the medical field by providing a detailed visualization of vital patient anatomy that is not perceptible to the human eye alone. Despite these innovations, modern imaging technology continues to rely on high-quality images and skilled practitioners to accurately interpret and identify potential ailments [242]. An important development occurred approximately 50 years ago when AI capabilities expanded beyond data analysis and problem-solving to include image recognition and interpretation with a lower error rate compared to radiologists [243, 244]. However, it is crucial to dispel public apprehension, as AI does not aim to replace the expertise of radiology professionals with robotic systems; rather, it complements their skills within this discipline. The integration of AI in radiology has gained significant attention, and is expected to enhance the diagnostic process by supplementing radiologists with AI algorithms. This approach aims to streamline operations, reduce redundancy, and improve accuracy in image interpretation [245]. During the COVID-19 pandemic, AI proved invaluable in detecting asymptomatic individuals infected with SARS-CoV-2 on CT scans, allowing radiologists to confidently rule out the disease [246, 247]. The use of AI visual recognition tools has played a crucial role in preventing transmission through false negative results. As shown in Figure 2.6, there has been a noticeable surge of interest among researchers studying the applications of AI technology to medical imaging in recent years [248].

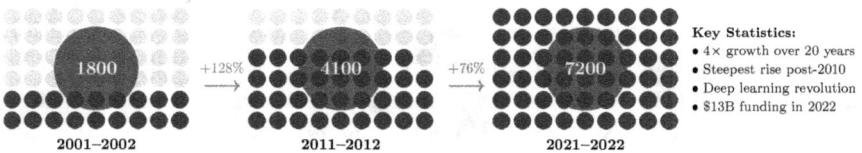

Figure 2.6: Trends in the number of PubMed-indexed publications on AI in medical imaging. The visualization shows dramatic growth from 1,800 publications (2001–2002) to 7,200 publications (2021–2022), representing a fourfold increase driven by technological advances in deep learning, increased funding, and expanding clinical adoption. Each dark circle represents approximately 100 publications, while light circles show the broader research landscape.

AI plays a vital role in automating echocardiographic analysis, aiding in the diagnosis of cardiovascular diseases. A recent literature review discussed AI algorithms used in various stages of analysis, including image acquisition, view classification, cardiac chamber segmentation, and quantification of cardiac structure and function [249, 250]. The authors found that such AI models demonstrate high accuracy in comparison to human experts. The same review explored the potential benefits and limitations of AI in healthcare, such as the need for larger datasets and to address algorithm biases to allow for wider clinical adoption.

Endoscopic ultrasound (EUS) has emerged as a widely utilized diagnostic tool for digestive diseases. With the gradual recognition of AI in health-care, its superiority in the field of EUS has become increasingly evident. Research findings demonstrate that EUS-AI exhibits superiority, or at least equivalence, to conventional methods of diagnosis, prognosis, and quality control for subepithelial lesions, early esophageal cancer, early gastric can-cer, and various pancreatic diseases, including pancreatic cystic lesions, autoimmune pancreatitis, and pancreatic cancer [251]. The implementation of EUS-AI has opened up new avenues for individualized precision medicine while introducing innovative approaches to diagnosing and treating digestive diseases.

2.4.7   AI's Role in Pandemics

The COVID-19 pandemic has underscored the potential of AI in effectively addressing healthcare challenges. It spurred the adoption and integration of AI technologies into medical practices, showcasing their ability to facili-tate rapid response, accurate diagnosis, efficient treatment, and extensive research endeavors [252]. The increased application of AI in healthcare is evident through the noticeable surge in academic publications, as de-picted in Figure 2.3. Importantly, this rise coincided with the onset of the COVID-19 pandemic. Throughout this crisis period, various applications of AI played a crucial role in diverse aspects such as pandemic response management, patient care enhancement, and innovative research initiatives. One of the key areas where AI can be utilized during pandemics is in the management of pandemic responses [253]. AI has proved instrumental in disease cluster identification, monitoring patients, determining mortality risk, disease diagnosis and management, contact tracing through geotagging, resource allocation, and data management. The following sections offer an elaboration on these key areas.

Diagnosis and Screening

In recent years, significant progress has been made in the development of AI-powered diagnostic tools designed to support healthcare professionals in identifying cases of COVID-19 using medical images. These advanced tools utilize convolutional neural networks (CNNs) to carefully examine chest X-rays and CT scans for potential indications of the virus within lung tissue. By analyzing large datasets containing both infected and non-infected images, these AI algorithms are trained to detect subtle patterns that could suggest the presence of COVID-19. This valuable assistance enables radiologists and clinicians to make faster and more precise diagnoses, particularly in regions where PCR testing (i.e., Polymerase Chain Reaction testing, the "gold standard" for COVID-19 tests) may be limited or subject to delays. The ability of AI systems to swiftly process medical images plays a pivotal role in facilitating early detection and treatment plans, ultimately influencing patient outcomes positively and helping to mitigate the spread of the virus [13]. Moreover, AI technology has proven to be beneficial in predicting the progression of COVID-19 cases. By analyzing patterns in symptoms and clinical data, AI algorithms can generate predictive models that help healthcare professionals anticipate how a patient's condition may develop over time. These predictions guide medical professionals in making informed decisions regarding the appropriate course of treatment and allocation of resources.

Drug Discovery and Vaccine Development

The integration of AI has significantly transformed the field of drug discovery. By utilizing AI algorithms, scientists are now able to simulate and predict the interactions between potential drugs and viral proteins. This is achieved through molecular docking, a technique that assesses how a drug molecule binds to its target protein. In addition to molecular docking, AI-enhanced molecular dynamics simulations provide valuable insights into the behavior of drug–protein complexes over time. These simulations aid researchers in selecting promising candidates for further testing by offering detailed information on their stability and efficacy. Moreover, AI models have been instrumental in vaccine development [254]. Through advanced prediction techniques, these models can accurately define viral protein structures and analyze potential epitopes that can trigger immune responses. By leveraging such predictions, researchers can design vaccines with greater precision that efficiently elicit strong and protective immune reactions against targeted pathogens. Consequently, this approach has substantially reduced the time required for developing viable vaccine candidates compared to traditional methods. AI has revolutionized the field of drug discovery by enabling researchers to accurately predict drug–protein interactions and efficiently design lead compounds [255]. Furthermore, AI has improved the process of drug development by automating various tasks and reducing the cost and time associated with preclinical and clinical trials.

Epidemiological Forecasting

AI-powered epidemiological models incorporate intricate data streams for predicting the transmission of the virus. These models analyze factors such as infection rates, hospitalization rates, population density, and human mobility. Machine learning algorithms play a role in refining these models by adapting them to real-world data. By simulating different scenarios based on varying intervention strategies, these models offer policymakers valuable insights into the potential consequences of their actions. Consequently, they aid in resource allocation decisions, inform the implementation of public health measures, and help to mitigate stress on healthcare systems during periods of high demand. AI-powered epidemiological models have become invaluable tools in predicting the transmission of viruses, including COVID-19. Furthermore, AI-based techniques can be utilized to track and monitor the spread of viruses at different scales, ranging from individual to population levels [253].

Remote Monitoring and Telehealth

AI-enabled remote monitoring tools have emerged as a valuable solution for facilitating patient care from the comfort of home. Through the use of wearable devices, vital signs and symptoms can be continuously tracked to generate streams of data. These extensive datasets are then subjected to AI algorithms that accurately identify any deviations from baseline levels, allowing healthcare providers to promptly address potential declines in patients' conditions. Additionally, telehealth platforms employ sophisticated chatbots driven by AI capabilities that aid patients in conducting symptom assessments, providing them with relevant information and determining the urgency required for medical attention. By leveraging these advanced systems, healthcare professionals can effectively enhance patient care while simultaneously mitigating unnecessary face-to-face interactions, an especially crucial measure during times such as widespread pandemics [257].

Data Analysis and Decision Support

The COVID-19 pandemic resulted in a significant influx of data, ranging from the number of cases to hospitalizations to genomic sequences. AI systems have played a crucial role in analyzing these datasets to uncover patterns that contribute to decision-making processes. Machine learning algorithms specifically help to identify risk factors correlated with severe outcomes and demographic trends regarding infections and to evaluate the effectiveness of interventions. The insights derived from these analyses can assist public health officials and policymakers in making well-informed choices, effectively allocate resources, and tailor interventions to cater to specific populations [258].

Natural Language Processing

Natural language processing techniques facilitate the comprehension and interpretation of human language by AI. In light of the COVID-19 pandemic, NLP tools empowered by AI are capable of systematically sifting through an expansive repertoire of scientific literature to extract significant insights. By summarizing research discoveries and identifying emerging patterns, these advanced tools assist researchers in promptly accessing pertinent information [259]. Furthermore, NLP drives the development of chatbots that deliver precise information to the general public, effectively addressing concerns and countering false or misleading narratives [260].

Contact Tracing

AI-powered contact tracing applications utilize smartphone technologies such as Bluetooth to monitor and record interactions among individuals. Advanced algorithms powered by machine learning assess the likelihood of disease transmission by considering factors such as proximity, duration, and contextual information [261]. To uphold privacy standards, these apps employ decentralized data storage and cryptographic techniques that safeguard sensitive data from unauthorized access. Through the implementation of AI technology, public health agencies can effectively trace potential infection routes, control outbreaks, and promptly notify individuals who may be at risk [262]. However, it is important to address privacy concerns that arise with the use of AI-powered contact tracing applications. One way to address privacy concerns in AI-powered contact tracing applications is by incorporating privacy-by-design principles [263]. Privacy-by-design principles ensure that privacy is considered at every stage of the design and development process of AI-powered contact tracing applications. By incorporating privacy-by-design principles, contact tracing apps can prioritize user privacy and data protection [264]. Additionally, contact tracing apps can adopt a decentralized approach to data storage. This means that personal data are stored locally on users' smartphones rather than being collected and stored centrally. This approach enhances privacy, as it minimizes the risk of unauthorized access to sensitive information. Furthermore, adopting an opt-in system for contact tracing apps can help to address privacy concerns. Adopting an opt-in system for contact tracing apps means that users have the choice to voluntarily participate in the app's functionality. This empowers individuals to make informed decisions about their privacy and control the collection and use of their personal data. Overall, the use of AI-powered contact tracing applications presents significant benefits for public health agencies in controlling disease transmission. However, the collection of personal data and potential surveillance associated with these apps continue to raise valid privacy concerns.

Patient Triage and Resource Allocation

AI-driven triage systems utilize advanced algorithms to assess patient information such as medical history, symptoms, and laboratory findings in order to anticipate the probability of severe illness [265]. These machine learning models detect early signs of complications, allowing healthcare professionals to prioritize individuals requiring urgent care. In situations where resources are scarce, AI technologies facilitate the efficient allocation of resources by considering predicted patient outcomes; this ensures optimal utilization of critical supplies like ventilators. In addition to patient triage, AI-based systems play a crucial role in resource allocation within hospitals and on a larger scale. By accurately predicting disease severity and patient outcomes, AI-driven triage systems aid in clinical decision-making as well as in the planning and allocation of resources across hospital systems and at the state/country level [266]. Moreover, the use of AI in patient triage and resource allocation becomes particularly vital during pandemics. During the COVID-19 pandemic, AI algorithms demonstrated their effectiveness in predicting patient outcomes and identifying individuals at high risk for severe illness. These AI-powered systems consider a wide range of factors, including pre-existing conditions, laboratory results, and in-hospital data.

2.4.8   Medical Training

The effectiveness of medical education is closely linked to a doctor's ability to provide proper care for their patients while minimizing the risk of irreversible errors or harm. As a result, physicians undergo extensive training over several years to acquire a well-rounded set of skills encompassing cognitive, psychomotor, and affective domains. In the past, medical education primarily emphasized the retention of large volumes of complex information for long periods. However, this task has become increasingly challenging in light of the vast amount of new knowledge being generated daily, which surpasses human capacity [267]. The rapid advancement of AI in the medical field has demonstrated the ability to effectively store, analyze, and retrieve medical data, saving clinicians valuable time and energy in patient management and treatment. This integration of cutting-edge technology necessitates a reformation in the education of future healthcare providers in order to align with these recent advancements, particularly the incorporation of AI into medical practice.

One benefit of incorporating AI into medical education is its ability to enhance the efficiency of learning and studying. This in turn reduces the workload for students and provides them with more opportunities to improve their fundamental clinical skills [268]. In an increasingly demanding healthcare industry, it is crucial for medical professionals to have proficient information recall and analysis abilities as well as to possess effective communication skills, manual dexterity in performing clinical tasks, cultural sensitivity, and empathy toward patients. The integration of AI technologies offers a valuable educational resource that streamlines the didactic components of medical training. Consequently, this allows students to prioritize developing their clinical expertise and interpersonal competencies while promoting a compassionate approach within the field of medicine [269]. Additionally, AI in medical education can facilitate the acquisition of practical skills through real-world use of technologies [270]. This can be achieved by incorporating AI-based tools such as intelligent tutoring systems that simulate interactive scenarios for students to practice their clinical decision-making and problem-solving skills

The integration of AI in medical training offers the potential for a more personalized educational experience tailored to meet the individual needs of students, thereby enhancing their overall performance [271]. The utilization of AI has proven effective in analyzing students' progress and identifying specific areas where knowledge gaps exist. This enables immediate and customized feedback, empowering students to learn at a pace that suits their abilities and preferences [271]. Additionally, AI-powered tools can provide valuable resources for medical education, such as computer-based models, virtual reality simulations, and personalized learning platforms [272]. These resources allow students to experience real-world scenarios in a safe and controlled environment, enabling them to develop practical skills and apply theoretical knowledge.

The incorporation of AI-based virtual reality simulations in medical education can offer significant benefits by providing a safer learning environment for students to refine their clinical skills before entering real-world patient care. This approach allows for practice in common scenarios such as suturing or conducting physical examinations while enabling preparation for rare yet potentially impactful catastrophic events. For example, research has demonstrated the feasibility of simulating Operating Rooms using AI technology, which proved effective in analyzing healthcare professionals' response to such emergencies and delivering appropriate training on how to handle these unique situations safely and effectively [273]. Furthermore, AI-driven virtual reality simulations have the potential to revolutionize radiology education [274]. With the integration of AI intelligence, radiology simulations in virtual environments can reproduce real-world scenarios and provide learners with immersive, interactive, and realistic training experiences that closely mimic clinical practice.

The incorporation of AI in the field of medicine is yet to be fully realized, resulting in a knowledge and skills gap among clinicians regarding its application in their day-to-day practice. This lack of familiarity with AI hinders clinicians from harnessing its numerous benefits within the medical sector. This is not due to a lack of interest in becoming proficient at utilizing AI on their part; rather, it can be attributed to the limited availability of educational resources for both students and practicing clinicians. A recent experimental study that introduced an AI course specifically designed for fourth year medical students demonstrated promising outcomes, as evidenced by an average score of 97% achieved by the participants [275]. These findings validate the effectiveness of online modules focusing on AI and emphasize the pressing need for additional educational opportunities within current medical training programs. The integration of AI into medical practice requires a thorough understanding of its potential benefits and limitations. This prompts medical educators to teach the best practices of AI as a tool while understanding its limitations [276]. To bridge the knowledge gap and enhance the understanding of AI among medical professionals, medical educators need to develop standardized AI content and incorporate it into medical training pathways [277]. This approach will ensure that medical students and clinicians are equipped with the necessary knowledge and skills to effectively utilize AI in their practice.

2.5   Considerations of AI Applications

The integration of AI in the healthcare sector has the potential to greatly enhance patients' overall experience with medical care. As previously mentioned, AI can be implemented across various areas within medicine [278]. However, it is important to address certain considerations such as biases and public awareness surrounding AI.

2.5.1   Ethical and Legal Considerations around AI

There are a number of relevant ethical and legal issues that need to be carefully considered moving forward. (a) Accountability and Liability: as AI systems take on increasingly complex tasks, determining responsibility for mistakes becomes a challenge. If an AI-driven diagnosis leads to harmful medical errors, it is uncertain where the liability rests; is it the healthcare provider, the developers of the AI system, or the machine itself? This legal conundrum needs to be addressed with comprehensive regulations addressing accountability and liability in AI applications in healthcare. (b) Privacy Protection: with AI systems processing vast amounts of sensitive patient information, ensuring data privacy becomes paramount. Patient data can be misused or fall into the wrong hands, making it crucial to have strong data protection measures in place. The legal frameworks regarding data privacy in the context of AI should adhere to principles of data minimization, purpose limitation, and secure data processing methods. (c) Bias and Discrimination: AI systems can unintentionally perpetuate existing biases present in healthcare data, leading to unequal treatment or inaccurate diagnoses for certain groups. Case studies on issues such as racial bias present in healthcare AI algorithms underline the importance of anti-bias measures in the development and deployment of these systems.

Regulatory bodies must enforce guidelines that ensure fairness and accuracy in the operation of AI systems. (d) Transparency and Explainability: the 'black-box' nature of many AI systems can significantly complicate healthcare delivery. When an AI system's decision-making process is not transparent, healthcare professionals may find it difficult to trust the system's outputs, affecting implementation. Regulations emphasizing transparency and explainability can facilitate better understanding and acceptance of AI tools in medical practice. (e) Consent: patient consent is another crucial issue when dealing with AI systems. Data used to train AI systems should be collected only after obtaining explicit and informed consent from the patients. Legal requirements need to specify the nature of consent required for different kinds of data usage. (f) Balancing Innovation and Regulatory Oversight: while regulations are necessary to maintain ethical standards, they should not stifle innovation. Policymakers need to ensure that regulatory frameworks provide enough space for the development and application of AI technologies while ensuring patient safety, privacy, and fair treatment.

As the healthcare industry experiences an increased workload resulting from heightened patient demand, digital health technology has garnered more attention as a potential solution. However, this advancement introduces concerns regarding patient privacy and the monitoring of sensitive information. Furthermore, due to the current absence of comprehensive regulations in place, AI systems raise legal and ethical issues such as liability attribution and privacy protection. The challenge lies in identifying responsibility when machines are capable of operating under non-rigid rules and independently acquiring new behavioral patterns [279]. This ambiguity poses a legal conundrum, and accountability for these actions remains uncertain. From an ethical standpoint, safeguarding an individual's privacy is closely intertwined with their right to autonomy and personal identity within the medical context. Consequently, maintaining strict confidentiality measures while ensuring robust security protocols for AI-based data management is imperative in order to minimize potential breaches or violations of patient privacy. Moreover, the integration of AI in healthcare raises concerns about algorithmic bias and the potential for discriminatory practices [280].

Another issue that may arise is the collection of patient data without informed consent. An example of this can be seen with AI devices gathering and transmitting data from older adults in their homes without their knowledge; these services may provide the collected data to AI developers

without patients' consent [281]. While this has the potential to benefit
healthcare through AI implementation, it raises concerns about breaching
patient privacy and eroding healthcare trust. Therefore, as mentioned
earlier, it is crucial to establish guidelines that set boundaries for how AI
utilizes patient data while allowing flexibility for unforeseen circumstances.
Integrating ethical and accountable AI solutions into organizational planning
is crucial for responsible AI [282]. This ensures the maintenance of trust,
minimizes privacy invasion, and meets stakeholder expectations and regulations. Although in its early stages, responsible AI aims to strike a balance
between patient needs and long-term economic value in healthcare [283, 284].
While leading researchers primarily focus on quantitative evaluation metrics,
physicians prioritize trustworthiness, ethics, and providing meaningful ex-
planations for decisions made by deep networks according to data protection
laws [285].

The American Medical Association (AMA) has released seven principles
for the use of AI in healthcare [286]. The aim is to create a uniform
governance framework for the advancement of AI in the industry. The
principles stress the importance of comprehensive policies to minimize
potential risks associated with AI technologies for patients and physicians.
According to the AMA, these principles will aid in optimizing the benefits of
AI in healthcare and reducing potential harms. Key aspects within the AMA
principles include favoring comprehensive governance for risk management
in healthcare AI and promoting transparency with legal requirements in AI
design, development, and deployment. In addition, the principles call for
privacy-centric AI design, secure handling of personal data, clear disclosure
around when AI impacts patient care, and development of policies to address
potential negative impacts before deploying generative AI. Furthermore,
the AMA urges early identification and mitigation of bias in AI algorithms
and advocates for limiting physician liability in the use of AI-enabled
technologies while aligning with current medical liability legal frameworks.
In the following section, bias and transparency in AI are assessed in more
detail.

2.5.2   Bias and Transparency of AI

Often, AI algorithms are developed and trained using healthcare datasets.
When these datasets contain inherent biases, the resulting AI system can
replicate or even magnify existing disparities. For example, if a dataset

used to train a disease prediction algorithm predominantly contains data from certain demographic groups, the algorithm might perform poorly when used on other demographics. This could lead to unequal treatment or misdiagnosis. Bias in decision making is another concern. AI algorithms often replicate the decision-making processes of the health professionals who trained them. If those professionals carry inherent biases, the AI systems might reflect these same biases. As an instance, a study by Obermeyer et al. found that a healthcare algorithm showed racial bias because it was designed to predict healthcare costs rather than sickness [287]. This bias manifested as lower referral rates for black people compared to other racial groups with similar health conditions. To ensure more equitable AI development, efforts must be made to use diverse datasets that accurately represent all population groups. Datasets must be interrogated for potential bias prior to training the algorithms. Furthermore, AI systems should be regularly validated on multiple datasets to ensure that they maintain high performance across diverse populations. AI's capacity in healthcare depends largely on how the ethical issue of algorithmic bias is addressed. Multidisciplinary efforts involving clinicians, data scientists, ethicists, and policy makers should be enforced to ensure the development and use of equitable and unbiased AI systems in healthcare. AI is meant to improve healthcare accessibility and inequality, not to inadvertently exacerbate existing disparities.

Certain diseases have a higher prevalence in specific genders, which presents a challenge when implementing AI for accurate solutions tailored to certain groups. Gender bias represents one of the obstacles encountered during the deployment of AI systems in medical imaging. For instance, a study by Larrazabal et al. revealed that an imbalanced dataset with unequal representation of males and females led to significantly lower performance averages across all diseases within the minority group, suggesting the presence of gender bias [288]. This highlights the need to consider gender bias when providing data for AI algorithms and to incorporate additional mechanisms that can effectively account for this bias to ensure precise outputs. It is important to address and mitigate bias in AI algorithms, as it can have negative impacts on health, particularly in under-resourced or racial/ethnic minority populations [289].

Obermeyer et al. investigated the potential racial bias present in healthcare AI algorithms used for managing the care of high-risk patients in the United States [287]. These algorithms are responsible for setting up special care management programs mandated by the Affordable Care Act designed

to provide extra resources to patients with complex medical needs with
the aim of preventing costly medical emergencies. Despite race not being
an explicit input into the algorithm, the research found significant racial
bias in the algorithm's predictions. Black patients were substantially less
likely to be selected by the algorithm as needing extra care compared to
their White counterparts, even when they were just as sick. This disparity
mainly stemmed from the algorithm's focus on health care costs as a proxy
for health needs and complexity, which overlooked the fact that less money
is spent on Black patients who have the same level of need. The consequent
under-identification of high-risk Black patients for care programs has significant implications on the equitable distribution of healthcare resources.
These findings suggest the need for careful scrutiny in the design and implementation of healthcare algorithms to ensure that they do not inadvertently
propagate systemic biases.

The use of AI in diagnosing various diseases is gaining popularity across
multiple medical specialties. AI has demonstrated high accuracy in the
diagnosis of dermatological skin lesions. A study conducted at Stanford
University in 2017 trained a convolutional neural network using a dataset of
over 100,000 images and 2000 diseases. The results showed that the CNN
had comparable performance to that of 21 board-certified dermatologists
when it came to classifying different types of skin cancer [290]. A study on
patient inclinations towards the utilization of AI for identifying skin cancer
pathways documented a positive attitude regarding the potential application
of AI for this objective [291]. However, it is important to recognize that bias
related to skin tone could impact the use of AI in this context. Inadequate
representation of varying skin tones in training AI/ML models can lead to
erroneous interpretations, especially for marginalized communities. A recent
review conducted in 2021 on the use of AI in dermatology examined 70
studies and found that only 10% included skin tone as part of the dataset.
Furthermore, it was revealed that darker skin tones were underrepresented
in these studies [292]. This highlights a potential flaw when using datasets
for diagnosing skin conditions, and emphasizes the need to address this
issue. Nonetheless, despite this limitation, incorporating AI into the field
of dermatological disorders has significant potential to provide accurate
diagnoses and effective treatments.

The transparency of AI has experienced significant growth in recent
years. This rapid advancement holds promise for enhancing public awareness
and understanding of AI's applications in healthcare. Addressing the need

for clarity on various aspects of AI can foster trust on the part of the public around the integration of AI into medical practice. An important factor in establishing this trust lies in developing a comprehensive understanding of how AI systems interpret information. Lack of knowledge about the inner workings and decision-making processes of these systems creates a gap, particularly among healthcare professionals who may struggle to comprehend their operations within the context of patient care. The difficulty of implementing AI in clinical settings and the clinical translation gap of AI-based tools are well described, and are driven in part by a lack of education and knowledge among clinicians [293]. Improving education and understanding regarding AI applications on the part of healthcare professionals could effectively address the current knowledge gap [294]. This educational initiative would aid in legislation, verification, and system improvement while fostering trust between the individuals involved [295]. It is crucial to focus on comprehending how AI-generated results are interpreted as well as on addressing legal and ethical considerations in order to bolster public confidence in healthcare AI. Furthermore, incorporating cultural constructs and values within the clinical environment is another critical obstacle to overcome in implementing AI in healthcare.

2.5.3 Cybersecurity

The implementation of EHR systems in hospitals worldwide has led to an increased need for cybersecurity measures to ensure patient safety and protect confidential information. There are two crucial reasons why cybersecurity is imperative in modern healthcare: the digital storage of sensitive patient data, and the vulnerability of electronic systems to remote access by hackers due to inadequate defenses [296]. Instances of cybercrime within the healthcare sector include ransom attacks, theft of patient health data, and unauthorized control over implanted medical devices, all of which pose serious risks to individuals' well-being. Additionally, cybersecurity plays a critical role in maintaining privacy and trust on the part of patients [297]. One main issue with cybersecurity in healthcare is the abundance of valuable data, including personal and medical information. The other issue is the weak defenses that are typically found in healthcare systems, making them easy targets for cyberattacks. The reliance on electronic health records and other core systems in healthcare means that an effective cybersecurity framework is necessary to protect these systems from threats [298]. In contrast to physical breaches, which involve accessing patient records directly, a single medical device can serve as an entry point into the health record software of any hospital [299]. The use of AI introduces new opportunities for attackers to compromise patient privacy and undermine healthcare security, which is already vulnerable; therefore, it is crucial to develop legislation that protects patient information and to implement effective digital safeguards before the widespread adoption of AI algorithms in medicine [300]. Fortunately, there is potential for AI itself to contribute to maintaining patient privacy through computational text de-identification algorithms, which may offer a faster and more cost-effective solution compared to human experts [301].

2.5.4 Public Opinion around AI in Healthcare

The implementation of AI in healthcare is progressing rapidly, and it is crucial to consider public opinion on its integration. While there are vast possibilities for AI to enhance the healthcare sector, it is important to acknowledge that public perception can significantly impact how AI technologies are adopted. This includes the public perspective on various aspects, such as data collection during early stages of medical care, as well as acceptance and trust in using AI for diagnoses and treatments later on [302]. It is clear that the public's perception of AI in healthcare is not homogeneous and that there are varying levels of acceptance and apprehension. Recent surveys conducted by Pew Research have assessed public sentiment across multiple categories, including reliance on and impact of AI in medical care, knowledge about diagnosis and treatment methods, utilization of surgical procedures and pain management techniques, and the use of chatbots for mental health support [303]. In general, the majority of individuals express discomfort with providers relying solely on AI for medical care. There is a divide in opinion regarding whether this reliance improves, worsens, or has no significant impact on overall healthcare outcomes. The public's perception of AI in healthcare is influenced by factors such as education, knowledge about AI, and previous experiences [304]. Similarly, the findings presented in Figure 2.7 indicate that individuals with higher education and knowledge about AI tend to have greater confidence in its capacity to enhance patient outcomes within the healthcare sector. Hence, individuals with higher education tend to perceive AI as a valuable tool in enhancing patient care, facilitating early detection and diagnosis, optimizing treatment plans, and improving overall healthcare outcomes. However, according to the survey findings the majority of respondents expressed reservations about using AI for determining pain medication after surgery or relying on surgical robots for procedures. Furthermore, most participants believed that incorporating AI into pain management would either exacerbate their symptoms or yield no significant differences. Similarly, a significant majority indicated an unwillingness to utilize an AI chatbot for mental health support unless they were concurrently seeing a therapist [305]. These opinions held true both among those familiar with chatbots and those who had no previous knowledge of them. Overall, this survey found that while there is an increasing awareness and interest in AI's potential in healthcare, there was also skepticism and concern among the public. This skepticism and concern may stem from a lack of understanding or familiarity with AI as a concept as well as apprehension about data privacy and control [303]. To address this, it is important to conduct comprehensive research that takes into account the public's perspective from various qualitative and quantitative studies even though public perceptions of AI in healthcare are not limited to concerns about trust and reliance on technology.

The survey findings indicate a strong association between knowledge of AI and belief in its potential to have a positive impact on healthcare. Participants who demonstrated a higher level of understanding were more inclined to embrace the integration of AI into their overall medical treatment. However, this correlation weakened when it came to specific areas such as mental health, where individuals may have been less receptive towards incorporating AI into their treatment for these conditions. Nevertheless, AI has diverse applications in mental healthcare beyond the scope of chatbots alone. While patients may show decreased interest in using AI for treating their mental health issues, it can offer benefits for diagnostic purposes. For example, AI-based speech analysis techniques have been developed to identify depression [306] and wearable AI devices have the potential to detect anxiety, although their current level of advancement does not yet allow for clinical use [307].

The surveys reveal an overarching lack of awareness among the general public regarding AI in healthcare settings, emphasizing the necessity for targeted efforts aimed at educating and informing individuals about its capabilities within this domain. Addressing this knowledge gap is crucial for fostering effective collaboration between AI initiatives and healthcare practices in order to enhance patient care outcomes and optimize the use of resources in the healthcare system. Additionally, it can be inferred that

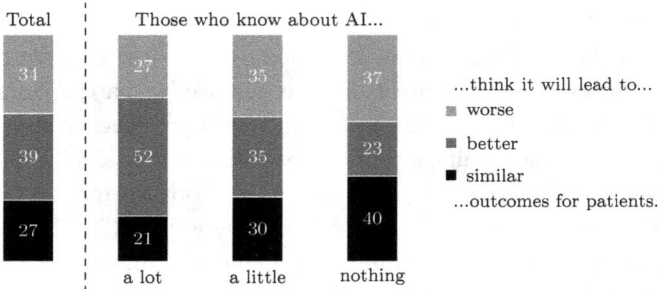

Figure 2.7: Public perception of AI's impact on patient outcomes, stratified by respondents' self-reported AI knowledge levels (Source: Pew Research Center [303]). The leftmost bar shows the total distribution across all respondents, while the three bars to the right represent responses from individuals with different levels of AI familiarity ('a lot,' 'a little,' and 'nothing'). Each bar is segmented into three categories: worse outcomes (dark blue, top), better outcomes (medium blue, middle), and similar outcomes (light blue, bottom), with percentages shown within each segment. The data reveals a clear correlation between AI knowledge and optimism about its healthcare impact. Those with high AI familiarity ('a lot') predominantly expect positive outcomes, with 52% believing AI will lead to better patient outcomes. In contrast, this optimism diminishes with decreasing AI knowledge. Among those with no AI knowledge, responses polarize towards either negative impacts (37%) or no difference in outcomes (40%), with only 23% expecting improvements. Similarly, those with little AI knowledge show a more balanced but still cautious view. This pattern suggests that deeper understanding of AI technologies tends to foster more positive expectations of its healthcare benefits, while limited knowledge appears to breed either skepticism or concerns about potential harmful effects on patient care.

healthcare specialists who have a deeper understanding of AI are more inclined to embrace and utilize this technology in their professional roles to enhance patient care.

While the general sentiment towards the utilization of AI in healthcare remains predominantly positive, it is crucial to acknowledge and address certain prevailing challenges that demand increased attention. Merely focusing on algorithmic concerns is insufficient; it is imperative to delve deeper into the practical implementation of legislation and guidelines to ensure the incorporation of principles such as fairness, accountability, transparency, and ethics within AI systems deployed in healthcare settings [308]. This comprehensive approach will contribute to safeguarding the integrity and responsible use of AI technology in healthcare.

2.6   Discussion

As the digital revolution continues to accelerate, it is clear that AI is becoming increasingly integral to healthcare. Its benefits, which include enhancing diagnostic accuracy, personalizing treatments, and increasing operational efficiency, have the potential to profoundly improve patient outcomes and reduce the burden on healthcare systems around the world. However, it is important to acknowledge that successful integration of AI into healthcare practices demands more than just technical proficiency. The ethical and social implications of AI usage in healthcare present considerable challenges. There is an urgent need to address issues such as data privacy, algorithmic bias, and accountability. Ensuring fairness, reliability, and transparency should be a priority in AI development. Moreover, collaboration between AI specialists, healthcare professionals, policy makers, and patients is key to developing AI tools that can truly meet the needs of all stakeholders. Additionally, due to the complex nature of medical decision-making, the role of AI should be envisioned as a support tool for clinicians rather than a replacement for human judgment. The human element in healthcare, which encompasses empathy, complex reasoning, and understanding of individual patient needs, cannot be replicated by an algorithm. Lastly, it is necessary to shift focus towards education and public awareness about AI in healthcare. Encouraging public understanding and dialogue about AI will be crucial for building trust and acceptance in the system. With a balanced and thoughtful approach, AI has the capacity to transform healthcare, bringing enormous benefits to both patients and providers. The rapidly evolving field of AI in healthcare will continue to offer exciting opportunities for further exploration and discovery in future work.

The field of AI has experienced rapid advancements and is now being utilized across various industries. Originally designed as a large computer for deciphering war signals, AI has evolved into a sophisticated cloud-based neural network. It functions as an adaptable tool that enhances complex human tasks in different sectors. In the medical domain specifically, the implementation of AI shows immense potential for future applications [309]. By demonstrating proficiency in surgical procedures, administrative responsibilities, diagnostics, imaging techniques, medical education, and patient management, AI can significantly alleviate healthcare burdens while fostering greater efficiency. This collaborative approach ensures that AI algorithms work alongside clinicians to enhance health outcomes and quality of care without posing any threat to job security or replacing human expertise in the healthcare field.

Collaboration among clinicians, educators, researchers, and developers is essential for the successful integration of AI into healthcare in the coming decade. Despite the impressive advancements made by AI, there remain many important considerations that need to be addressed. These include addressing biases and ensuring transparency as well as tackling legal and ethical challenges. Additionally, it is imperative to take into account public opinion and awareness regarding the incorporation of AI in medicine, as this will greatly influence progress within the field. Nonetheless, despite the need for these challenges to be resolved over time, AI has already demonstrated numerous promising capabilities that have tremendous potential for improving healthcare delivery and shaping the future of medicine. It should be emphasized that while AI shows immense promise, it necessitates rigorous validation processes along with ongoing collaboration between experts in AI and medical professionals to ensure safe implementation practices yielding effective results.

In light of the aforementioned challenges associated with AI in healthcare, the AMA has introduced guidelines pertaining to the advancement and application of AI in the healthcare sector. These guidelines aim to tackle critical concerns, including data privacy, cybersecurity, and the utilization of AI by insurance providers [286]. The report emphasizes the "quadruple aim" for AI systems: to enhance patient care and outcomes, improve population health, reduce healthcare costs while increasing value, and support the wellbeing of healthcare professionals. The guidelines further stress the need for regulatory oversight, transparency, data protection, and the avoidance of exacerbating inequities in healthcare while aiming to ensure AI tools meet both physician and patient needs.

2.7   Conclusions

An essential point to underscore is the collaborative potential between AI and healthcare professionals. AI is best viewed not as a replacement for healthcare professionals but as an adjunct tool, that is, a partner that can handle extensive data analysis, provide diagnostic support, and free up more time for healthcare professionals to spend on direct patient care. The successful implementation of AI would enable healthcare providers to leverage their unique skills of empathy, complex decision-making, and direct patient communication that AI cannot emulate. Rather than eliminating jobs, AI is more likely to transform them, shifting healthcare professionals' emphasis to duties that complement AI technologies. Nevertheless, it is worth noting that along with the exciting advancements and numerous advantages there are challenges that need to be tackled. Key among these are the legal and ethical complexities inherent in AI's integration into healthcare. Moving forward, there is significant potential for AI in healthcare; however, realizing this potential will require continued research, cross-disciplinary cooperation, and open dialogue among AI developers, healthcare professionals, and ethical and legal experts. Combining AI's capabilities with the human elements of healthcare professionals will lead to more personalized, effective, and efficient patient care.

Chapter 3

Foundations of ML Evaluation

Medicine is entering an era defined by digital transformation, with artificial intelligence (AI), especially machine learning (ML), rapidly reshaping how clinicians diagnose, prognosticate, and treat disease. AI-powered diagnostic tools now analyze medical images, predict patient risk, and even propose personalized treatment plans; often with a speed and accuracy that rivals or exceeds human performance in controlled studies.

Yet, the promise of AI in healthcare is matched by its complexity and potential pitfalls. A tool that boasts "99% accuracy" may, in reality, miss the very patients who most need care, or perform well in one hospital but fail catastrophically in another due to hidden biases or technical shortcuts. As future physicians and stewards of patient safety, medical trainees must become more than passive users of these technologies. They must learn to critically evaluate AI systems, understanding not just their advertised benefits, but also their limitations, sources of error, and the ethical ramifications of their deployment.

3.1 Introduction

This chapter aims to equip medical students and practitioners with the foundational skills needed to appraise AI-assisted diagnostics. We will explore why traditional metrics like accuracy can be misleading, delve into the dangers of overfitting, underfitting, and data leakage, and provide frameworks for asking the right questions of AI vendors and researchers. By developing critical evaluation skills, clinicians can ensure that AI tools augment, rather than undermine, clinical judgment; delivering safer, more equitable, and more effective care in the age of digital medicine.

It is vital to recognize that ML is not meant to replace physicians, but to augment clinical expertise. The most promising future for medicine is one of collaboration, where human judgment and AI work together to improve patient care. As future clinicians, a foundational understanding of ML will empower you to interpret, critically evaluate, and responsibly deploy these technologies in practice; ensuring that the benefits of digital transformation are realized safely and equitably.

3.2   Foundations of ML in Medicine

Medicine is undergoing a profound technological transformation, and at its core lies ML, i.e., a form of AI that is enhancing our approach to disease detection, diagnosis, and treatment. ML enables computers to learn from vast amounts of data, much like a senior physician develops clinical intuition through years of experience, but on a scale and speed previously unimaginable [310].

3.2.1   The Main Branches of ML

Machine learning is not a single technique, but a collection of approaches, each suited to different types of problems in medicine. The three primary branches (namely, supervised learning, unsupervised learning, and reinforcement learning) mirror familiar processes in clinical reasoning and patient care. Table 3.1 summarizes these branches, their definitions, and clinical analogies to help ground these concepts in everyday medical practice.

Supervised learning is the most common in healthcare, where algorithms are trained on datasets with known outcomes (such as disease/no disease) and then used to predict outcomes for new patients. Unsupervised learning, by contrast, seeks to uncover hidden patterns in data without predefined labels; useful for discovering new disease subtypes. Reinforcement learning is inspired by behavioral psychology, where algorithms learn optimal strategies through feedback, much like clinicians refine treatment plans based on patient outcomes.

Branch	Definition	Clinical Analogy
Supervised Learning	Algorithm learns from labeled data (input-output pairs)	Learning from known patient cases with established diagnoses
Unsupervised Learning	Algorithm finds patterns in unlabeled data	Noticing clusters of symptoms in patients with an unknown syndrome
Reinforcement Learning	Algorithm learns by trial and error, receiving rewards or penalties	Adjusting a treatment plan based on patient response over time

Table 3.1: The three main branches of machine learning and their clinical analogies.

3.2.2 Common ML Algorithms in Healthcare

ML algorithms are rapidly becoming indispensable tools in modern medicine, offering clinicians a "magnifying glass" to detect patterns and make predictions from vast and complex datasets that would be impossible to analyze manually. As a medical student, you are trained to synthesize clues from patient histories, physical exams, and lab results. ML algorithms extend this detective work, learning from thousands or even millions of examples to spot subtle relationships and trends that can inform diagnosis, prognosis, and treatment decisions.

While the mathematics behind these algorithms can be intricate, the core ideas are intuitive and closely parallel clinical reasoning. Understanding these foundational algorithms will help you interpret their outputs, recognize their limitations, and collaborate effectively with data scientists and engineers. Table 3.2 summarizes several of the most widely used ML algorithms in healthcare, explaining their underlying concepts and providing concrete clinical examples.

These algorithms are the building blocks of many AI-powered tools now being integrated into electronic health records, diagnostic imaging platforms, and clinical decision support systems. For example, linear regression is used for predicting continuous outcomes like lab values, while logistic regression is suited for binary classification tasks such as disease detection. Decision trees and random forests are valued for their interpretability and robustness, and support vector machines excel at distinguishing between complex patient groups. The field of ML in healthcare is evolving at a breathtaking pace, with new algorithms and applications emerging rapidly. Deep learning,

Algorithm	Concept	Healthcare Example
Linear Regression	Finds a straight-line relationship between inputs and a continuous output	Predicting blood pressure based on age and weight
Logistic Regression	Predicts the probability of a binary outcome using a sigmoid curve	Predicting disease presence (yes/no) from lab results
Decision Trees	Asks a series of yes/no questions to reach a decision	Clinical algorithms for chest pain evaluation
Random Forests	Aggregates many decision trees for robust predictions	Risk prediction for cardiovascular events
Support Vector Machines	Finds the optimal boundary separating two groups	Classifying responders vs. non-responders to a treatment

Table 3.2: Common machine learning algorithms and their healthcare applications.

natural language processing, and reinforcement learning are already making their mark in areas such as medical imaging, genomics, and personalized medicine.

As a future physician, staying informed about these advances will be vital; not only to leverage their benefits, but also to ensure their safe and ethical use in patient care. By understanding the strengths and limitations of these foundational algorithms, you will be better equipped to critically evaluate AI tools, interpret their outputs, and advocate for technologies that truly enhance patient care.

3.2.3 Applications of ML in Medicine

The impact of ML in healthcare is already visible across a range of domains. Table 3.3 highlights key application areas, describing how ML is transforming clinical practice and research.

For instance, ML algorithms can rapidly analyze radiological images to assist in the detection of tumors or strokes, often matching or exceeding human performance in controlled settings. In personalized medicine, ML helps integrate genetic, lifestyle, and environmental data to tailor prevention and treatment strategies. Drug discovery is being accelerated by ML models that predict which compounds are most likely to succeed, and predictive

Application Area	Description	Example
Medical Imaging	Automated analysis of images for disease detection	Identifying tumors in CT scans
Personalized Medicine	Tailoring risk prediction and treatment to the individual	Using genomics to guide cancer therapy
Drug Discovery	Accelerating identification of new drug candidates	Predicting drug efficacy and side effects
Predictive Analytics	Forecasting patient risk using EHR data	Early warning for sepsis or heart failure

Table 3.3: Key applications of machine learning in healthcare.

analytics are enabling earlier interventions for high-risk patients by mining patterns in electronic health records.

3.3   Data Splitting and Cross-Validation

The foundation of reliable ML evaluation rests upon the proper division of available data into distinct subsets for training, validation, and testing. This fundamental step, referred to as data splitting, determines whether a model's reported performance reflects genuine predictive capability or merely an artifact of methodological flaws. In clinical applications, where patient safety depends on accurate predictions, the choice of validation methodology can mean the difference between a robust diagnostic tool and a dangerous overconfident algorithm.

The most common approach in machine learning is the three-way split, where the dataset is divided into training (typically 60-80%), validation (10-20%), and test (10-20%) subsets. The training set serves as the foundation for model learning, allowing algorithms to identify patterns and relationships within the data. The validation set provides an independent dataset for hyperparameter tuning and model selection during the development process, helping to optimize performance while avoiding overfitting to the training data. Finally, the test set remains completely untouched throughout the entire development process, serving as the ultimate arbiter of model performance and providing an unbiased estimate of real-world effectiveness (see Table 3.4). This three-way approach offers the advantage of maintaining strict separation between model development and final evaluation, thereby reducing the risk of optimistic bias in performance estimates.

Subset	Purpose	When Used	Data Access Level	Typical Size
Training	Model fitting/learning	During training	Full access: model learns directly from this data	60–80%
Validation	Hyperparameter tuning	During development	Indirect access: performance feedback guides model decisions	10–20%
Test	Final evaluation	After development	No access: completely held out during all development stages	10–20%

Table 3.4: Data split proportions, purposes, and access levels in machine learning.

However, clinical datasets are often constrained by limited sample sizes, particularly for rare diseases or specialized patient populations where data collection is challenging and expensive. In such scenarios, dedicating 20-40% of already scarce data to validation and testing may leave insufficient examples for robust model training. When datasets are too small to support reliable three-way splits without compromising statistical power, researchers must consider alternative validation strategies. The two-way split approach, dividing data only into training and test sets, represents one such alternative, but this method sacrifices the independent validation set that guides model development decisions. Without a separate validation set, researchers risk inadvertent overfitting to the test set through repeated model adjustments, ultimately leading to overly optimistic performance estimates.

Cross-validation emerges as the preferred solution when dataset limitations preclude effective three-way splitting. In k-fold cross-validation, the available data is divided into k roughly equal subsets, with k-1 subsets used for training and the remaining subset reserved for validation (as demonstrated in Figure 3.1). This process repeats k times, with each subset serving as the validation set exactly once, allowing every data point to contribute to both training and validation across the complete procedure. The final performance estimate represents the average across all k validation rounds, providing a more robust and less variable assessment than single train-test splits, particularly crucial when working with limited clinical data.

The choice of k in cross-validation involves balancing computational efficiency with statistical reliability. Five-fold cross-validation (k=5) offers a reasonable compromise for most clinical applications, providing meaningful

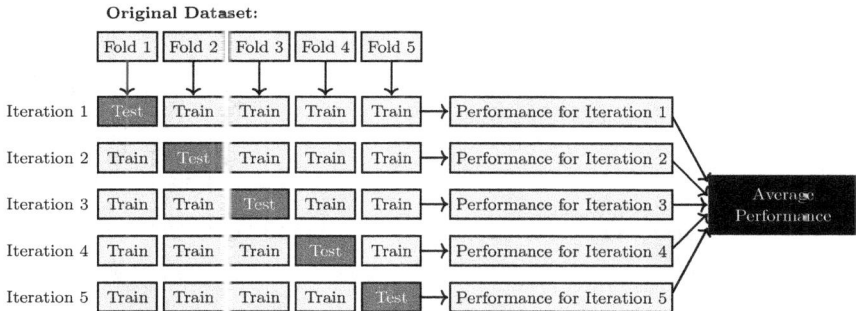

Figure 3.1: Illustration of 5-fold cross-validation methodology. The dataset is partitioned into 5 equal folds, and the process iterates 5 times. In each iteration, one fold serves as the validation set while the remaining 4 folds constitute the training set. This ensures that every data point is used for validation exactly once, maximizing data utilization while maintaining rigorous evaluation standards.

performance estimates while maintaining manageable computational requirements. Each fold uses 80% of the data for training and 20% for validation, similar to traditional three-way splits but with the advantage of utilizing all data for both purposes across iterations. Ten-fold cross-validation (k=10) provides even more robust estimates by using 90% of data for training in each iteration, though at increased computational cost. The choice between k=5 and k=10 often depends on dataset size, computational resources, and the criticality of obtaining precise performance estimates.

The decision framework for choosing validation methodology should prioritize both statistical validity and practical feasibility within clinical constraints. When datasets contain sufficient samples to support meaningful three-way splits (generally requiring hundreds to thousands of examples per class), this approach provides the cleanest separation between model development and evaluation phases. However, when sample sizes are limited, k-fold cross-validation offers superior utilization of available data while maintaining rigorous evaluation standards. The specific value of k should reflect the trade-off between bias and variance: smaller values of k (such as k=5) provide less biased estimates of model performance but with higher variance, while larger values (such as k=10) reduce variance but may introduce slight upward bias in performance estimates

Regardless of the chosen validation strategy, the fundamental principle remains constant: the evaluation methodology must provide an honest assessment of how the model will perform on genuinely unseen clinical

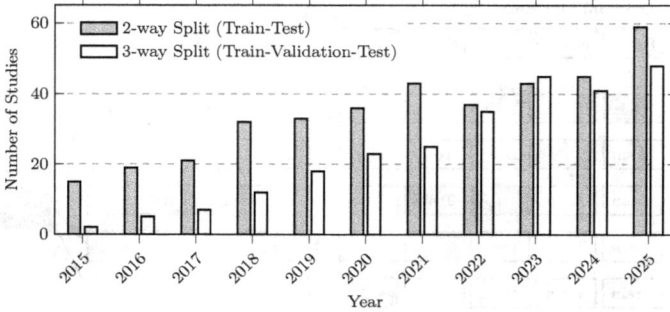

Figure 3.2: Annual count of PubMed-indexed machine learning classification studies (2015–2025) using 2-way (train-test) and 3-way (train-validation-test) data splits. The data for this figure was synthesized by reviewing abstracts and full texts of PubMed search results for the keywords "machine learning" and "classification" (search conducted in September 2025). Studies were categorized based on explicit descriptions of their data splitting strategies. While some articles did not specify their approach, only those with clearly identified split strategies were included in the counts presented here.

data. This requires careful attention to temporal aspects of data collection, ensuring that validation sets reflect the intended deployment scenario rather than artificially favorable conditions. In clinical settings, this often means evaluating models on data from different time periods, institutions, or patient populations to assess true generalizability beyond the development cohort.

The Figure 3.2 highlights a growing adoption of the 3-way split approach over the past decade, reflecting increased awareness of the importance of robust model evaluation. Whenever feasible, researchers should strive to use a 3-way split separating training, validation, and test sets. This practice helps ensure unbiased hyperparameter tuning and performance assessment, reducing the risk of overfitting and improving the generalizability of machine learning models in biomedical research.

3.4   Evaluating ML Algorithms

The evaluation of ML algorithms in medicine requires a rigorous and nuanced approach. While the promise of ML lies in its ability to detect patterns and make predictions from complex datasets, the true value of an algorithm is only realized when its performance is critically appraised in a clinical context. Traditional metrics such as accuracy, while intuitively appealing, can be misleading; especially in scenarios involving imbalanced datasets, where the prevalence of disease is low. For instance, an algorithm that always predicts the absence of a rare disease may achieve high accuracy but fail to identify any true cases, rendering it clinically useless.

In clinical medicine, the application of ML most often centers on classification tasks. These tasks involve sorting patients into clinically meaningful categories, such as distinguishing between healthy and diseased individuals (binary classification), or further differentiating among multiple disease types or severity levels (multi-class classification). For example, an ML model may be tasked with predicting whether a patient has pneumonia or not, or with classifying the stage of diabetic retinopathy based on retinal images. The ultimate goal is to support clinical decision-making by providing accurate, actionable categorizations that align with real-world diagnostic and treatment pathways.

Predicted

	Disease	No Disease
Disease	True Positive (TP)	False Negative (FN)
No Disease	False Positive (FP)	True Negative (TN)

Actual (row label spanning Disease / No Disease)

Term	Clinical Interpretation
TP	Correctly identified disease
FP	False alarm
FN	Missed diagnosis
TN	Correctly identified healthy

$\text{Accuracy} = (TP+TN)/(TP+TN+FP+FN)$
$\text{Precision} = TP/(TP+FP)$
$\text{Recall} = TP/(TP+FN)$
$\text{F1-score} = 2\times(\text{Precision}\times\text{Recall})/(\text{Precision}+\text{Recall})$

Figure 3.3: Confusion matrix showing the four possible outcomes in binary classification with clinical interpretations.

Because the majority of ML use cases in healthcare revolve around these classification problems, the evaluation of algorithmic performance must be tailored accordingly. The confusion matrix is a foundational tool in this process (see Figure 3.3). It provides a detailed breakdown of the model's predictions compared to the actual clinical outcomes, categorizing results into true positives (correctly identified cases), false positives (incorrectly flagged cases), true negatives (correctly identified non-cases), and false negatives (missed cases). This matrix is not only applicable to binary classification but can be extended to multi-class scenarios, where it summarizes the model's ability to distinguish among several disease categories or severity levels.

Relying solely on overall accuracy can be dangerously misleading, especially in medicine where disease prevalence is often low. For instance, in a screening context for a rare cancer, a model that always predicts "no cancer" could achieve high accuracy simply by virtue of the disease's rarity, yet fail to identify any true cases. Thus, rendering it clinically useless. The confusion matrix enables the calculation of more informative metrics such as sensitivity (recall), specificity, precision, and the area under the receiver operating characteristic (ROC) curve (AUC). Each of these metrics provides unique insights into the strengths and weaknesses of an algorithm, and their relative importance varies depending on the clinical context. For example, high sensitivity is crucial for screening tools to minimize missed cases, while high specificity is essential in diagnostic settings to avoid unnecessary interventions.

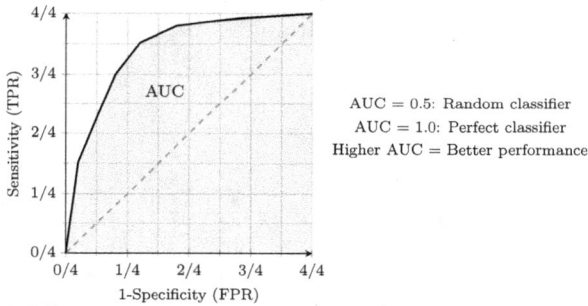

Figure 3.4: ROC curve illustrating the trade-off between sensitivity and specificity, with the area under the curve (AUC) representing overall discriminative ability.

Figure 3.4 presents an example of an ROC curve, which is a widely used tool for evaluating the performance of classification models in medicine. The x-axis of the ROC curve is labeled as "1-Specificity" (FPR), where FPR stands for *False Positive Rate*. This is because the false positive rate is mathematically defined as FPR $= \frac{FP}{FP+TN}$, and it is equivalent to $1 - $ Specificity, where specificity measures the proportion of true negatives correctly identified. Thus, as you move to the right along the x-axis, the model is making more false positive errors, i.e., incorrectly labeling healthy individuals as diseased. The y-axis is labeled as "Sensitivity" (TPR), or *True Positive Rate*, which is the proportion of actual disease cases correctly identified by the model (TPR $= \frac{TP}{TP+FN}$). Plotting TPR against FPR at various thresholds allows us to visualize the trade-off between correctly detecting disease and avoiding false alarms. The ideal model would achieve high sensitivity (TPR close to 1) while maintaining a low false positive rate (FPR close to 0), corresponding to the top-left corner of the plot. This visualization helps clinicians and researchers understand how changing the decision threshold affects both types of errors, which is vital for clinical decision-making.

3.4.1 Overview of Terminology

The evaluation of classification algorithms is, unfortunately, complicated by the diversity of terminology used across different fields and publications. Terms such as accuracy, precision, recall, sensitivity, and F1-score are frequently encountered, yet their definitions and relationships are not always presented consistently (see all the variations summarized in Table 3.5).

Primary Term	Alternative Names	Source of Confusion
Recall	Sensitivity, True Positive Rate (TPR)	Medical literature favors "sensitivity" while computer science uses "recall" for identical metric
Precision	Positive Predictive Value (PPV)	Medical contexts often use "positive predictive value" instead of "precision"
Sensitivity	Recall, True Positive Rate (TPR)	Same metric as recall but terminology varies by field, creating apparent differences
F1-score	F-measure, F-score	Harmonic mean notation varies but refers to same precision-recall balance metric
Accuracy	Overall Accuracy, Classification Accuracy	Generally consistent terminology but can be misleading metric in imbalanced datasets

Table 3.5: Common terminology variations and sources of confusion in machine learning evaluation metrics.

Accuracy is the most general metric, representing the proportion of all correct predictions (both positive and negative) among the total number of cases evaluated. While intuitively straightforward, accuracy alone may not provide meaningful insight in clinical contexts where class imbalance is common, as previously discussed.

Precision and recall are more nuanced metrics that focus specifically on the model's performance with respect to the positive (diseased) class. Precision, also known as positive predictive value, quantifies the proportion of cases labeled as positive by the model that are truly positive. In contrast, recall (also referred to as sensitivity or true positive rate) measures the proportion of actual positive cases that are correctly identified by the model.

The use of both "recall" and "sensitivity" to describe the same concept is a frequent source of confusion; in medical literature, "sensitivity" is the preferred term, whereas "recall" is more common in computer science and information retrieval.

The F1-score provides a single summary metric that balances precision and recall. It is defined as the harmonic mean of precision and recall, and is particularly useful when the costs of false positives and false negatives are both significant, or when class distributions are imbalanced. By combining these two metrics, the F1-score offers a more comprehensive assessment of a model's ability to correctly identify positive cases without over-predicting them.

Hence, while accuracy offers a broad measure of correctness, precision and recall (sensitivity) provide more clinically relevant insights into a model's strengths and weaknesses in identifying disease. The F1-score further synthesizes these aspects into a single value, facilitating comparison between models. Recognizing the equivalence of recall and sensitivity, and understanding the distinct roles of each metric, is essential for the rigorous evaluation of machine learning algorithms in medicine.

3.5   Beyond Accuracy: Understanding Key Metrics and Their Limitations

Relying solely on accuracy as a measure of ML performance can obscure critical deficiencies, particularly in medical applications where the cost of errors is high. Sensitivity (recall) measures the proportion of actual positives correctly identified, making it vital for applications where missing a diagnosis could have severe consequences. Specificity, on the other hand, quantifies the proportion of true negatives, helping to avoid unnecessary treatments or anxiety for healthy individuals. Precision, or positive predictive value, reflects the likelihood that a positive prediction is correct, which is essential for building clinical trust in AI recommendations.

The area under the ROC curve (AUC) provides a single summary statistic of a model's ability to discriminate between classes, but it too has limitations, especially in highly imbalanced datasets. In such cases, precision-recall curves may offer a more informative assessment. Ultimately, the choice of metric should be guided by the clinical context and the relative consequences of false positives and false negatives.

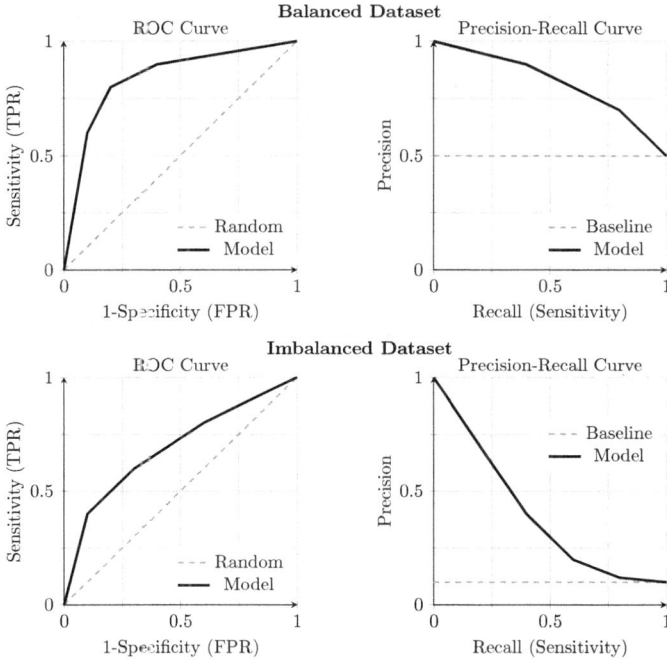

Figure 3.5: Comparison of ROC and precision-recall curves for a model evaluated on balanced versus imbalanced datasets. The top row shows results for the balanced dataset, while the bottom row shows results for the imbalanced dataset. Note how the ROC curve may appear similar in both cases, while the precision-recall curve reveals the impact of class imbalance on model performance.

Figure 3.5 illustrates how ROC and precision-recall curves behave under balanced and imbalanced class distributions. In the top row, both the ROC and precision-recall curves for the balanced dataset show strong model performance, with the ROC curve bowing toward the top-left and the precision-recall curve maintaining high precision across a range of recall values. In contrast, the bottom row demonstrates the effect of class imbalance: while the ROC curve for the imbalanced dataset still appears reasonably good (better than guessing), the corresponding precision-recall curve drops sharply, revealing a substantial decline in precision as recall increases. This discrepancy highlights a key limitation of ROC curves in imbalanced settings: they may overstate model performance by not reflecting the low prevalence of the positive class. Precision-recall curves, on the other hand, are more sensitive to class imbalance and provide a clearer picture of a model's ability to correctly identify positive cases without being overwhelmed by false positives. Therefore, when evaluating models on imbalanced datasets, precision-recall curves often offer a more informative assessment than ROC curves, especially in applications where the minority class is of primary interest.

3.6 Algorithmic Bias and Ensuring Equity

Algorithmic bias represents one of the most significant ethical and practical challenges in the deployment of ML in healthcare. Bias can originate from unrepresentative training data, flawed labeling, or the use of proxies that inadvertently encode social or demographic disparities. For example, an algorithm trained predominantly on data from one demographic group may perform poorly when applied to others, exacerbating existing health disparities. Similarly, using healthcare costs as a proxy for illness severity can perpetuate systemic inequities, as historically marginalized groups may have lower healthcare expenditures despite similar levels of illness.

To ensure equity, it is vital to scrutinize the composition of training datasets and demand performance metrics stratified by key demographic variables such as race, sex, and age. Transparent reporting and ongoing monitoring are necessary to identify and mitigate bias, ensuring that ML tools serve all patient populations fairly.

The SOURCE Consortium's 2025 multicenter study represents a relevant study on the application of ML to clinical ophthalmology, specifically in predicting which patients with glaucoma are likely to progress to the point of requiring surgical intervention [311]. Leveraging a large, diverse electronic health record (EHR) dataset from multiple institutions, the researchers developed and validated several ML models to forecast glaucoma progression and the need for surgery. The study found that while the models achieved strong overall predictive performance, there were notable differences in sensitivity and specificity across demographic groups, as illustrated in Figure 3.6. For example, sensitivity was highest among White and Asian patients, but substantially lower for Black patients, particularly Black females, highlighting the presence of algorithmic bias. Clinically, high sensitivity means that most patients at risk are detected by the model, minimizing missed cases (false negatives). Specificity measures the model's ability to correctly identify patients who do not have the condition, i.e., those who will not require surgery. High specificity means the model avoids incorrectly labeling

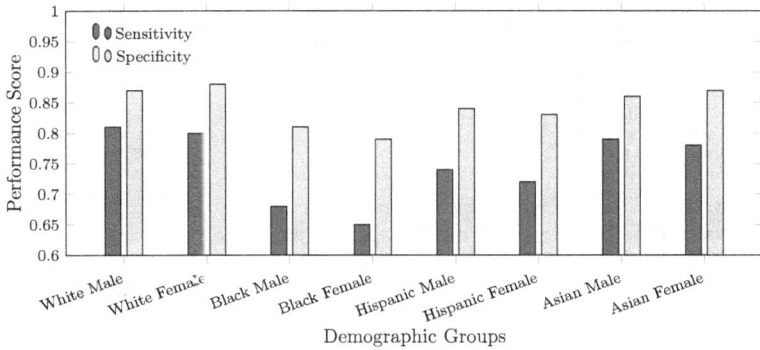

Figure 3.6: Performance of a machine learning model for predicting glaucoma surgery risk, stratified by demographic group. Bars show sensitivity (darker) and specificity (lighter) for each intersectional subgroup (race and gender), based on results from the SOURCE Consortium's multicenter study of glaucoma progression prediction using electronic health record data [311].

healthy patients as at risk (false positives), which helps prevent unnecessary anxiety, further testing, or treatment.

These disparities underscore the critical need for equity-aware modeling and rigorous subgroup analysis in clinical ML research. The findings have important implications for the deployment of AI in healthcare: without careful attention to demographic performance, ML models risk perpetuating or even exacerbating existing health disparities. The SOURCE Consortium's work demonstrates both the promise and the challenges of integrating AI into clinical practice, emphasizing the necessity of ongoing efforts to ensure fairness, transparency, and generalizability in predictive healthcare models [311].

3.7   Validation: From Model Development to Real-World Clinical Impact

Validation is the process by which the generalizability and clinical utility of an ML model are established. Internal validation, performed on data from the same source as the training set, is a necessary first step but is insufficient for clinical adoption. While internal validation methods such as cross-validation or split-sample testing can help guard against overfitting, they cannot guarantee that a model will perform well outside the specific

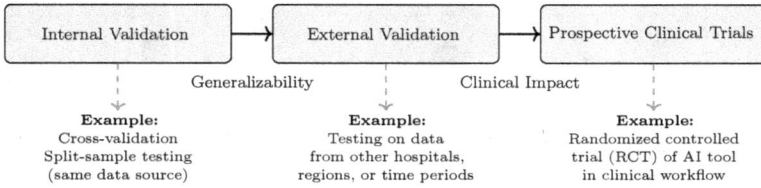

Figure 3.7: Flowchart illustrating the stages of machine learning model validation: internal validation (e.g., cross-validation within a single dataset), external validation (testing on independent datasets from other institutions or populations), and prospective clinical trials (randomized controlled trials assessing real-world clinical impact).

context in which it was developed. This is because internal validation may inadvertently capture and reinforce patterns, biases, or artifacts unique to the original dataset, rather than true underlying clinical relationships.

The stages of model validation (including internal validation, external validation, and prospective clinical trials) are summarized in Figure 3.7. This flowchart illustrates the progression from initial model development to real-world clinical impact, emphasizing the central role of external validation in establishing generalizability and the ultimate importance of prospective evaluation for clinical adoption.

External validation is a critical step in the evaluation pipeline. By testing the model on data from different institutions, populations, or time periods, researchers can assess whether the model's performance is robust and truly generalizable. External validation provides evidence that the model is not simply memorizing idiosyncrasies of the training data, but is instead capturing clinically meaningful patterns that hold across diverse settings. Without external validation, there is a significant risk that a model will fail when deployed in real-world clinical environments, where patient populations, data collection practices, and disease prevalence may differ substantially from those in the original study. In fact, external validation is often considered the minimum standard for demonstrating that a model is ready for broader clinical use.

However, in some cases, external validation may not be immediately feasible; such as when access to independent datasets is limited, or when the model is being developed for a rare disease with few available data sources. In these situations, it is still possible to gain insight into the likely generalizability of the model by conducting a rigorous assessment of the training dynamics, as described in this chapter. Careful monitoring of learning curves, evaluation of model performance across different subgroups within the training data, and the use of techniques such as repeated cross-validation can help identify overfitting and provide early warnings about potential generalization failures. While these approaches cannot fully substitute for true external validation, they offer valuable information about the stability and reliability of the model's predictions.

Ultimately, the highest standard of validation is achieved through prospective studies and randomized controlled trials (RCTs), which directly measure the impact of an ML tool on patient outcomes in real-world clinical settings. These studies provide the strongest evidence that the use of an AI tool leads to measurable improvements in care, such as reduced mortality or shorter hospital stays. Without such rigorous validation, even the most technically impressive models may fail to deliver meaningful clinical benefits.

3.8   Spotting Red Flags

This section equips the reader with practical diagnostics for detecting methodological red flags that can undermine clinical ML results and clarifies what healthy training and evaluation should look like. It begins by characterizing overfitting and underfitting and by showing how to read learning curves to distinguish healthy convergence from pathologies such as memorization, excessive regularization, or data leakage, preparing you to interpret the visual patterns that follow. It then examines the major forms of data leakage (namely, temporal, patient-level, preprocessing, and label-related) using clinical timelines and workflow schematics to illustrate how leakage arises and how to prevent it in practice. Finally, it demonstrates subset-wise performance trends across train, validation, test, and external cohorts, explaining why a monotonic, gradual decline on increasingly challenging data indicates true generalization, whereas erratic jumps or reversals signal overfitting or leakage. Throughout, it is emphasized that headline metrics are insufficient without transparent training dynamics and that rigorous reporting of curves and subset-wise behavior is vital for credible, clinically useful models.

3.8.1   Overfitting, Underfitting

Overfitting, underfitting, and data leakage are critical pitfalls that can undermine the reliability of ML models in healthcare. Overfitting occurs when a model learns the training data (including noise and irrelevant details) too well, resulting in poor generalization to new data. This is often indicated by a large gap between training and validation accuracy. Underfitting, conversely, arises when a model is too simplistic to capture the underlying patterns, leading to uniformly poor performance.

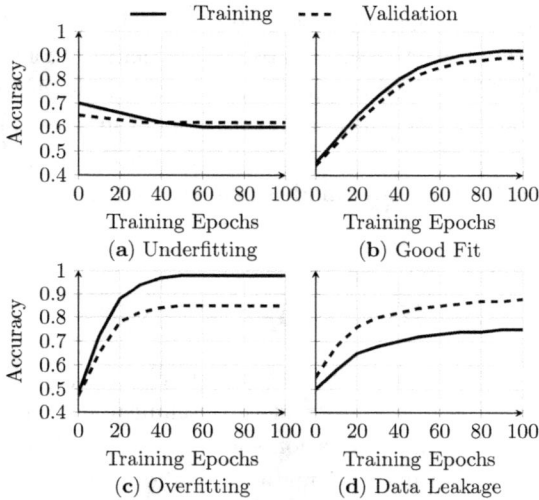

Figure 3.8: Learning curves illustrating four fundamental training scenarios: underfitting (a) where both curves remain low due to insufficient model complexity, good fit (b) where curves converge with a small gap indicating proper generalization, overfitting (c) where a large persistent gap reveals poor generalization despite high training accuracy, and data leakage/excessive regularization (d) where validation accuracy exceeds training accuracy, indicating methodological issues that require investigation.

A nuanced understanding of learning curves, as depicted in Figure 3.8, is vital for diagnosing the root causes of poor model performance. In the underfitting scenario (Figure 3.8a), both the training and validation accuracy curves remain low and fail to improve meaningfully with additional training epochs. This pattern signals that the model lacks sufficient complexity or capacity to capture the underlying structure of the data, resulting in uniformly poor performance on both seen and unseen cases. In contrast, a well-fitted model (Figure 3.8b) demonstrates both curves rising and plateauing at high values, with only a small, stable gap between them, i.e., an indicator of effective learning and generalization. Overfitting (Figure 3.8c) is characterized by a training curve that continues to climb while the validation curve stagnates or even declines, creating a widening gap that betrays the model's reliance on memorizing training examples rather than extracting generalizable patterns. Notably, if the validation accuracy curve ever rises above the training curve (Figure 3.8d), this may point to issues such as excessive regularization, data leakage, or an unrepresentative training set. Such a crossing is atypical and should prompt careful investigation, as it often reflects methodological flaws rather than genuine model superiority on unseen data.

Of particular interest is the scenario depicted in Figure 3.8d, where the validation accuracy curve consistently exceeds the training accuracy. While this pattern is a classic indicator of data leakage, where information from the validation set inadvertently influences the model during training, it can also arise from other methodological issues. For example, excessive regularization may suppress training performance more than validation performance, or a significant class imbalance may cause the validation set to be easier than the training set by chance. Regardless of the cause, such a crossing is atypical and should prompt careful investigation, as it often reflects flaws in experimental design or data handling rather than genuine model superiority on unseen data.

Thus, the interplay and relative positions of these curves provide critical insights into whether a model is learning, memorizing, or failing to capture the task altogether, and should be a routine part of model evaluation in clinical machine learning research.

Learning Curves and Model Convergence

A critical aspect of evaluating ML models for clinical tasks is the careful monitoring of performance metrics throughout the training process. Learning curves, i.e., plots of model performance (e.g., accuracy) on both training and validation datasets as a function of training set size or epochs, are indispensable tools for diagnosing model health and generalizability.

The Figure 3.9 presents two sets of learning curves, each representing a different training scenario:

Triangle Curves (Healthy Model Training): The curves with triangle markers (shown in black and gray) illustrate a model that is learning appropriately. As the training set size increases, both the training and validation accuracy curves rise together, eventually converging and plateauing at similar values. Importantly, a small, stable gap is maintained between the two curves. This pattern indicates that the model is learning generalizable pat-

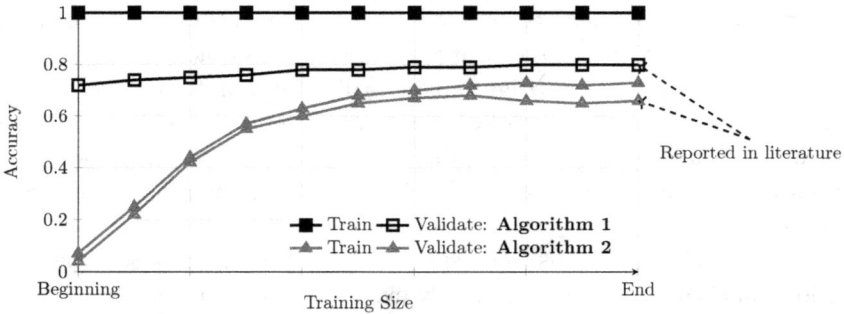

Figure 3.9: Learning curves comparing healthy model training (Algorithm 2, triangles) versus problematic training (Algorithm 1, squares). The triangular markers show both training and validation accuracy rising together and converging with a small gap, indicating good generalization. The square markers show high, flat training accuracy with much lower validation accuracy, indicating overfitting and poor generalization.

terns from the data, rather than memorizing the training set. The small gap reflects a healthy balance between fitting the training data and maintaining the ability to generalize to unseen cases, i.e., a hallmark of robust, clinically reliable ML.

It is important to note that, in healthy model training, the small gap between the training and validation curves should be most evident at the end of training, once both curves have plateaued. This final gap reflects the model's generalization ability after learning has stabilized. Additionally, the training curve should consistently remain above the validation curve, as the model is always expected to perform slightly better on data it has seen during training compared to unseen validation data. These features (i.e., small, stable gap at the plateau and correct curve order) are key indicators of robust model convergence and generalizability.

Square Curves (Unhealthy/Pathological Training): In contrast, the curves with square markers (shown in black) represent a model whose training and validation accuracy remain nearly constant throughout the entire training process. The training accuracy is very high and flat, while the validation accuracy is much lower and also flat, resulting in a large, persistent gap between the two curves. This scenario suggests that the model is not learning new or meaningful patterns as training progresses. The large gap is a classic sign of overfitting: the model has essentially memorized the training data but fails to generalize to new, unseen data. Such a model is unreliable for clinical deployment.

Implications for Clinical ML Research

Despite the diagnostic value of learning curves, many published ML studies in the medical literature do not report or analyze training dynamics. Instead, they often present only final performance metrics (such as accuracy or AUC) on a hold-out test set. This omission is problematic: without insight into the training process, it is impossible to determine whether reported results reflect genuine learning or are artifacts of overfitting, data leakage, or other methodological flaws.

As the figure demonstrates, a model can achieve superficially high accuracy on the training set while failing to generalize; a pitfall that can go undetected without learning curve analysis. Inadequate reporting of training dynamics means that published results may be the product of poor ML practice rather than true clinical utility.

The arrows in Figure 3.9 highlight two values (final validation accuracies) that are often the only results reported in the literature. In some studies, a three-way split is used, and the final accuracy on a separate test (hold-out) set is reported instead. However, even when a test set is used, relying solely on this final metric can be misleading. If one were to judge only by these reported values, Algorithm 1 might appear preferable, as its final accuracy is higher than that of Algorithm 2. This would be a critical mistake: Algorithm 1's persistently large gap between training and validation accuracy reveals severe overfitting, indicating that it cannot be trusted to generalize to new patients. In clinical practice, such a model would be essentially useless, as its apparent performance is an artifact of memorizing the training data rather than learning generalizable patterns. No matter how high the final test or validation accuracy appears, serious conclusions about clinical utility cannot be drawn from a model that has not demonstrated healthy training dynamics and convergence. This example underscores the danger of accepting published results at face value without scrutinizing the underlying training process. Only by examining the full learning curves can we distinguish between models that are truly robust and those likely to fail in real-world clinical settings.

Many studies in the literature fail to assess or report these training dynamics, leading to a risk that their results are simply artifacts of poor ML training rather than evidence of real-world clinical performance. This lack of transparency undermines the credibility of reported findings and can result in the adoption of models that are not fit for clinical use. Recognizing this gap, recent FDA guidance on AI/ML in healthcare explicitly addresses the need for standardized validation frameworks that include the monitoring of training dynamics and learning curves [312]. The FDA guidance emphasizes that high in-domain accuracy alone is insufficient; robust model development requires transparent reporting of how models learn and converge during training, and mandates the inclusion of learning curve analysis as part of regulatory submissions.

Property	Alg. 1	Alg. 2	Evidence from Figure 3.9
Training Progression	Static, no learning	Dynamic learning	Algorithm 1: Training accuracy remains flat at 100% throughout. Algorithm 2: Training accuracy rises from 7% to 73%, showing clear learning progression.
Validation Trajectory	Stagnant performance	Parallel improvement	Algorithm 1: Validation accuracy flat at $\sim$80% with no improvement. Algorithm 2: Validation accuracy rises from 4% to 66%, tracking training curve.
Convergence Pattern	No convergence	Healthy convergence	Algorithm 1: Large persistent gap (20%) between curves with no closing trend. Algorithm 2: Curves converge with small final gap ($\sim$7%).
Learning Dynamics	Memorization behavior	Genuine learning	Algorithm 1: Perfect training + poor validation suggests memorization. Algorithm 2: Parallel curve progression indicates pattern recognition.
Generalization Gap	Large, persistent	Small, stable	Algorithm 1: 20% gap maintained throughout training. Algorithm 2: Gap remains small, increasing from $\sim$3% to a stable $\sim$7%.
Clinical Reliability	Unreliable deployment	Suitable for deployment	Algorithm 1 patterns indicate poor generalization to new patients. Algorithm 2 shows predictable, stable performance characteristics.

Table 3.6: Learning curve characteristics comparison demonstrating healthy versus pathological training behaviors (Figure 3.9).

Failure to assess and report learning curves should be viewed as a significant red flag. Robust ML evaluation must go beyond final metrics to include a thorough analysis of training dynamics. Only by ensuring that both training and validation curves converge and plateau together (with a small, stable gap) can we be confident that a model is suitable for clinical use. Hence, learning curves are not just technical artifacts; they are critical indicators of model health and generalizability. Their absence from published studies should prompt skepticism, and their inclusion is now a best practice endorsed by regulatory authorities. By adopting these standards, the medical AI community can move toward more trustworthy, clinically meaningful ML applications.

To demonstrate the importance of learning curve analysis in clinical ML evaluation, Table 3.6 and Figure 3.9 present a detailed comparison of two algorithms exhibiting fundamentally different training behaviors. This comparison illustrates how learning curves can reveal essential characteristics about model reliability and generalizability that traditional final performance metrics alone cannot capture. Algorithm 1 exemplifies a pathological training pattern commonly observed in clinical ML research: achieving perfect training accuracy while maintaining a consistently poor and stagnant validation performance, creating a large, persistent gap that indicates severe overfitting and memorization rather than genuine learning. Algorithm 2 demonstrates the hallmarks of healthy model training: as training progresses, both the training and validation curves converge and plateau, with the training curve remaining above the validation curve and the gap between them being small and stable.

It is not necessary for both the training and validation curves to start from low initial values or to rise together. What matters is that, at convergence, this pattern of a small, stable gap and proper curve order is achieved, as it indicates healthy model training and good generalization. The training curve may start at a much higher value than the validation curve, especially if the model can easily fit the training data from the outset or if the initial training set is small or not representative. The key diagnostic feature is not the starting point, but how the curves evolve and where they settle as training progresses. Healthy learning curves are characterized by both curves plateauing at some value, with the training curve consistently above the validation curve. The gap between them should be small and stable at convergence, indicating good generalization. A large, persistent gap suggests overfitting, while curves that cross (where the validation curve overtakes the training curve) may indicate underfitting or data leakage.

In clinical applications where model reliability across diverse patient populations is paramount, this distinction between memorization and true learning is not merely theoretical; it directly determines whether a model can be safely deployed in real-world healthcare settings where patient safety depends on consistent, predictable performance.

3.8.2 Data Leakage

Data leakage is a critical concern in ML, particularly within clinical applications. It arises when information that would not be available at the time of prediction (such as future data or post-diagnosis variables) inadvertently influences model development. This phenomenon can lead to artificially inflated performance metrics during model validation, which often fail to translate into reliable results when the model is deployed in real-world settings. As a result, rigorous scrutiny of data handling procedures and validation strategies is vital to ensure the integrity and generalizability of ML models.

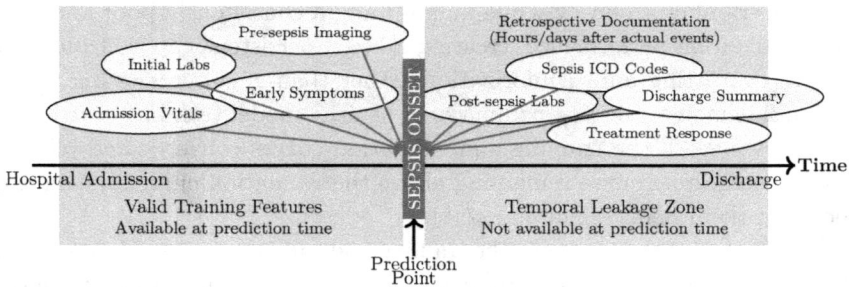

Figure 3.10: Temporal leakage in sepsis prediction models. Valid training features (left) are available before sepsis onset, while post-diagnosis data (right) represents temporal leakage when used in ML training, artificially inflating model performance that cannot be replicated in real-world deployment where such future information is unavailable.

Several distinct forms of data leakage can undermine the validity of clinical machine learning studies. Temporal leakage is among the most prevalent, occurring when models are trained using data that would not be available at the intended time of prediction. For example, a model designed to predict sepsis may inadvertently incorporate laboratory values or vital signs recorded after the onset of sepsis, or diagnostic codes assigned days after the clinical decision point. The complexity of temporal ordering in electronic health records, often due to retrospective documentation, further complicates the detection of this type of leakage. Figure 3.10 illustrates how temporal leakage occurs in sepsis prediction, showing the critical distinction between valid training features available before sepsis onset and problematic post-diagnosis data that creates artificially inflated model performance.

Patients	Medical Scans	Dataset
Patient A	Scan 1 Scan 2 Scan 3	Train
Patient B	Scan 1 Scan 2 Scan 3	Train
Patient C	Scan 1 Scan 2 Scan 3	Validate
Patient D	Scan 1 Scan 2 Scan 3	Validate
Patient E	Scan 1 Scan 2 Scan 3	Test
Patient F	Scan 1 Scan 2 Scan 3	Test

Patients	Medical Scans	Dataset
Patient A	Scan 1 Scan 2 Scan 3	Mixed!
Patient B	Scan 1 Scan 2 Scan 3	Mixed!
Patient C	Scan 1 Scan 2 Scan 3	Mixed!
Patient D	Scan 1 Scan 2 Scan 3	Mixed!
Patient E	Scan 1 Scan 2 Scan 3	Mixed!
Patient F	Scan 1 Scan 2 Scan 3	Mixed!

Figure 3.11: Patient-level data leakage in medical imaging studies. Left: Proper data splitting ensures all scans from the same patient remain in the same dataset split (train, validate, or test). Right: Inappropriate splitting allows the same patient's scans to appear in both training and test sets, leading to data leakage and overoptimistic performance estimates that fail to generalize to new patients.

Patient-level data leakage represents another critical form of leakage, particularly common in medical imaging and longitudinal studies. This occurs when data from the same patient appears in both training and test sets, allowing the model to learn patient-specific patterns rather than generalizable disease characteristics. Figure 3.11 demonstrates this problem in medical imaging studies, where improper data splitting can place multiple scans from the same patient across different dataset splits. This violation of independence between training and test data leads to overoptimistic performance estimates that fail to translate to new, unseen patients in clinical deployment.

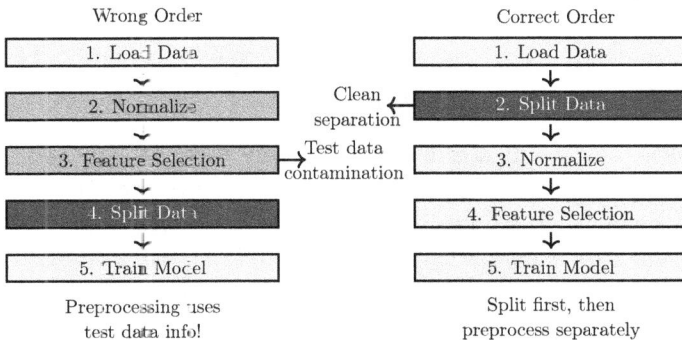

Figure 3.12: Preprocessing leakage occurs when data preprocessing steps (normalization, feature selection) are performed before train-test split, allowing information from the test set to influence preprocessing parameters. The correct approach splits data first, then applies preprocessing separately to each subset.

Preprocessing leakage is a subtle yet pervasive threat to the validity of machine learning pipelines, particularly in clinical research. This form of leakage arises when data preprocessing steps (such as normalization, feature selection, or imputation) are performed prior to splitting the dataset into training and test sets. As a result, information from the test set can inadvertently influence the parameters or features selected during preprocessing, leading to overly optimistic model performance estimates. Figure 3.12 illustrates this issue by contrasting two workflows: the incorrect approach, where preprocessing precedes data splitting and contaminates the test set, and the correct approach, where the data is first split and all preprocessing is conducted independently within each subset. Adhering to the latter strategy is vital to preserve the independence of the test set and ensure that model evaluation accurately reflects real-world deployment scenarios.

Preventing data leakage necessitates strict enforcement of temporal ordering, ensuring that all features used for prediction are available prior to the prediction time point. This requires careful consideration of clinical workflows and documentation practices. The use of independent validation datasets from different time periods or institutions is recommended to assess generalizability. Feature auditing processes should involve clinical domain experts to identify potentially problematic variables. Cross-validation strategies must be adapted for temporal data, employing techniques such as time-series splits or walk-forward validation rather than random k-fold approaches. Preprocessing pipelines should be designed to prevent information leakage, with all transformation parameters computed exclusively on training data and applied consistently to validation and test sets.

Implications for Clinical ML Research

Data leakage is not only a technical pitfall but also a profound challenge for the integrity of clinical ML research. The ease with which leakage can occur (whether by accident or, in rare cases, by design) means that researchers may end up with models that report inflated performance metrics. This is especially problematic in clinical contexts, where the stakes are high and decisions based on faulty models can have real-world consequences, as summarized in Table 3.7.

One of the most insidious aspects of data leakage is its ability to produce results that appear "too good to be true." As humans, we are naturally inclined to celebrate strong results and may subconsciously avoid scrutinizing them for fear of uncovering errors that would force us to discard

Leakage Type	Primary Risk	Detection Focus	Key Features and Prevention Strategies
Temporal Leakage	Model failure in deployment	Temporal validation	Uses data unavailable at prediction time (post-diagnosis labs, retrospective documentation). Prevention: Strict temporal validation, clinical workflow mapping, careful feature selection.
Patient-level Leakage	Poor generalization	Patient-level splitting	Same patient in train/test sets, model memorizes patient traits. Prevention: Patient-level data splitting, unique patient IDs, cross-validation at patient level.
Preprocessing Leakage	Test contamination	Pipeline auditing	Preprocessing performed before data split, test information leaks to training. Prevention: Split data before preprocessing, pipeline automation, audit preprocessing steps.
Label Leakage	Misleading conclusions	Feature correlation analysis	Features derived from or highly correlated with target label (treatment codes, discharge summaries). Prevention: Exclude label-derived features, clinical feature review, importance analysis.

Table 3.7: Summary of data leakage types, risks, and prevention strategies in clinical machine learning applications.

promising findings. This cognitive bias can be particularly pronounced in ML research, where complex pipelines and large datasets make it easy to overlook subtle sources of leakage. As reviewers, how often do we pause to ask: *How exactly was the input processed? Was there any step that could have introduced leakage?* The nuances are many, and the risk of oversight is high; especially in healthcare, where data is often messy, temporally complex, and retrospectively documented.

Moreover, the interdisciplinary nature of clinical ML research means that collaboration between medical professionals and ML developers is essential. Without clinical expertise, it is easy for ML developers to make mistakes in data handling (such as including post-diagnosis variables or improperly splitting patient data) that lead to misleadingly high performance metrics. Conversely, clinicians may not be familiar with the technical subtleties of ML pipelines that can introduce leakage. Therefore, training and fostering communication between these groups is critical to ensure that models are both technically sound and clinically relevant.

Ultimately, vigilance against data leakage must become a core part of the culture in clinical ML research. This includes not only rigorous technical checks but also a willingness to question and verify results, even when they are favorable. Only through such diligence can we ensure that ML models deliver genuine value in clinical practice, rather than illusory gains that evaporate upon deployment.

3.8.3   Subset-wise Performance Trends

In machine learning, it is standard practice to divide the available dataset into three distinct subsets: the training set, the validation set, and the test set. This division is fundamental to ensuring that the model is both well-trained and properly evaluated, and it helps to prevent methodological issues such as overfitting and data leakage. The training set is the portion of the data used to fit the model. During this phase, the model learns the underlying patterns and relationships present in the data. Typically, the majority of the data (often around 60–80%) is allocated to the training set, as a larger volume of examples enables the model to learn more robustly and generalize better to new data. The validation set is a separate subset, commonly comprising 10–20% of the data, which is used during the model development process to tune hyperparameters and make decisions regarding model architecture or feature selection. The model does not learn from this data directly; instead, it is used to provide an unbiased evaluation of the model's performance during training. This helps to identify and mitigate overfitting, as it offers insight into how well the model generalizes to data it has not seen before. The test set is another distinct subset, also typically 10–20% of the data, which is reserved for the final evaluation of the model after all training and hyperparameter tuning are complete. The test set is strictly held out from all stages of model development to provide an unbiased estimate of the model's real-world performance. This ensures that the reported performance metrics are not artificially inflated by repeated exposure to the same data during development.

A vital yet often overlooked aspect of model evaluation is the analysis of performance metrics across progressively challenging data subsets. This approach provides a more granular view of model generalizability and robustness, especially in clinical machine learning, where real-world deployment often involves data distributions that differ from the original training set. Subset-wise performance metric analysis involves partitioning the clinical data into a series of increasingly challenging or "unseen" subsets. For each subset, standard performance metrics (such as accuracy, sensitivity, specificity, F1-score, etc., typically derived from confusion matrices) are computed. The expectation is that as the subsets become more challenging (typically by including data that is less similar to the training set or represents more difficult cases) the model's performance should decrease.

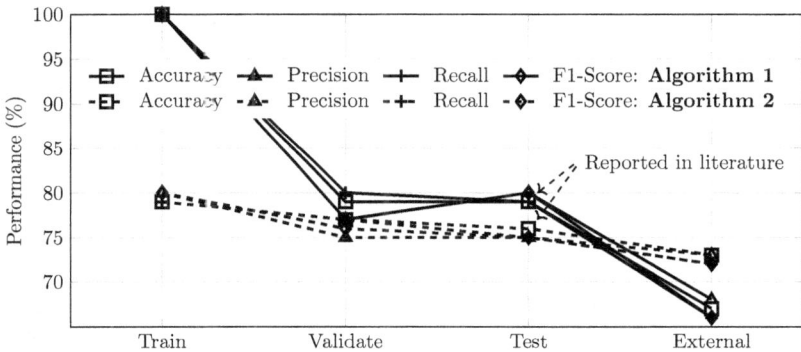

Figure 3.13: Performance comparison of two algorithms across training, validation, test, and external datasets. Algorithm 1 (solid lines) demonstrates severe overfitting with perfect training performance (100%) followed by substantial degradation on unseen data, dropping to 66-68% on external validation. Algorithm 2 (dashed lines) shows more robust and consistent performance across all datasets (72-80%), indicating better generalization capability. Arrows highlight the accuracies usually reported in existing literature. While Algorithm 2 exhibits lower reported accuracy, its consistent generalizability across data subsets provides significantly greater clinical value than Algorithm 1's inflated accuracy metrics.

With each subsequent subset, the algorithm has access to less familiar or more challenging data. Therefore, it is natural and desirable for all performance metrics to decrease as the subsets progress. If a model's metrics do not decrease, or if they even improve on harder subsets, this may indicate data leakage, overfitting, or methodological flaws. Conversely, a steep drop-off in performance may signal that the model lacks robustness and is not suitable for deployment in diverse clinical settings.

The Figure 3.13 illustrates this principle. Each line represents a different performance metric (e.g., accuracy, precision, recall, F1-score) plotted across a series of data subsets, from easiest (left) to hardest (right). The green lines (representing a robust model) show a gradual, consistent decrease in all metrics as the data becomes less familiar. The blue lines (representing a problematic model) show erratic or steep drops, or even increases in performance on harder subsets; clear red flags for methodological issues. What to watch for:

– Performance should decrease: As the model is evaluated on increasingly challenging subsets, the performance metrics should show a downward trend. This is clearly illustrated in Figure 3.13: for Algorithm 2 (dashed lines), all metrics (accuracy, precision, recall, and F1-score) decrease gradually and consistently from the training set through to the external set, reflecting proper generalization and the expected effect of encountering less familiar data. In contrast, Algorithm 1 (solid lines) exhibits erratic behavior: for example, its precision and F1-score actually increase from the validation to the test set (77% to 80%), before dropping sharply on the external set. Such non-monotonic trends (where metrics go down and then up) are a red flag, suggesting overfitting, data leakage, or methodological flaws. Only Algorithm 2 demonstrates the desirable, consistent decrease across all subsets, indicating robust and reliable model performance.

– The decrease should not be too steep: A gradual decline suggests the model is robust and generalizes well. A sharp drop indicates overfitting or lack of generalizability. In Figure 3.13, Algorithm 2 (dashed lines) demonstrates this ideal behavior, with all metrics (accuracy, precision, recall, and F1-score) declining gently from the training set (79–80%) to the external set (72–73%). This indicates that Algorithm 2 maintains reasonable performance even as the data becomes less familiar, reflecting good generalizability. In contrast, Algorithm 1 (solid lines) shows a dramatic drop: all metrics plummet from perfect scores on the training set (100%) to the high 60s on the external set (66–68%). Such a steep decline is a hallmark of overfitting, where the model has memorized the training data but fails to perform on new, unseen data. This pattern signals that Algorithm 1 is not robust and would likely perform poorly in real-world or clinical deployment.

– Monitor all performance metrics, not just accuracy: It is vital to observe the trends in sensitivity, specificity, F1-score, and other metrics derived from the respective confusion matrices, as a robust model should exhibit a consistent, gradual decrease across all these measures. Figure 3.13 highlights this point: for Algorithm 2, all metrics decrease in parallel, reinforcing the conclusion that its generalization is not limited to a single aspect of performance. However, Algorithm 1 displays inconsistent trends; precision and F1-score, for example, actually increase from the validation to the test set before dropping again, while recall and accuracy remain flat or decrease. Such inconsistencies suggest that Algorithm 1's apparent strengths may be misleading, and that relying on a single metric (like accuracy) could mask underlying weaknesses. Comprehensive monitoring across all metrics is essential to ensure true model robustness and reliability.

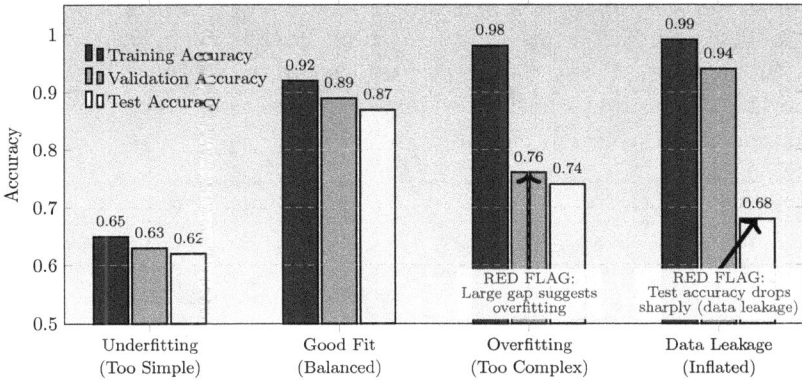

Figure 3.14: Subset-wise accuracy across four AI model scenarios: underfitting, good fit, overfitting, and data leakage. Each scenario shows training, validation, and test accuracy. The "Good Fit" scenario demonstrates balanced, high performance across all subsets. The "Overfitting" scenario shows a large gap between training and validation/test accuracy, while the "Data Leakage" scenario shows inflated validation accuracy but a sharp drop on test dataset. Colored bands indicate performance quality, and red arrows highlight methodological red flags.

Figure 3.14 provides a complementary visualization of subset-wise performance trends by comparing training, validation, and test accuracy across four common AI model scenarios: underfitting, good fit, overfitting, and data leakage. The bar chart highlights how a well-balanced model maintains high and consistent accuracy across all subsets, while overfitting is characterized by a large gap between training and validation/test accuracy. The data leakage scenario is particularly problematic, as it shows artificially high validation accuracy but a dramatic drop on test dataset; an indicator of methodological flaws such as improper data partitioning. Colored background bands denote regions of high, moderate, and poor performance, and red arrows draw attention to critical red flags. This figure reinforces the importance of subset-wise analysis for diagnosing overfitting and data leakage, and for ensuring robust model generalization in clinical machine learning.

Implications for Clinical ML Research

Incorporating subset-wise performance metric analysis into model evaluation provides a useful diagnostic tool for identifying overfitting, data leakage, and lack of robustness. It complements learning curve analysis by offering a direct assessment of how well a model handles increasingly unfamiliar data. This approach is especially important in clinical applications, where patient populations and data distributions can vary widely. Transparent reporting of subset-wise metrics should be considered a best practice and a requirement for claims of clinical utility.

Property	Alg. 1	Alg. 2	Evidence from Figure 3.13
Overfitting Behavior	Severe overfitting	Minimal overfitting	Algorithm 1: 100% training performance drops to 66–68% external. Algorithm 2: 79–80% training to 72–73% external.
Performance Consistency	Erratic, inconsistent	Stable, consistent	Algorithm 1 shows large metric variations and non-predictable patterns. Algorithm 2 exhibits parallel declining trends across all metrics.
Monotonic Decrease	Non-monotonic trends	Proper monotonic	Algorithm 1: Precision/F1-score increase from validation (77%) to test (80%). Algorithm 2: All metrics decrease consistently across subsets.
Decline Steepness	Steep drop	Gradual decline	Algorithm 1: 32–34% performance drop from training to external. Algorithm 2: 6–8% performance drop across same transition.
Generalization Capability	Poor, memorization	Good, true learning	Algorithm 1 curves suggest data memorization with failure on unseen data. Algorithm 2 curves show maintained reasonable performance across all subsets.

Table 3.8: Algorithm performance properties demonstrated across training, validation, test, and external datasets (Figure 3.13).

To illustrate these principles in practice, Table 3.8 and Figure 3.13 present a detailed comparison of two hypothetical clinical machine learning algorithms evaluated using the subset-wise performance framework. This comparison demonstrates how the same performance evaluation methodology can reveal dramatically different characteristics between algorithms that might appear similar when assessed using traditional single-dataset metrics. Algorithm 1 represents a common but problematic pattern in clinical ML research: achieving perfect or near-perfect performance on training data while exhibiting severe degradation on external validation, suggesting overfitting and poor generalizability to real-world clinical settings. Algorithm 2 exemplifies the desired behavior: demonstrating consistent, gradual performance decline across increasingly challenging data subsets, indicating robust learning and reliable generalization. In clinical applications, where models must perform reliably across diverse patient populations, hospital systems, and data acquisition protocols, the distinction between these two patterns is not merely academic; it directly impacts patient safety and clinical utility. The analysis reveals that Algorithm 2, despite showing lower reported accuracy in traditional evaluation frameworks, provides significantly greater clinical value due to its predictable and stable performance characteristics across varied deployment scenarios.

3.9   Class Imbalance in Clinical Evaluation

Although the challenges of class imbalance have been discussed previously, it is necessary to reiterate its central significance in clinical prediction tasks. Many clinical prediction tasks, such as screening or early detection, are characterized by low event prevalence (i.e., class imbalance). In these settings, overall accuracy can be misleading: trivial classifiers that always predict the majority class may achieve high accuracy while failing to identify cases of greatest clinical importance. Therefore, evaluation should emphasize confusion matrices, per-class metrics (precision, recall, F1), and Precision–Recall (PR) analysis, with explicit attention to prevalence and decision thresholds. While ROC–AUC remains informative for discrimination, PR–AUC is often more sensitive to prevalence and aligns more closely with clinical harms under skewed class distributions.

For example, in a screening task with 5% positives and 95% negatives, the class distribution is highly imbalanced: out of 1,000 patients, only 50 are positive and 950 are negative. This imbalance highlights why accuracy alone is insufficient; confusion matrices, per-class metrics, and PR–AUC are recommended. Figures 3.15 and 3.16 illustrate the "accuracy paradox" and the differential behavior of ROC vs. PR under imbalance.

3.9.1   Accuracy Paradox and Thresholded Performance

When positives are rare, a classifier that always predicts "negative" can achieve high accuracy but zero clinical benefit (recall = 0). Confusion-matrix–based metrics (recall, precision, F1) reveal patient-impacting errors that accuracy obscures. PR curves are more informative than ROC curves in imbalanced settings because precision directly reflects the false-positive burden at a given recall, which becomes salient as prevalence falls. Figure 3.15 depicts the all-negative classifier; Figure 3.16 shows why PR curves separate models more clearly under imbalance (similar to Figure 3.5), even when ROC curves appear similar.

Predicted

	Positive	Negative
Actual Positive	TP = 0	FN = 50
Actual Negative	FP = 0	TN = 950

$$\text{Accuracy} = \frac{0+950}{1000} = 95\%$$

$$\text{Recall} = \frac{0}{50} = 0; \text{F1} = 0 \text{ (no clinical utility)}$$

Figure 3.15: A trivial "all-negative" classifier achieves 95% accuracy at 5% prevalence but misses all true cases. Confusion-matrix–based metrics and PR analysis reveal clinical utility that accuracy obscures.

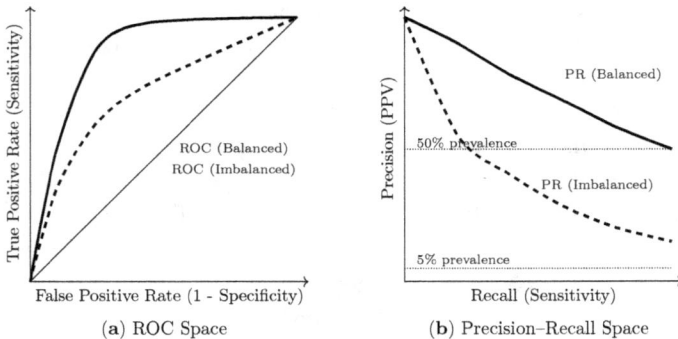

(a) ROC Space

(b) Precision–Recall Space

Figure 3.16: ROC curves can look similar under balance and imbalance, but PR curves and PR–AUC expose precision loss as recall increases at low prevalence. PR–AUC and confusion matrices are recommended for imbalanced problems.

3.9.2 Mitigation Strategies

Mitigation strategies for class imbalance operate at multiple levels. Table 3.9 provides a structured overview of practical strategies for addressing class imbalance in clinical prediction tasks. From a clinical perspective, the strategies summarized in Table 3.9 are vital for ensuring that predictive models are both safe and effective in real-world healthcare settings. In clinical practice, the cost of missing a true positive (e.g., failing to detect a disease) is often much higher than the cost of a false positive (e.g., unnecessary follow-up testing). Therefore, models must be evaluated and tuned with these asymmetric clinical harms in mind. The table's emphasis on endpoint-weighted utilities and per-class metrics directly addresses this need, supporting decision-making that prioritizes patient safety and resource allocation.

Level	Primary Strategies	Advanced Techniques	Key Implementation Considerations
Data-level	Stratified splitting to preserve minority proportion	Random under/over-sampling; synthetic sampling (SMOTE) with noise cleaning (SMOTE–ENN)	Apply resampling within folds only to prevent leakage; maintain class distribution across train/validation/test splits
Algorithm-level	Class-weighted or cost-sensitive losses	Focal loss for hard example mining; threshold optimization for PPV/recall trade-offs	Ordinal/endpoint-aware utilities when clinical harms are asymmetric; tune class weights based on clinical costs
Evaluation-level	Report confusion matrices; include PR–AUC and per-class metrics	Calibration and decision-/utility-curve analysis	External validation essential; subgroup (fairness) analyses across patient demographics and clinical settings

Table 3.9: Summary of mitigation and reporting practices for imbalanced clinical classification. Data, algorithm, and evaluation choices should be coordinated with strict leakage control and external validation; endpoint-weighted utilities reflect asymmetric clinical costs.

3.9.3　Reporting, Validation, and Leakage Avoidance

When dealing with class imbalance, transparent reporting should describe the class distributions within the dataset, present full confusion matrices, and provide per-class metrics such as precision, recall, and F1 scores to ensure that performance is accurately characterized for each class. Additionally, it is important to report both ROC–AUC and PR–AUC values, as these metrics offer insight into model performance, particularly in imbalanced settings where traditional accuracy may be misleading. Finally, documenting training dynamics, such as learning curves, is vital for diagnosing issues like overfitting and understanding how the model's performance evolves during training.

External validation on independent cohorts (by institution, geography, or time) is required to establish generalizability and avoid optimistic bias. Subset-wise reporting (e.g., by sex, race/ethnicity, age) is necessary to assess equity and algorithmic fairness. Strict prevention of data leakage (temporal, patient-level, preprocessing) is imperative, as leakage can inflate performance, especially when class prevalence is skewed.

Chapter 4

Imaging Classification

This chapter focuses on the application of machine learning (ML) algorithms in the classification of medical images related to cardiovascular disorders. It highlights the intricate process involved in selecting the most suitable ML algorithm for predicting specific heart-related conditions, emphasizing the critical role of real-world data in testing and validation. The paper navigates through various ML methods utilized in the cardiovascular healthcare field, including Supervised Learning, Unsupervised Learning, Self-Supervised Learning, Deep Neural Networks, Reinforcement Learning, and Ensemble Methods. The challenge lies not only in selecting an ML algorithm but also in identifying the most appropriate one for specific cardiovascular tasks, given the vast array of options available. Each unique dataset related to cardiovascular imaging necessitates a comparative analysis to determine the best-performing algorithm. However, testing all available algorithms is impractical. This paper examines the performance of various ML algorithms in recent studies, focusing specifically on their application across different imaging modalities for diagnosing cardiovascular diseases. It provides a summary of these studies, serving as a starting point for researchers and practitioners seeking to select the most suitable ML algorithm for cardiovascular disorders and their corresponding imaging techniques.

4.1 Introduction

The selection of a machine learning (ML) algorithm for predicting specific cardiovascular disorders is a complex process that necessitates careful consideration of various factors [313]. This selection is typically guided by the algorithm's performance relative to other ML algorithms [314], evaluated txhrough a series of tests and validations using real-world cardiovascular data [315]. Different ML algorithms exhibit varying effectiveness depending on the type of data being analyzed [316]. For example, Convolutional Neural Networks (CNNs) are particularly well-suited for processing image data, making them a popular choice for tasks in cardiovascular medical imaging. CNNs are designed to automatically and adaptively learn spatial hierarchies of features from input images, which is particularly advantageous in the realm of cardiovascular imaging, where the data is often complex and high-dimensional [317].

Conversely, algorithms like Support Vector Machines (SVMs) or Random Forests may prove to be more effective when analyzing structured, tabular data related to cardiovascular disorders. These algorithms excel at handling high-dimensional data and are less prone to overfitting, making them particularly suitable for tasks such as predicting disease outcomes based on patient records, including risk assessments for conditions like coronary artery disease or heart failure. The specific cardiovascular disorder in question significantly influences the choice of an ML algorithm, as certain diseases may exhibit distinct patterns or characteristics that are more readily detected by specific algorithms. Therefore, the selection of the most appropriate algorithm is contingent upon the specific task, the nature of the data, and the cardiovascular disease (CVD) being addressed.

Performance metrics are a crucial factor in the decision-making process for selecting machine learning algorithms for cardiovascular disorders [318]. These metrics provide a quantitative assessment of an algorithm's effectiveness in detecting and diagnosing CVDs. Common metrics include accuracy, precision, recall, and the Area Under the Receiver Operating Characteristic Curve (AUC-ROC). The choice of metric often depends on the specific task and the relative importance of different types of errors. For example, in scenarios where false negatives can have severe consequences–such as in the detection and classification of CVDs–recall may be prioritized over overall accuracy to ensure that critical cases are not overlooked.

This review highlights a variety of ML algorithms utilized for processing medical images specifically aimed at diagnosing and predicting cardiovascular disorders. These algorithms include Decision Trees (DT), Support Vector Machines (SVM), K-Nearest Neighbors (KNN), Logistic Regression (LR), Deep Learning techniques, Convolutional Neural Networks (CNN), LightGBM, Linear Discriminant Analysis (LDA), Google Teachable Machine, Naive Bayes (NB), Random Forests (RF), XGBoost, and AdaBoost. Each algorithm possesses unique strengths and is selected based on the specific requirements of the cardiovascular diagnostic task at hand. The integration of these algorithms in cardiovascular medical diagnostics holds great promise for enhancing both accuracy and efficiency in the detection of heart-related diseases.

4.2 Medical Imaging Modalities for Cardiovascular Disorders

Medical imaging plays a pivotal role in the diagnosis, management, and treatment of CVDs. Non-invasive and minimally invasive imaging techniques provide valuable insights into the structure and function of the heart and blood vessels, enabling healthcare professionals to accurately diagnose conditions, assess disease progression, and plan appropriate interventions.

The mind map presented in Figure 4.1 showcases the key imaging modalities commonly used in the assessment of CVDs, including X-rays, ultrasound, and MRI. This diverse landscape of medical imaging modalities is intricately linked to various medical conditions, offering a comprehensive overview that will inform our subsequent exploration of this complex field and its intersection with ML.

The development of medical imaging modalities has transformed the landscape of cardiovascular healthcare, offering insights into various cardiovascular disorders and facilitating accurate diagnoses. These advanced imaging techniques have become essential in understanding the complexities of conditions such as coronary artery disease, heart failure, and arrhythmias. With the emergence of ML, the potential to enhance these imaging modalities is immense, promising to elevate diagnostic capabilities and redefine the future of cardiovascular diagnostics.

Each of the cardiovascular disorders previously mentioned, ranging from coronary artery disease and heart failure diagnosed through advanced imaging techniques to arrhythmias identified via echocardiography, can now

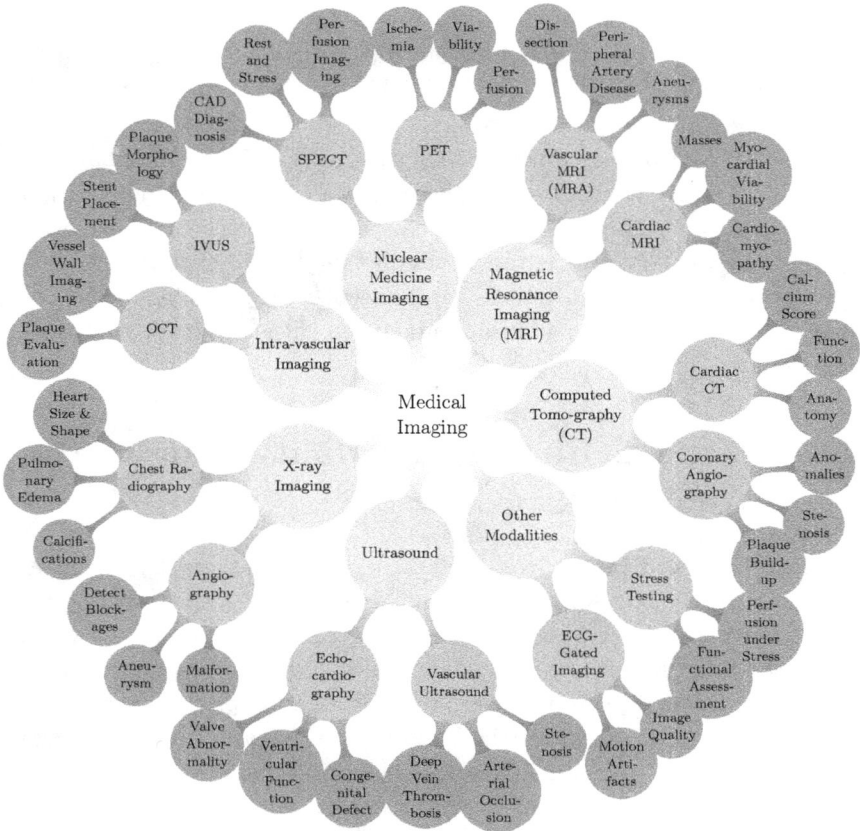

Figure 4.1: This mind map illustrates the various modalities of medical imaging utilized in the diagnosis and management of CVDs. At the center of the diagram is the overarching category of Medical Imaging, which branches out into seven primary imaging techniques, each represented by distinct colors for clarity. Overall, this mind map serves as a comprehensive overview of the diverse imaging techniques available in the field of cardiovascular medicine, highlighting their specific applications and relevance in clinical practice.

be detected with greater speed and precision. This enhanced capability is achieved through the integration of ML algorithms with these imaging modalities, enabling the analysis of vast amounts of data and the identification of patterns that may be overlooked by the human eye, ultimately leading to more accurate diagnoses and improved patient outcomes.

4.3   Inclusion Criteria

This chapter includes recent studies on cardiovascular disorders that used metrics such as the Area Under the Curve (AUC) and accuracy to evaluate the performance of ML models designed to predict disease presence. These metrics assess different aspects of model performance and are applied in various contexts within CVD prediction. Accuracy is a straightforward metric commonly used in binary classification problems, such as determining whether a patient has a CVD or not. It calculates the proportion of correct predictions–both true positives (diseased patients correctly identified) and true negatives (healthy patients correctly identified)–out of all predictions made. However, accuracy can be misleading in cases where there is a significant class imbalance, which is often the case in medical datasets. For example, if 95% of patients do not have a particular cardiovascular condition (Class A) and only 5% do (Class B), a model that always predicts "no disease" will achieve an accuracy of 95%. Despite this seemingly high accuracy, the model fails to identify any actual cases of the disease, rendering it ineffective for diagnostic purposes.

AUC, on the other hand, is derived from the Receiver Operating Characteristic (ROC) curve, which plots the true positive rate against the false positive rate at various threshold settings. The AUC measures the model's ability to distinguish between classes across all thresholds, providing an aggregate performance metric that is not sensitive to class imbalance. In the context of CVD prediction, where positive cases are relatively rare compared to negative cases, AUC offers a more reliable assessment of a model's discriminative ability. It's important to note that a model can have high accuracy but low AUC, and vice versa. For instance, a model that predicts every patient as healthy (the majority class) may have high accuracy due to the prevalence of healthy individuals but will have a low AUC because it cannot distinguish between patients with and without the disease. Conversely, a model that effectively ranks patients by their risk of CVD may achieve a high AUC but might have lower accuracy if the classification threshold is not optimally set for prediction purposes.

Therefore, while both AUC and accuracy are useful metrics in evaluating machine learning models for cardiovascular disorders, they provide different insights into model performance. Accuracy reflects the overall rate of correct predictions but can be misleading in imbalanced datasets. AUC assesses the model's ability to distinguish between diseased and healthy patients across all thresholds and is better suited for evaluating performance when positive cases are scarce. The choice of metric should align with the specific objectives of the study and consider the class distribution within the dataset to ensure that the model is effective in identifying patients with CVDs.

4.4 Guided Selection of Machine Learning Models

While each dataset is distinct, this section outlines the process for selecting an appropriate machine learning algorithm tailored for predicting specific cardiovascular conditions based on various medical imaging modalities. The table below (Table 4.1) summarizes recent relevant studies published between 2015 and 2024. However, in prioritizing studies for inclusion in this review, preference was given to the most recent publications. Most of these studies performed comparative analyses of multiple machine learning models to identify the most effective ones, and only the top-performing algorithms are included in the table.

These studies focus on particular CVDs and utilize specific imaging techniques, capturing essential details such as the disease being investigated and the imaging modality employed. The table also presents key performance metrics, including accuracy and AUC, for the validation cohort; however, metrics for the testing cohort are not included. The validation set, which is used for model tuning and selection, serves as a more reliable indicator of the model's expected performance on new, unseen data.

Accuracy measures the model's overall ability to correctly classify cases, while AUC evaluates its discriminative power–both metrics are crucial for assessing a model's effectiveness on unseen data. It is important to note that some studies have reported either accuracy or AUC, which is a significant oversight. Since both metrics provide complementary insights into model performance, they should be reported together to enable a thorough and reliable evaluation. Future studies should ensure that both accuracy and AUC are included in their findings to deliver a complete assessment of model performance and facilitate accurate comparisons across different machine learning approaches.

The following guidelines delineate how physicians or researchers can utilize this summary to select the most appropriate machine learning model for diagnostic purposes, contingent upon the specific medical condition and the imaging modality employed:

- Step 1 (Identify the Cardiovascular Disease): Determine the specific CVD that necessitates diagnosis. For example, when diagnosing coronary artery disease, it is essential to focus on the entries in Table 4.1 that pertain to this condition.

- Step 2 (Identify the Imaging Modality): Ascertain the imaging modality that is available for use. This may include modalities such as computed tomography (CT), magnetic resonance imaging (MRI), or ultrasound. In Table 4.1, examine the rows that correspond to both the identified medical condition and the available imaging modality.

- Step 3 (Refer to Comparative Analysis): Consult the comparative analysis presented in Table 4.1. This table details the machine learning models that have been employed for the specified medical condition and imaging modality, along with their associated performance metrics, including accuracy and area under the curve (AUC).

- Step 4 (Choose the ML Model): Select the machine learning model based on the comparative analysis. For instance, if the diagnosis pertains to coronary artery disease and the imaging modality is CT, one would consider models such as linear discriminant analysis (LDA) and logistic regression (LR), which exhibit comparable accuracy and AUC. If the imaging modality is MRI, the choice may be between logistic regression and XGBoost. In the case of ultrasound, the study referenced in the last column indicates that convolutional neural networks (CNN) are the most effective algorithm.

- Step 5 (Apply the Chosen ML Model): After selecting the appropriate machine learning model, proceed to implement it within the diagnostic process.

   The Table 4.1 provides a summary of comparative analyses of various ML models applied to different CVDs and imaging modalities. It eliminates the necessity for conducting new comparative evaluations each time a diagnosis is needed for a cardiovascular condition. By referencing this table, physicians and researchers can swiftly identify the most suitable ML algorithm for predicting specific cardiovascular conditions using a designated imaging modality. This approach streamlines the decision-making process and enhances the efficiency of diagnostics.

   A considerable number of the studies reviewed lack external prospective validation, and several demonstrate significant issues related to data leakage.

Medical Condition	Imaging Modality	ML Algorithm	Accuracy	AUC	Ref.	Year
Coronary artery disease	Stress Echo-cardiogram	SVM	N/A	0.934	[319]	2022
		RF	N/A	0.934	[319]	2022
		LR	N/A	0.934	[319]	2022
	Echo-cardiogram	Gradient boosting	85.2%	0.852	[320]	2023
		LGBoost	>80%	0.824	[320]	2023
		RF	>80%	0.817	[320]	2023
		Catboost	>80%	0.829	[320]	2023
		XGBoost	>80%	0.824	[320]	2023
	Cardiac CTA	Boosted Ensemble	N/A	0.790	[321]	2016
		SVM	94%	0.940	[322]	2015
		DL	76%	0.780	[323]	2019
	PET	CNN	N/A	0.900	[324]	2024
Cardio-myopathy	Echo-cardiogram	RF	~75%	0.900	[325]	2023
		LR	~75%	0.925	[325]	2023
		XGBoost	~75%	0.934	[325]	2023
	Cardiac MRI	BRL	80.72%	0.796	[326]	2015
Adverse cardiovascular events	Risk factors	KNN	85.94%	N/A	[327]	2020
		LR	87.5%	N/A	[327]	2020
		SVC	86.72%	N/A	[327]	2020
		DT	71.88%	N/A	[327]	2020
		MLP	62.5%	N/A	[327]	2020
		RF	86.72%	N/A	[327]	2020
		LightGBM	79.69%	N/A	[327]	2020
		Gradient boosting	83.59%	N/A	[327]	2020
Cardiomegaly	X-ray	CNN	81.2%	0.900	[328]	2024
Cardiac Function Assessment	Echo-cardiogram	CNN	97.8%	0.996	[329]	2017
		DL	98.8%	N/A	[330]	2021
		DL	92.5%	N/A	[330]	2021
		DeepNN	N/A	0.880	[331]	2021
Hypertrophic cardio-myopathy	Cardiac MRI	3D CNN	98%	N/A	[332]	2019

Table 4.1: Summary of ML algorithms utilized in cardiovascular imaging classification tasks described following this table. (Note that the reported values may be overly optimistic when generalized to a broader patient population due to inherent limitations within the studies.)

These limitations raise concerns regarding the accuracy values reported, suggesting they may be overly optimistic when generalized to a broader patient population. External prospective validation is an essential component in the assessment of machine learning models, as it entails evaluating the model on a completely independent dataset that was not utilized during the training or internal validation phases [149]. This independent dataset is typically gathered in a different context or at a later time, thereby providing a more realistic assessment of the model's performance in real-world scenarios. The absence of such validation in many studies listed in Table 4.1 casts doubt on the generalizability of their findings across diverse clinical settings.

Data leakage, conversely, occurs when information from outside the training dataset is inadvertently incorporated into the model, resulting in inflated performance metrics [148]. This situation can arise when features from validation or test sets are utilized during the training process, granting the model access to information that would not be available in actual clinical practice. The presence of significant data leakage issues in several studies further undermines the reliability of their reported accuracy values, thereby compromising the true diagnostic potential of the models [333].

While the selection of an appropriate ML algorithm for medical image classification is undeniably critical, it is equally important to first clearly define the clinical question at hand. This initial step not only informs the choice of algorithm but also guides decisions regarding data collection, feature selection, and the evaluation metrics employed in the study [334]. Furthermore, despite the aggregation of numerous studies, it is essential to acknowledge that each dataset possesses unique characteristics and complexities. These inherent differences can significantly influence the selection of the most suitable ML algorithm.

In medical imaging, the choice of algorithm can profoundly affect the performance and accuracy of image analysis. Specific attributes of the imaging dataset, such as its size, complexity, and type, must be considered when determining the appropriate algorithm. Additionally, the nature of the data (whether structured or unstructured) can play a decisive role in guiding the algorithm selection process. Tailoring the ML approach to the specific characteristics of the dataset is important for achieving optimal diagnostic outcomes.

Figure 4.2 illustrates a flowchart that delineates the process of selecting and implementing an ML algorithm specifically for the classification of CVDs. The flowchart commences with the initial input conditions, which encompass the specific cardiovascular condition being addressed and the selected imaging modality. Subsequently, the process advances to the selec-

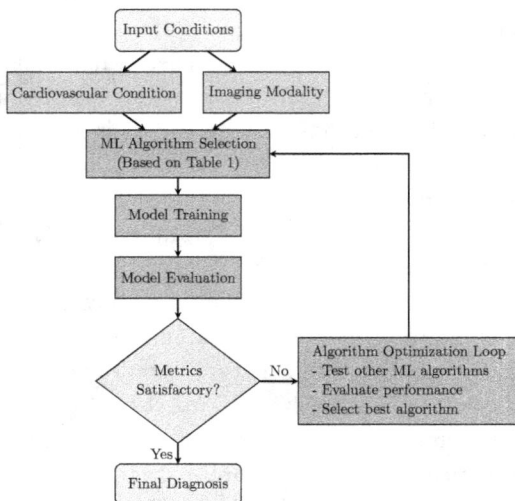

Figure 4.2: Flowchart for the selection and implementation of ML algorithms in the classification of cardiovascular diseases. This process integrates the specific cardiovascular condition, the chosen imaging modality, and the performance metrics of the algorithms to guide the selection and optimization of ML models for diagnostic tasks.

tion of an appropriate ML algorithm, based on the information summarized in Table 4.1.

Following that, the model undergoes training and evaluation, leading to a critical decision point where performance metrics are assessed. If the performance metrics meet the established thresholds, the process proceeds to the final diagnostic step. Conversely, if the metrics are deemed unsatisfactory, the process enters an algorithm optimization loop. During this phase, alternative ML algorithms are tested and evaluated before returning to the model training stage for further refinement. This iterative approach ensures the selection of the most effective algorithm for accurate and reliable classification of CVDs.

In Figure 4.2, "satisfactory metrics" refers to the performance measures of the ML model, such as accuracy, AUC, sensitivity, and specificity, that are considered adequate for the intended diagnostic application in CVDs. The precise threshold for what constitutes "satisfactory" varies based on the specific cardiovascular condition being addressed and the imaging modality employed. To evaluate whether the metrics are satisfactory, researchers and clinicians can compare their model's performance to the metrics reported in

Table 4.1 for similar studies focused on CVDs. This comparative analysis enables them to assess their model's efficacy in relation to other published work within the same domain. The process entails identifying studies in Table 4.1 that concentrate on the same cardiovascular condition and imaging modality as the current research, and subsequently comparing the model's accuracy and AUC (when available) to those reported in analogous studies.

Several factors should be considered when evaluating whether the performance metrics of a model for CVD classification are satisfactory:

- Contextual Relevance: A model with slightly lower performance metrics may still be deemed satisfactory if it offers additional advantages, such as reduced processing time or lower computational demands, which can be critical in clinical settings.

- Clinical Significance: Even if a model's metrics fall below those reported in some published studies, they may still be acceptable if they meet the minimum thresholds for clinical utility specific to CVD diagnostics.

- Dataset Characteristics: If the dataset utilized is more complex or diverse than those employed in previous studies, achieving metrics comparable to those reported in the literature could be considered satisfactory.

- Performance Trade-offs: A minor reduction in one metric (e.g., accuracy) may be acceptable if it results in substantial improvements in another critical metric (e.g., AUC) that is particularly relevant for CVD applications.

By comparing a model's performance to the metrics reported in Table 4.1 and taking these factors into account, researchers can make informed decisions regarding the adequacy of the model's metrics for their specific CVD classification tasks. This approach facilitates a more nuanced evaluation that reflects the current state of the art in the field.

4.5 Evaluating ML Studies for Image Classification

The application of ML in cardiovascular imaging is necessitating a critical evaluation of the validity and reliability of these studies. A thorough understanding of how to assess ML studies is essential to ensure that their results are trustworthy and that the models developed are robust and generalizable. This section focuses on methods to evaluate ML studies in medical imaging classification, emphasizing the identification of potential issues such as overfitting or underfitting, evaluating performance metrics, and recognizing the significance of proper data splitting and validation strategies.

4.5.1 Data Splitting Strategies

A fundamental aspect of developing and evaluating ML models is the division of data into distinct subsets: training, validation, and testing sets. Proper data splitting is crucial to prevent overfitting and to ensure that the model's performance is generalizable to new, unseen data. The training set is used to train the ML model, allowing it to learn patterns from the data. The validation set is used during model development to tune hyperparameters and make decisions about model architecture, providing an unbiased evaluation of the model's performance during training. The testing set is used to provide an unbiased evaluation of the final model's performance after training and validation and should only be used once the model is fully trained.

Potential data splitting strategies include hold-out validation, where the dataset is split once into training, validation, and testing sets. Common proportions for this split include 60% training, 20% validation, and 20% testing; however, other ratios such as 70% training, 15% validation, and 15% testing, or 80% training, 10% validation, and 10% testing are also frequently used, depending on the size of the dataset and the specific requirements of the study. Another strategy is k-fold cross-validation, where the dataset is partitioned into k equal-sized folds. The model is trained and validated k times, each time using a different fold as the validation set and the remaining folds as the training set, maximizing the use of available data. Additionally, stratified splitting ensures that each subset has the same class distribution as the original dataset, which is particularly important in cases of class imbalance. Proper data splitting techniques are essential to prevent information leakage between datasets, which can artificially inflate performance metrics and lead to overly optimistic conclusions about a model's capabilities.

4.5.2 Learning Curves and Model Convergence

Learning curves are valuable tools for diagnosing the learning behavior of ML models. They plot the model's performance on the training and validation sets over successive iterations or epochs, providing insights into how well the model is learning and whether it is overfitting or underfitting. The training curve illustrates the model's performance on the training data, while the validation curve reflects the model's performance on the validation data.

Healthy learning curves for a converged ML classification task typically exhibit convergence, where both training and validation curves approach a plateau, indicating that the model's performance is stabilizing. A small gap between the training and validation performance suggests good generalization, and plateauing values indicate that further training may not significantly improve performance. Signs of overfitting include the training curve showing high performance while the validation curve lags behind or declines, indicating that the model is learning noise specific to the training data and not generalizing well. Underfitting is indicated when both training and validation curves show poor performance and do not improve with more training, suggesting that the model is too simple to capture the underlying patterns in the data. Analyzing learning curves helps in assessing whether the model has been appropriately trained and whether it is likely to perform well on new data.

4.5.3   ROC Curves and Performance Metrics

The Receiver Operating Characteristic (ROC) curve is an important tool for evaluating classification models, especially in medical diagnostics where the balance between sensitivity and specificity is critical. The ROC curve plots the true positive rate (sensitivity) against the false positive rate (1 minus specificity) at various threshold settings. The Area Under the ROC Curve (AUC) is a scalar value summarizing the model's performance across all classification thresholds; a higher AUC indicates better discriminative ability.

Interpreting ROC curves for validation and testing sets involves looking for consistent performance, where similar ROC curves and AUC values for the validation and testing sets suggest that the model generalizes well. Discrepancies between curves, such as significant differences in ROC curves between validation and testing sets, may indicate overfitting, where the model performs well on validation data but poorly on unseen testing data. Large differences in AUC between validation and testing sets suggest overfitting, while consistently low AUC values on both sets indicate underfitting.

4.5.4 Confusion Matrices and Model Performance

A confusion matrix provides a detailed breakdown of a model's classification performance, showing the counts of true positives, true negatives, false positives, and false negatives. Analyzing confusion matrices entails comparing the validation and testing sets; the confusion matrix for the testing set should show performance metrics slightly lower than but close to those of the validation set. Significant discrepancies may indicate overfitting. Consistency in errors, such as similar patterns of errors across validation and testing sets, suggests that the model reliably captures data patterns.

Expected differences between validation and testing performance include a slight decrease in performance on the testing set, which is normal due to its nature as completely unseen data. A large drop in performance may indicate that the model has not generalized well and may have overfitted to the training and validation data.

4.5.5 Importance of External Validation

External validation involves testing the model on data from different settings or populations than those used in training and validation, providing insight into the model's generalizability. Benefits of external testing include assessing generalizability, demonstrating that the model performs well across different populations, imaging devices, or clinical settings, and enhancing credibility, as models validated externally are more likely to be trusted by the medical community.

Challenges in obtaining external data involve data access difficulties due to privacy concerns, data sharing restrictions, and lack of standardized data formats, as well as variability in data due to differences in data acquisition protocols, equipment, and patient demographics. While external validation is ideal, its absence necessitates careful consideration of the model's generalizability and applicability to broader clinical practice.

4.5.6 Understanding the Model and Methodology

A thorough understanding of the model and its methodology is critical for evaluating ML studies. Key considerations include knowledge of the model architecture, understanding the type of model used (e.g., neural networks, decision trees) and the rationale behind its selection, details about hyperparameters, optimization algorithms, and data augmentation strategies providing insight into model development, and transparency and reproducibility, including availability of code, detailed methodology, and sufficient information for replication.

4.5.7 Identifying High-Quality Machine Learning Studies

In the assessment of ML studies within medical imaging classification, it is essential to identify the characteristics that distinguish robust models from those susceptible to overfitting or underfitting. Recognizing these indicators aids in evaluating the validity, reliability, and generalizability of the ML models presented. Tables 4.2 and 4.3 provide a comprehensive summary of key aspects to consider when determining whether an ML study represents a healthy model or exhibits signs of overfitting or underfitting. This table serves as a practical guide for researchers and practitioners to critically appraise ML studies and ensure the integrity of their findings.

Red flags indicating potential issues include lack of validation or testing data, with studies reporting results only on training data likely overestimating performance. Unrealistically high performance, such as exceptionally high accuracy without corresponding validation on external data, may indicate overfitting. Insufficient methodological details, such as missing information on model training or evaluation, hinder assessment of validity.

Critical evaluation of ML studies in cardiovascular imaging classification is essential to ensure that models are reliable, valid, and generalizable. By understanding data splitting strategies, interpreting learning curves and performance metrics, and assessing methodological rigor, it is possible to make informed judgments about the trustworthiness of reported results. As ML continues to advance in the medical field, such scrutiny plays an important role in effectively and responsibly translating these technologies into clinical practice.

Aspect	Robust ML Study	Overfitting	Underfitting
Data Splitting	Proper division into training, validation, and testing sets with no data leakage; appropriate proportion and stratification if necessary	Possible improper splitting or data leakage leading to artificially inflated performance on validation set	May have insufficient data or improper splitting, leading to poor learning of patterns
Performance Metrics	Consistent and high metrics (e.g., accuracy, precision, recall) across training, validation, and testing sets; metrics reflect true performance	Metrics are high on training and validation sets but substantially lower on testing set; indicates over-reliance on training data	Low metrics across all datasets; model fails to perform above baseline levels
Learning Curves	Training and validation curves converge and plateau at similar performance levels; small gap between curves indicating good generalization	Training curve shows high performance (e.g., low loss), but validation curve lags behind or worsens; large gap between curves indicating model is not generalizing	Both training and validation curves show poor performance; curves may plateau at low performance levels, indicating model is too simple
ROC Curves and AUC	Similar ROC curves and AUC values for validation and testing sets; high AUC indicating good discriminative ability	High AUC on validation set but significantly lower AUC on testing set; ROC curves differ markedly, suggesting model has learned noise from training data	Low AUC values on both validation and testing sets; ROC curves indicate poor ability to distinguish between classes
Confusion Matrices	Testing set confusion matrix shows slightly lower but comparable performance to validation set; errors are consistent across sets	Significant drop in performance from validation to testing set; confusion matrix shows model performs poorly on unseen data	Poor performance on both validation and testing sets; high misclassification rates indicating inability to capture patterns

Table 4.2: Technical Evaluation Metrics for Robust, Overfitting, and Underfitting ML Studies

Aspect	Robust ML Study	Overfitting	Underfitting
Generalization Ability	Model generalizes well to unseen data; performs reliably across different datasets	Model does not generalize; performs well on training data but poorly on new, unseen data	Model cannot capture underlying patterns; fails to generalize due to oversimplification
Model Complexity	Appropriate complexity matching the problem; neither too simple nor too complex; uses regularization techniques if necessary	Model is overly complex; may have too many parameters leading to memorization of training data	Model is too simple; lacks the capacity to learn the necessary patterns in data
External Validation	Includes external validation using independent datasets from different settings; confirms model's generalizability	Lacks external validation; performance may be inflated due to overfitting on internal data	May not reach stage of external validation due to poor performance on internal data
Methodological Rigor	Detailed and transparent reporting of methods; proper use of cross-validation; avoidance of data leakage; reproducible results	Insufficient methodological details; potential data leakage; lack of transparency hindering assessment of validity	Methodology may be inadequate; poor model selection and training procedures

Table 4.3: Conceptual and Methodological Aspects for Robust, Overfitting, and Underfitting ML Studies

4.6   Discussion

Selecting an appropriate ML algorithm for predicting specific cardiovascular conditions is a multifaceted process that involves several challenges unique to the cardiovascular domain. These challenges include the need for large, annotated datasets specific to cardiovascular imaging modalities, ensuring the model's generalizability across diverse patient populations with varying cardiovascular risk profiles, and addressing issues related to overfitting and underfitting in model development.

One of the primary obstacles in developing robust ML models for CVD prediction is the requirement for extensive, high-quality datasets. Cardiovascular imaging data, such as echocardiograms, cardiac MRI, and CT scans, require detailed expert annotation to capture the nuances of cardiovascular pathology. The availability of such datasets is often limited due to privacy concerns, the labor-intensive nature of data annotation, and the need to represent diverse populations with different CVD patterns. This limitation can lead to models that perform well on training data but fail to generalize to new, unseen patient populations, highlighting the risk of overfitting.

Out of all the studies cited in this review, only two–Lee et al. and Ambale-Venkatesh et al.–utilized multicenter data, enhancing the generalizability of their findings. Lee et al. conducted a retrospective, multicenter cohort study assessing the predictive performance of various risk scores in an BrS population, including an intermediate-risk subgroup [335]. By incorporating data from multiple centers, this study addressed the variability inherent in patient populations and reduced the risk of overfitting the model to a single-center dataset. Similarly, Ambale-Venkatesh et al. assessed the ability of random survival forests to predict six cardiovascular outcomes using data from the MESA, comparing its performance to traditional cardiovascular risk scores [336]. The multicenter nature of the MESA dataset allowed for a more diverse representation of CVD manifestations, enhancing the robustness and applicability of the ML model across different populations.

Recognizing robust ML studies is crucial for clinicians and researchers aiming to apply these models in practice. Robust studies often include key features such as the use of multicenter data, appropriate data splitting strategies to prevent data leakage, thorough validation using separate testing datasets, and external validation when possible. Overfitting and underfitting are significant red flags in ML studies. Overfitting occurs when a model learns the noise in the training data rather than the underlying pattern, leading to poor performance on new data. Underfitting happens when a model is too simplistic to capture the complexity of the data, resulting in poor performance both on training and unseen data.

Evaluating ML studies in cardiovascular imaging requires careful scrutiny of their methodology. Studies should report comprehensive performance metrics, including both accuracy and AUC, to provide a complete picture of the model's predictive capabilities. The lack of reporting either metric, as noted in some studies within this review, can hinder the assessment of a model's true performance. Moreover, proper data splitting into training, validation, and testing sets is essential to avoid data leakage and ensure that the model's performance on unseen data is a reliable indicator of its real-world applicability. Cross-validation techniques and the use of external datasets for validation, especially from multiple centers, can enhance the model's credibility and generalizability.

The "black box" nature of complex ML models presents additional challenges in cardiovascular healthcare, where understanding the rationale behind a diagnostic decision is critical. Clinicians need transparent and interpretable models to trust and effectively integrate ML into patient care. Efforts to develop explainable AI and adhere to guidelines such as the INTRPRT framework [337] are necessary to bridge the gap between model complexity and clinical usability.

Hence, while ML has the potential to significantly advance CVD diagnosis and prediction, it is imperative to develop models that are robust, generalizable, and transparent. Collaborations between medical professionals and ML experts are essential to address the intricacies of model development, prevent issues like overfitting and underfitting, and ensure that models are evaluated rigorously. By focusing on these aspects, and giving particular attention to studies that utilize diverse, multicenter data, the cardiovascular field can better harness the power of ML to improve patient outcomes.

Chapter 5

Core Machine Learning Algorithms: Concepts and Examples

A wide range of ML algorithms are now routinely applied in medical research and clinical practice to support data analysis, classification, and prediction tasks. This chapter outlines the fundamental concepts underlying several core ML models, with emphasis on their typical applications in medicine. For each algorithm, a concise explanation is provided, accompanied by illustrative examples and summaries of relevant studies, to demonstrate their practical utility in medical data analysis and diagnostics.

It is important to recognize that the field of ML is rapidly evolving, and the landscape of available algorithms is vast and continually expanding. Beyond the core models discussed here, many more algorithms exist, each offering unique approaches to learning from data. Furthermore, each algorithm comes with its own set of input parameters and hyperparameters that can be tuned or enhanced to optimize performance for specific tasks. These parameters (ranging from tree depth in decision trees, kernel functions in support vector machines, to learning rates and regularization terms in neural networks) allow for extensive customization and adaptation to the nuances of different datasets and clinical problems. The options for algorithm selection and parameter optimization are virtually endless, enabling researchers to tailor models to the specific characteristics of their data and the clinical questions at hand.

Given this diversity, it is neither practical nor necessary to exhaustively evaluate every possible algorithm and parameter combination for each new medical application. Instead, this chapter offers an overview of some of the core algorithms that have been previously utilized in cardiovascular disease classification tasks, as these represent a well-established foundation for medical ML applications. For each algorithm, representative recent publications are described under the respective algorithm's section, providing concrete examples of how these models have been applied in real-world cardiovascular diagnostics and research.

By focusing on these core algorithms and their documented applications, this chapter aims to equip clinicians, researchers, and students with a practical understanding of the strengths, limitations, and typical use cases of ML in medicine. Readers are encouraged to view these models as starting points for their own investigations, while remaining mindful of the broader array of algorithms and parameter enhancements available as the field continues to advance. Ultimately, the goal is to foster informed, evidence-based adoption of ML tools that are both robust and clinically meaningful, supporting improved patient care and medical discovery

5.1   Decision Trees (DT)

Decision trees are hierarchical, flowchart-like structures that are commonly used in differential diagnosis. These trees provide a clear, systematic way to assess and classify patients, making them particularly effective in identifying risk factors for cardiovascular disorders. By mapping out possible outcomes at each decision point, decision trees help clinicians visualize complex relationships between various risk factors, such as age, lifestyle, medical history, and clinical symptoms.

Figure 5.1 illustrates the structure and operation of a machine learning decision tree model trained for myocardial infarction (MI) risk stratification. In this example, the decision tree algorithm automatically learns a sequence of decision rules from clinical data, such as troponin I levels, age, chest pain score, ECG changes, GRACE score, and the presence of diabetes and hypertension. At each node, the model selects the feature and threshold that best splits the patient population to maximize class separation, as measured by the Gini impurity. The tree recursively partitions the data, ultimately assigning patients to low, moderate, or high MI risk categories at

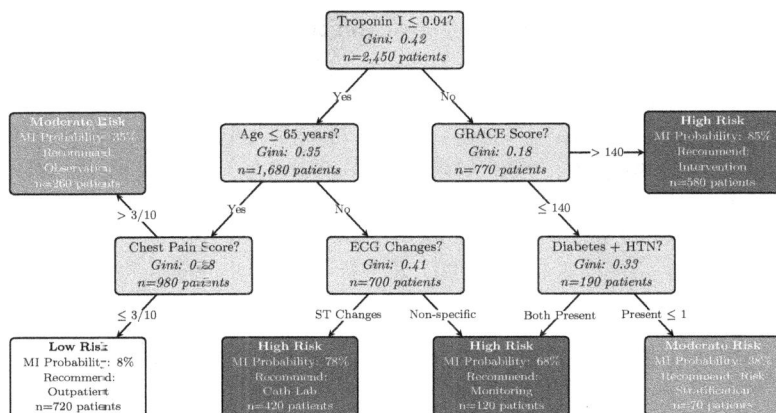

Figure 5.1: Illustrative decision tree for myocardial infarction (MI) risk stratification in suspected acute coronary syndrome. The structure and values are not taken from a published source, but similar ML approaches for MI risk prediction have been described in the literature (e.g., [338, 339]).

the leaf nodes. This process demonstrates how decision trees can be used in supervised learning to model complex, nonlinear relationships among clinical variables and generate interpretable, rule-based predictions for medical decision support. The structure and values in Figure 5.1 are illustrative and reflect typical applications of decision tree algorithms in clinical risk prediction.

A study conducted by Hsu et al. aimed to build a hemogram-based decision tree model to assess the relationship between current probability of metabolic syndrome and predictions of future CVD risk, hypertension, and type 2 diabetes mellitus [340]. A decision tree classification was performed to assess the presence or absence of MetS at baseline, using age, sex, and hemogram variables (white blood cell count, hemoglobin, and platelet count) as independent factors. The analysis was carried out on randomly assigned training (70%) and validation (30%) groups. Participants without MetS at baseline ($n = 25,643$) were subsequently followed to determine if they developed MetS, hypertension, type 2 diabetes, or CVD over time. The decision tree demonstrated modest accuracy in both the training and validation groups, with area under the curves of 0.653 and 0.652, respectively, suggesting that the results were reasonably generalizable. The predicted probability of baseline MetS was derived from the decision tree analysis. Participants without baseline MetS were divided into three equally sized groups based on their predicted probabilities. Those in the third tertile faced significantly higher risks for developing future MetS (hazard ratio 1.40, 95% CI 1.25–1.58), type 2 diabetes (1.46, 1.17–1.83), hypertension (1.14, 1.01–1.28), and CVD (1.21, 1.01–1.44), compared to those in the first tertile. This study concluded that performing a hemogram-based decision tree analysis can help identify elderly patients at high risk for developing hypertension, type 2 diabetes, and CVD, enabling early detection and timely management.

5.2   Support Vector Machine (SVM)

Support Vector Machines are extensively employed in the classification of medical images for the detection of CVDs, offering robust capabilities in various imaging modalities. In cardiac MRI and CT scans, SVMs play a pivotal role in identifying abnormalities such as coronary artery disease, myocardial infarction, and heart failure by effectively distinguishing between healthy and diseased tissues. In the realm of echocardiography, SVMs assist in diagnosing conditions like valve abnormalities, left ventricular dysfunction, and other structural heart diseases by analyzing detailed images of the heart's chambers and valves. They are equally valuable in the interpretation of chest X-rays, where they help detect signs of cardiovascular issues, such as aortic aneurysm or pulmonary edema. Moreover, while ECG signals do not strictly qualify as traditional "medical images," SVMs are applied to these signals to detect arrhythmias or ischemia, classifying distinctive signal patterns indicative of cardiovascular conditions. In each of these applications, SVMs establish decision boundaries between various categories of images or signals, enabling a more accurate, efficient, and automated diagnosis of CVDs. This makes SVMs an indispensable tool in the modern landscape of cardiovascular diagnostics, where their ability to handle complex datasets enhances the precision and speed of disease detection.

An illustrative example (Figure 5.2) presents a schematic illustration of a SVM applied to the classification of cardiovascular disease using clinical parameters. In this diagram, individual data points represent patients and are plotted according to their troponin I levels (x-axis) and left ventricular ejection fraction (y-axis). Healthy patients are depicted as white circles and are clustered in the region characterized by low troponin and high ejection fraction, while patients with cardiovascular disease are shown as black circles, occupying the area of high troponin and low ejection fraction. The SVM

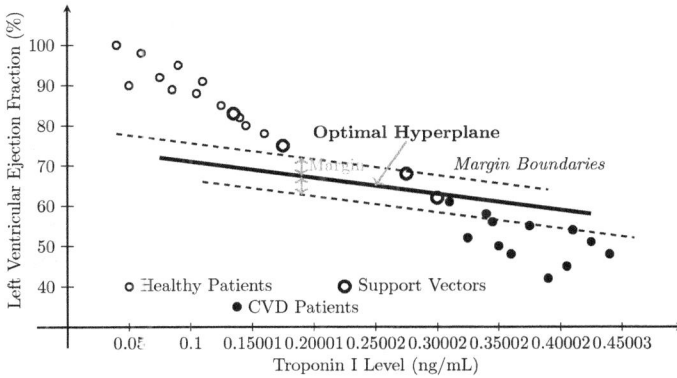

Figure 5.2: Illustrative Support Vector Machine for cardiovascular disease classification. The SVM establishes an optimal decision boundary (hyperplane) that maximally separates healthy patients from those with cardiovascular disease, using clinical parameters such as troponin I levels and left ventricular ejection fraction. Support vectors (highlighted points) define the margin boundaries and are critical for the classification model. The structure and values are illustrative, but similar SVM approaches for CVD risk prediction have been widely described in the literature.

algorithm identifies an optimal separating hyperplane, represented by a solid line, which maximizes the margin between the two groups. The margin boundaries are indicated by dashed lines, and the support vectors (critical data points that lie on these boundaries and influence the position of the hyperplane) are highlighted with thicker outlines. This visual representation underscores the fundamental mechanism by which SVMs achieve robust binary classification in medical diagnostics, specifically by maximizing the separation between classes based on clinically relevant features.

A study conducted by Lee et al. developed IVUS-based supervised ML algorithms to identify coronary lesions with a fractional flow reserve (FFR) ≤ 0.80, as compared to those with FFR > 0.80 [341]. A total of 1,328 patients with non-left main coronary lesions were randomized into training and test sets in a 4:1 ratio. Masked IVUS images were generated using an automatic segmentation model, and a set of 99 computed IVUS features, along with six clinical variables (age, gender, body surface area, vessel type, segment involvement, and proximal left anterior descending artery involvement), were used to train the ML models with 5-fold cross-validation. The diagnostic performance of various binary classifiers—L2 penalized logistic regression, artificial neural network, random forest, AdaBoost, CatBoost, and support vector machine—was evaluated on non-overlapping test samples.

For classifying lesions into FFR ≤ 0.80 versus > 0.80, the diagnostic accuracies for the test set were 82% with L2 penalized logistic regression, 80% with the artificial neural network, 83% with random forest, 83% with AdaBoost, 81% with CatBoost, and 81% with support vector machine (AUCs: 0.84–0.87). When excluding lesions with borderline FFR values (0.75–0.80), the overall accuracies for the test set were 86% with L2 penalized logistic regression, 85% with the artificial neural network, 87% with random forest, 87% with AdaBoost, 85% with CatBoost, and 85% with support vector machine. The study concluded that the IVUS-based ML algorithms demonstrated good diagnostic performance in identifying ischemia-producing lesions and could potentially reduce the need for pressure wire measurements.

5.3   K-Nearest Neighbor (KNN)

K-Nearest Neighbor is a widely used algorithm in the realm of medical diagnostics, particularly for predicting disease outcomes based on patterns observed in patient symptoms and clinical data. By analyzing the characteristics of a patient's condition in relation to the "neighbors" or closest cases in a dataset, KNN can predict the likelihood of disease progression or patient outcomes, making it particularly valuable in cardiovascular medicine.

The relationship between patient features and the KNN classification process is visually depicted in Figure 5.3. This figure presents a two-dimensional scatter plot where each point represents an individual patient, plotted according to exercise duration (minutes) on the x-axis and maximum heart rate (bpm) on the y-axis. Healthy patients are indicated by circles, while patients with cardiovascular disease are shown as diamonds. A star symbol marks the query point, representing a new patient whose classification is to be determined. The five nearest neighbors to this query point are highlighted with darker circles, and dashed concentric circles illustrate the distance-based neighborhood search. Arrows connect the query point to its five closest neighbors, visually emphasizing the selection process. This graphical representation demonstrates the core mechanism of the KNN algorithm, where the class of a new instance is inferred from the majority class among its nearest neighbors in the feature space, as commonly described in the literature

A study conducted by Lee et al. aimed to develop a machine learning-based algorithm to improve the diagnostic performance of a treadmill exercise test, which has a high false-positive rate and may lead to unnecessary inva-

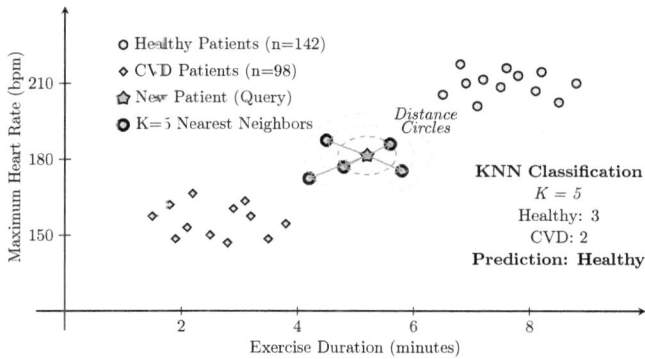

Figure 5.3: Illustrative KNN algorithm for cardiovascular disease classification. The algorithm classifies a new patient (star) by examining the K=5 nearest neighbors in the feature space defined by exercise duration and maximum heart rate achieved during stress testing. In this example, 3 of the 5 nearest neighbors are healthy patients, leading to a "healthy" classification. The distance circles visualize the neighborhood search process. The structure and values are illustrative, but similar KNN approaches for CVD risk prediction have been described in the literature.

sive coronary angiography [342]. KNN, along with support vector machine, logistic regression, random forest, and extreme gradient boosting, were used to build the predictive models, and the performance of each model was compared with that of conventional TET. Four out of the five models demonstrated similar diagnostic performance, outperforming traditional TET. The random forest algorithm achieved an AUC of 0.73, which improved to 0.74 when combined with clinical features. A key advantage of the algorithm is its ability to reduce the false-positive rate compared to conventional TET (55% vs. 76.3%), while maintaining comparable sensitivity (85%). This study concluded that by integrating an artificial intelligence-based model that includes KNN with data from conventional TET, a more accurate diagnosis can be achieved.

5.4   Logistic Regression (LR)

Logistic Regression is a widely utilized statistical method in the field of cardiovascular medicine, particularly for predicting patient readmissions and diagnosing a range of CVDs, including coronary artery disease, heart failure, myocardial infarction, and hypertension. This algorithm excels in binary classification tasks, where it categorizes outcomes into two distinct groups,

such as the presence or absence of a disease, by estimating the probability
of each possible outcome (see Figure 5.4).

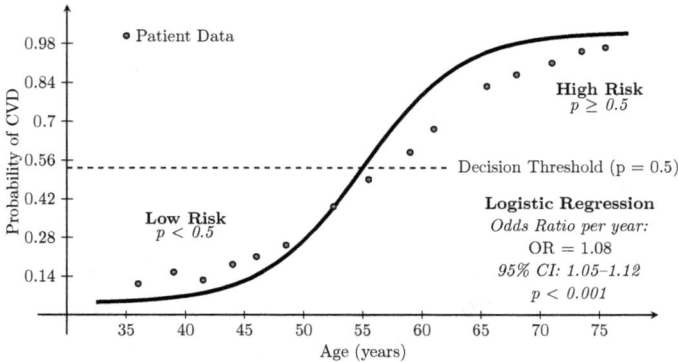

Figure 5.4: Illustrative Logistic Regression model for cardiovascular disease risk prediction. The sigmoid curve demonstrates how the probability of CVD increases with age, with a decision threshold at $p = 0.5$ separating low-risk from high-risk classifications. The logistic function provides smooth probability estimates between 0 and 1, making it particularly suitable for binary classification tasks in cardiovascular medicine. The structure and values are illustrative, but similar logistic regression approaches for CVD risk prediction are widely used in clinical practice.

Figure 5.4 presents a graphical illustration of a logistic regression model applied to cardiovascular disease risk prediction. The figure displays a sigmoid (S-shaped) curve that models the probability of cardiovascular disease as a function of patient age. Along the horizontal axis, age in years is plotted, while the vertical axis represents the estimated probability of developing cardiovascular disease. Individual patient data points are distributed along the curve, with younger patients clustering at lower probabilities and older patients at higher probabilities. A dashed horizontal line marks the decision threshold at a probability of 0.5, which separates individuals classified as low risk (below the threshold) from those classified as high risk (above the threshold). This visual representation underscores how logistic regression provides smooth probability estimates between 0 and 1, facilitating binary classification tasks such as distinguishing between the presence or absence of cardiovascular disease in clinical practice.

A study conducted by Cheng et al. aimed to analyze serum interferon health data in coronary heart disease using logistic regression and artificial neural network (ANN) models [343]. A total of 155 CHD patients diagnosed by coronary angiography between January 2017 and March 2020 were included in this study. The patients were randomly divided into a training set ($n = 108$) and a test set ($n = 47$). Logistic regression and ANN models were developed using the training set to identify predictive factors for coronary artery stenosis, and the models were evaluated using the test set. Health information, including serum levels of IFN-γ, MIG, and IP-10, was collected and measured using double antibody sandwich ELISA. Spearman correlation analysis revealed a positive correlation between the degree of stenosis and the levels of these serum markers. Both the logistic regression and ANN models identified MIG and IP-10 as independent predictors of the Gensini score (MIG: 95% CI: 0.876–0.934, $P < 0.001$; IP-10: 95% CI: 1.009–1.039, $P < 0.001$). No significant difference was found between the performance of the logistic regression and ANN models ($P > 0.05$). This study concluded that the logistic regression and ANN models exhibit comparable predictive performance for identifying risk factors of coronary artery stenosis in CHD patients. In these patients, the levels of IFN-γ, IP-10, and MIG are positively correlated with the degree of stenosis. Additionally, IP-10 and MIG are independent risk factors for coronary artery stenosis.

5.5   Convolutional Neural Network (CNN)

Convolutional Neural Networks represent a specialized class of neural networks primarily designed for image recognition tasks. In the context of cardiovascular medicine, CNNs are extensively employed to analyze and interpret medical images, including X-rays, MRIs, and CT scans, in order to identify a wide range of CVDs. These networks are particularly adept at automatically extracting hierarchical features from images, enabling them to detect subtle patterns and abnormalities that may not be immediately apparent to the human eye.

Figure 5.5 illustrates the architecture of a CNN designed for image recognition tasks. The network takes an input image and processes it through a series of convolutional and pooling layers, which automatically extract hierarchical features from the raw pixel data. The initial convolutional layer applies multiple filters to detect local patterns such as edges or textures, followed by pooling operations that reduce the spatial dimensions while retaining the most salient information. This process is repeated in subsequent layers, enabling the network to learn increasingly abstract and complex features relevant for distinguishing between different image categories. After the final convolutional and pooling stages, the extracted feature maps

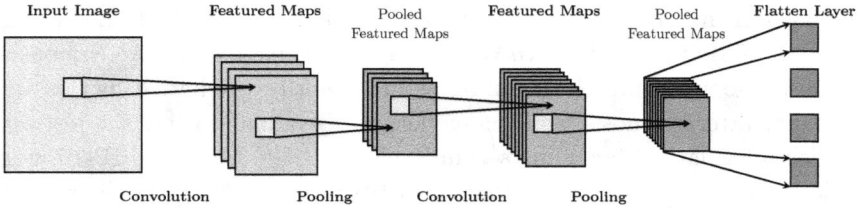

Figure 5.5: Architecture of a Convolutional Neural Network for image classification. The network processes a 36×36 input image through multiple convolutional and pooling layers, progressively extracting higher-level features while reducing spatial dimensions. Each convolutional layer applies multiple filters to create feature maps, followed by max-pooling operations that downsample the representations. The final layer produces class probabilities for classification. The highlighted squares alternate between upper and lower regions of each processing stage, with converging arrows illustrating the focused information flow through the network's receptive fields.

are flattened and passed through fully connected layers, which integrate the learned features to perform classification. The output layer produces a probability distribution over the possible image classes, enabling the network to assign the input image to the most likely category. The highlighted patch on the input image demonstrates the concept of a local receptive field, where each neuron in the convolutional layer processes information from a small, localized region of the input. This architectural approach allows the CNN to efficiently learn spatial hierarchies of features, making it highly effective for a wide range of image recognition applications.

A study conducted by Sun et al. aimed to develop an artificial intelligence-based approach for screening patients with a left ventricular ejection fraction (LVEF) of 50% or lower using only electrocardiogram (ECG) data [344]. They collected standard 12-lead ECG and transthoracic echocardiogram (TTE) data, including the LVEF value, then paired the ECG and TTE data from the same individual. In cases where multiple ECG-TTE pairs were available from a single individual, only the earliest pair was included. The ECG-TTE pairs were randomly divided into training, validation, and testing datasets in a 9:1:1 ratio for the development and evaluation of the CNN model. Finally, the screening performance was assessed using overall accuracy, sensitivity, specificity, positive predictive value, and negative predictive value. In the testing set, the CNN algorithm achieved an overall accuracy of 73.9%, with a sensitivity of 69.2%, specificity of 70.5%, positive predictive value of 70.1%, and negative predictive value of 69.9%. The study concluded that a well-trained CNN algorithm could serve as an affordable and noninvasive tool for identifying patients with left ventricular dysfunction.

A study conducted by Mamun et al. showed a hybrid one-dimensional convolutional neural network (1D CNN), which leverages a large dataset gathered from online surveys and selected features using feature selection algorithms, demonstrated superior accuracy compared to other contemporary machine learning algorithms and artificial neural networks [345]. The validation data for non-coronary heart disease (no-CHD) and coronary heart disease (CHD) achieved accuracy rates of 80.1% and 76.9%, respectively. The model was benchmarked against an artificial neural network, random forest, AdaBoost, and support vector machine. Overall, the 1D CNN outperformed these models in terms of accuracy, false negative rates, and false positive rates. Similar approaches were applied to four other heart conditions, with the hybrid 1D CNN consistently delivering better accuracy in all cases.

5.6 Light Gradient Boosting Machine (Light-GBM)

Light Gradient Boosting Machine is an advanced gradient boosting framework that leverages tree-based learning algorithms to produce highly effective predictive models. LightGBM is particularly well-suited for handling large, complex datasets, such as those encountered in cardiovascular image analysis. By constructing an ensemble of decision trees in a sequential manner, where each subsequent tree corrects the errors of the previous one, LightGBM excels at capturing intricate patterns and relationships within data.

Figure 5.6 demonstrates the sequential ensemble learning architecture of LightGBM, which forms the foundation of its powerful predictive capabilities in cardiovascular diagnostics. The algorithm begins with the original training data containing patient features and target outcomes, then constructs the first decision tree as a base model. Rather than training trees independently, LightGBM employs a gradient boosting approach where each subsequent tree is specifically trained to predict the residual errors of the previous ensemble. This iterative process, illustrated by the arrows showing the sequential progression, enables the model to progressively reduce prediction errors and capture increasingly complex patterns in the data. The darkly shaded nodes represent leaves that cannot be expanded further in the current iteration, while the white nodes indicate potential expansion points.

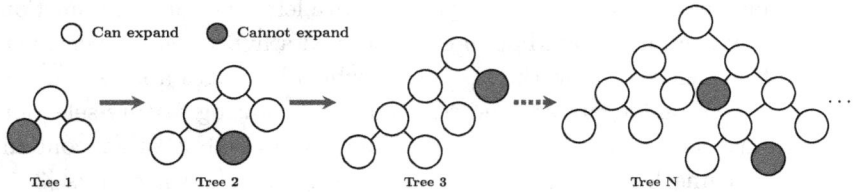

Figure 5.6: Progressive tree growth in LightGBM illustrating the leaf-wise expansion strategy. Each tree becomes increasingly complex as the algorithm focuses on splitting the most beneficial leaf nodes (shown as darkly shaded nodes) rather than growing level-wise. The arrows demonstrate the sequential nature of the boosting process, where each subsequent tree is built to correct the errors of the previous ensemble. This leaf-wise growth pattern allows LightGBM to achieve higher accuracy with fewer splits compared to traditional level-wise approaches.

This sequential error-correction mechanism allows LightGBM to achieve superior performance on cardiovascular prediction tasks by systematically addressing the weaknesses of previous iterations, making it particularly effective for identifying subtle relationships in complex medical datasets where traditional single-model approaches may fall short.

A retrospective, multi-center cohort study conducted by Lee et al. assessed the predictive performance of various risk scores in an Asian Brugada Syndrome (BrS) population, including its intermediate risk subgroup [335]. The study included consecutive BrS patients diagnosed between January 1, 1997, and June 20, 2020, in Hong Kong, with sustained ventricular tachyarrhythmias (VT/VF) as the primary outcome. Two novel risk scores and machine learning models such as LightGBM, random survival forest, AdaBoost classifier, Gaussian Naïve Bayes, random forest classifier, gradient boosting classifier, and decision tree classifier were developed, and the area under the receiver operating characteristic curve (AUC) was compared across the models. The cohort comprised 548 consecutive BrS patients (7% female, mean age at diagnosis 50 ± 16 years, mean follow-up 84 ± 55 months). For the entire cohort, the risk score developed by Sieira et al. performed best (AUC: 0.806 [0.747–0.865]), while a novel score, combining the Sieira score with additional variables identified through univariable Cox regression, showed improved performance (AUC: 0.855 [0.808–0.901]). A simpler score based on non-invasive measures alone had a comparable AUC (0.784 [0.724–0.845]), which improved further when applied to random survival forests (AUC: 0.942 [0.913–0.964]). Among the intermediate risk subgroup ($N = 274$), the gradient boosting classifier model provided the best performance (AUC:

0.814 [0.791–0.832]). This study concluded that a simple risk score based on clinical and electrocardiographic variables demonstrated good performance for predicting VT/VF, which was further enhanced using machine learning techniques.

5.7   General Linear Model Boosting (GLMB)

General Linear Model Boosting integrates general linear models with the boosting technique to enhance predictive accuracy by iteratively refining predictions. In cardiovascular imaging, GLM Boosting can optimize the analysis of complex medical images (e.g., CT scans, MRIs, echocardiograms), improving the detection of abnormalities, predicting disease risk, and aiding in the development of personalized treatment plans. By combining clinical and imaging data, it enhances diagnostic performance, enabling earlier and more precise identification of conditions such as coronary artery disease and heart failure. While it holds substantial promise for improving patient outcomes, challenges related to data quality, model interpretability, and computational demands must be addressed before it can be widely adopted in clinical practice.

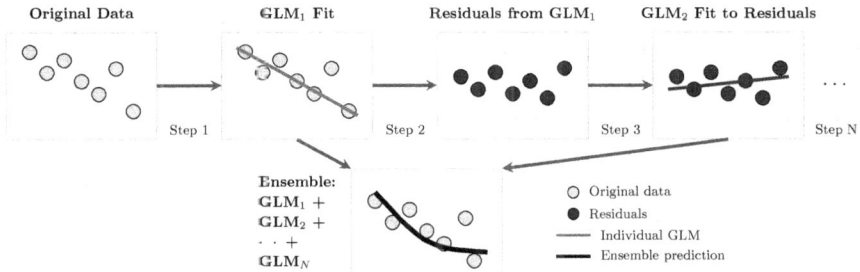

Figure 5.7: Sequential ensemble learning process in GLMB. The algorithm begins with the original dataset and fits the first generalized linear model (GLM_1) to capture the primary relationships. Subsequent models (GLM_2, GLM_3, ..., GLM_N) are sequentially fitted to the residuals of the previous ensemble, allowing each new model to focus on correcting the remaining prediction errors. The final ensemble combines all individual GLMs to produce a more accurate and robust prediction that captures complex nonlinear patterns through the additive combination of multiple linear components.

Figure 5.7 illustrates the iterative ensemble learning mechanism that underlies General Linear Model Boosting's effectiveness in cardiovascular image analysis applications. The algorithm initiates with the original training dataset containing patient features extracted from medical imaging data, then sequentially constructs generalized linear models where each subsequent model targets the residual errors left by the previous ensemble. This boosting approach, demonstrated by the step-wise progression from GLM_1 through GLM_N, enables the framework to capture complex nonlinear relationships in cardiovascular data through an additive combination of simpler linear components. Unlike traditional single-model approaches, GLMB's sequential error-correction strategy allows it to progressively refine predictions by having each new GLM focus specifically on the prediction errors that remain unexplained by the current ensemble. The final ensemble prediction, shown in the bottom subplot, demonstrates how this iterative process results in a more sophisticated model that can identify subtle patterns in cardiovascular imaging data, making it particularly valuable for applications such as automated detection of coronary artery stenosis, assessment of cardiac function parameters, and prediction of adverse cardiovascular events where traditional linear models alone may be insufficient.

A study conducted by Asadi et al. aimed to determine the most effective tree-based machine learning method for detecting CVD [346]. Data from 9,499 participants were analyzed, focusing on 38 different variables, with the presence of CVD as the target variable and villages as the cluster variable. The models compared included the standard decision tree, random forest, Generalized Linear Mixed Model tree (GLMM tree), and Generalized Mixed Effect Random Forest (GMERF). The performance of each model was evaluated using prediction power indices to identify the best method. The analysis revealed that five variables—age, LDL cholesterol levels, family history of cardiac disease, physical activity level, and the presence of hypertension—were most influential in predicting CVD. The models' area under the ROC curve (AUC) were 0.56 for the decision tree, 0.73 for random forest, 0.78 for GLMM tree, and 0.80 for GMERF. The GMERF model showed the best predictive performance overall. The study also highlighted that accounting for the clustered nature of the data using appropriate machine learning approaches can improve prediction accuracy and lead to more targeted prevention strategies for CVD.

5.8   Linear Discriminant Analysis (LDA)

Linear Discriminant Analysis is a technique widely used in cardiovascular diagnostics for both dimensionality reduction and classification tasks. By projecting high-dimensional data onto a lower-dimensional space, LDA simplifies the analysis of complex cardiovascular images while retaining critical discriminatory information. This enables more efficient classification of different disease states, such as distinguishing between healthy and diseased tissues in the context of conditions like coronary artery disease, heart failure, or myocardial infarction.

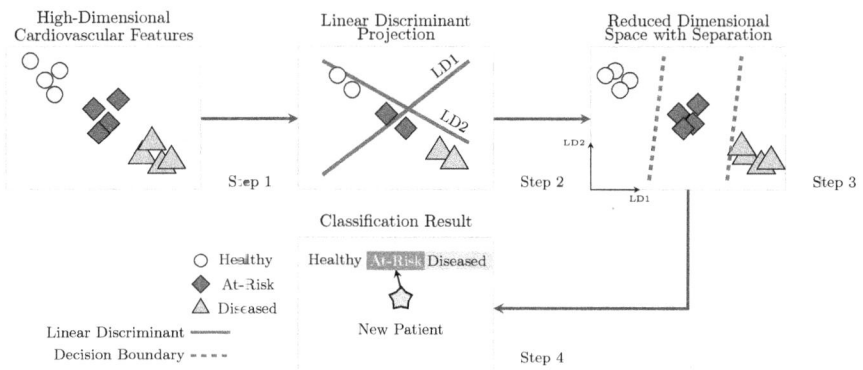

Figure 5.8: Linear Discriminant Analysis workflow for cardiovascular diagnosis classification. The algorithm begins with high-dimensional cardiovascular features extracted from medical imaging data (ejection fraction, wall thickness, perfusion indices, etc.) representing different patient categories. LDA identifies optimal linear discriminants (LD1, LD2) that maximize between-class separation while minimizing within-class variance. The projection onto these discriminants creates a lower-dimensional space where healthy, at-risk, and diseased patient groups are more distinctly separated. Decision boundaries in this reduced space enable efficient classification of new patients based on their projected coordinates, facilitating rapid and accurate cardiovascular diagnosis.

The process illustrated in Figure 5.8 provides an overview of how LDA is applied to cardiovascular diagnostic data. The figure is organized into four sequential panels, each representing a distinct stage in the analysis pipeline. Initially, high-dimensional cardiovascular features are collected from medical imaging, with each data point corresponding to a patient and characterized by multiple quantitative measurements. These data points are visually grouped according to patient categories, such as healthy, at-risk, and diseased.

The second panel demonstrates the application of LDA, where the algorithm identifies optimal linear discriminants that maximize the separation between the predefined patient groups. The original data are projected onto these new axes, labeled LD1 and LD2, which are specifically chosen to

enhance class separability. In the third panel, the result of this projection
is shown as a reduced-dimensional space in which the different patient
groups form distinct clusters. Decision boundaries are depicted to indicate
the regions associated with each class, thereby clarifying the separability
achieved through LDA.

The final panel presents the classification outcome in this reduced space.
Here, the regions corresponding to each patient category are delineated,
and the classification of a new patient is illustrated by projecting its data
point into the space and assigning it to the appropriate group based on its
position relative to the decision boundaries. Overall, Figure 5.8 encapsulates
the transformation of complex, high-dimensional cardiovascular data into
a form that enables efficient and accurate classification of patient health
status through LDA.

A study conducted by Morguet et al. assessed 15 patients (ages 36–
75, median age 59) with stable single-vessel disease ($\geq 70\%$ stenosis) and
regional wall-motion abnormalities using multiple diagnostic techniques and
analyzed with linear discriminant analysis [347]. The diagnostic techniques
included echocardiography to evaluate wall motion, Tl dipyridamole single-
photon emission computed tomography (SPECT) for perfusion imaging, and
quantitative F-fluorodeoxyglucose positron emission tomography (PET) to
evaluate myocardial viability in 16 left ventricular wall segments. MCG was
performed using a shielded 49-channel low-temperature superconducting
quantum interference device (SQUID) system, and various time and area
parameters were extracted from the baseline-corrected data. Of the 240
wall segments assessed, 117 were lesion-dependent, with 88 segments (75%)
deemed viable and 29 segments (25%) showing signs of scar tissue. The
patients were categorized based on the number of scar segments: five had no
scar, six had scar in 1–3 segments, and four had scar in ≥ 4 segments. Using
linear discriminant analysis, the three MCG parameters with the highest
selectivity were identified, and Fisher's discriminant functions successfully
classified all patients accurately (Wilks' lambda = 0.079). The results
suggest that MCG can effectively classify patients according to the extent
of myocardial scar and viability, indicating its potential value in assessing
myocardial viability in coronary artery disease. Further multicenter studies
are needed to confirm these findings.

A study conducted by Ciaccio et al. developed an algorithm to extract morphological components based on frequency, and its effectiveness in
distinguishing complex fractionated atrial electrograms (CFAE) was eval-

uated [348]. The study involved recording CFAE of 16 seconds from two sites each at the four pulmonary vein ostia (PV) and from the anterior and posterior left atrial free wall (FW) in nine patients with paroxysmal atrial fibrillation (AF) and ten with longstanding persistent AF. The dominant frequency (DF) was calculated for each of two 8-second CFAE segments within the 16-second recordings. Each CFAE segment was transformed into a set of basis vectors representing the electrogram morphology at each frequency. The dominant morphology (DM) was defined as the ensemble average of sequential signal segments, with the segment length matching the period at the DF. The DMs of the two 8-second pairs were correlated, and normalized correlation coefficients were calculated for all data, with separate analyses for the PV and FW sites. The means and coefficients of variation of the DM correlation coefficients were plotted, and a linear discriminant function was used to classify persistent versus paroxysmal AF. For comparison, the CFE-mean and interval confidence level (ICL) parameters were also calculated for both groups. The results showed that the mean DM correlation for persistent AF was 0.62 ± 0.22, compared to 0.50 ± 0.19 for paroxysmal AF ($p < 0.001$). At individual anatomical sites, the correlation was higher in persistent AF, with significant differences observed at the left superior ($p < 0.001$) and right superior ($p < 0.05$) PV. While spatial variation in the correlation coefficient was greater in paroxysmal AF, the difference was not statistically significant. Using the DF correlation coefficients, 17 out of 19 patients were correctly classified. Additionally, the CFE-mean parameter averaged 89.01 ± 20.99 ms in persistent AF versus 93.96 ± 33.81 ms in paroxysmal AF ($p < 0.05$), and the ICL averaged 94.54 ± 18.52 deflections/8 s in persistent AF versus 90.70 ± 19.28 deflections/8 s in paroxysmal AF ($p < 0.05$). This study concluded that the DM parameter showed greater temporal morphological variation in CFAE recordings from paroxysmal AF compared to persistent AF ($p < 0.001$), whereas the CFE-mean and ICL parameters showed only moderate significance in distinguishing the two types of AF ($p < 0.05$). The DM parameter thus offers a promising new measure for identifying both temporal and spatial variations in CFAE recordings, potentially aiding in the differentiation of paroxysmal versus persistent AF.

5.9   Naïve Bayes (NB)

The Naïve Bayes algorithm is a probabilistic classifier based on Bayes' theorem. It is particularly valuable in medical diagnosis due to its simplicity, efficiency, and ability to handle large datasets with numerous features. By assuming conditional independence between features, NB can quickly calculate the likelihood of a given outcome based on the available data. This makes it especially effective for tasks such as disease classification, where multiple variables, such as patient demographics, medical history, and imaging data, need to be considered simultaneously. Its computational efficiency and ability to scale to large datasets make NB a popular choice for applications in cardiovascular diagnostics, where fast, accurate predictions are essential.

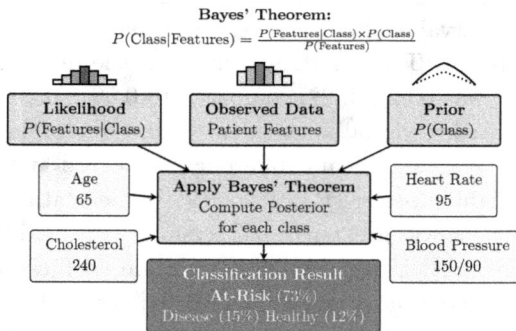

Figure 5.9: Illustration of the Naïve Bayes algorithm principle: the classifier estimates the probability of each class given observed features by applying Bayes' theorem, assuming conditional independence among features. The workflow begins by extracting relevant features from the input data, such as clinical measurements. For each class, the algorithm computes the likelihood of the observed features, multiplies this by the prior probability of the class, and normalizes across all classes to obtain posterior probabilities. The class with the highest posterior probability is then selected as the prediction.

The NB classifier is a probabilistic model that applies Bayes' theorem to perform classification tasks under the simplifying assumption that all input features are conditionally independent given the class label. This assumption, while rarely true in practice, enables the algorithm to efficiently compute the posterior probability of each class by multiplying the individual likelihoods of the observed features for each class with the prior probability of that class. The classifier then assigns the instance to the class with the highest posterior probability. The workflow, as depicted in Figure 5.9, begins by extracting relevant features from the input data, such as patient demographics or clinical measurements For each possible class, the algorithm calculates the likelihood of observing the given feature values, multiplies this by the prior probability of the class (often estimated from population statistics), and normalizes across all classes. The result is a set of posterior probabilities, from which the most probable class is selected as the prediction. This approach is computationally efficient and particularly well-suited for high-dimensional datasets, making it a popular choice in domains like medical diagnosis where rapid and interpretable predictions are essential.

A study conducted by Miranda et al. developed a mining model that uses a NB classifier to detect CVD and assess its risk level in adults [349]. The model was developed by analyzing medical records to identify key factors related to CVD and its associated risk levels. The primary risk factors considered include diabetes mellitus, blood lipid levels, coronary artery function, and kidney function. Based on these factors, class labels were assigned to indicate three risk levels. The evaluation of the model's performance was conducted using accuracy, sensitivity, and specificity measures, as well as feedback from cardiologists and internists. The results showed that the proposed model correctly predicted the risk level for more than 80% of the cases, and over 80% of the medical professionals who participated in the evaluation agreed that the model followed medical procedures and could support clinical decision-making related to CVD. This study concluded that the NB classifier model performs well in detecting CVD and identifying its risk levels.

5.10   Random Forests (RF)

Random Forests are ensembles of decision trees that provide robust performance and valuable insights into feature importance. By combining multiple decision trees, each trained on different subsets of the data, they enhance predictive accuracy and reduce the risk of overfitting. In medical diagnostics, Random Forests are extensively used due to their ability to handle large and complex datasets, which often involve numerous variables such as patient characteristics, clinical data, and imaging features. Their versatility and high accuracy make them particularly effective for classifying cardiovascular conditions, while their ability to assess the importance of different features offers additional interpretability, aiding clinicians in understanding which factors most significantly influence disease outcomes.

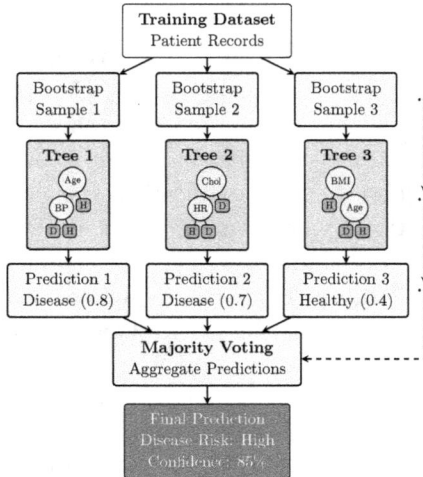

Figure 5.10: Illustration of the Random Forests algorithm: the ensemble method combines multiple decision trees trained on different bootstrap samples of the data to produce robust predictions. Each tree uses a random subset of features at each split, and the final prediction is determined through majority voting for classification tasks. The diagram shows how bootstrap sampling creates diverse training sets, leading to different tree structures that capture various patterns in the data, ultimately improving generalization performance.

Random Forests represent a powerful ensemble learning technique that leverages the collective intelligence of multiple decision trees to enhance predictive performance and reduce overfitting. As illustrated in Figure 5.10, the algorithm begins by creating multiple bootstrap samples from the original training dataset, where each sample is generated through random sampling with replacement. Each bootstrap sample is then used to train an individual decision tree, with the additional constraint that at each node split, only a random subset of available features is considered for determining the optimal splitting criterion. This dual randomization (in both data sampling and feature selection) ensures that each tree in the forest captures different aspects of the underlying data patterns, promoting diversity within the ensemble. Once all trees are trained, new instances are classified by passing them through each tree in the forest to obtain individual predictions. The final classification is determined through majority voting, where the class receiving the most votes across all trees becomes the ensemble's prediction. This aggregation process not only improves accuracy by reducing the variance associated with individual trees but also provides natural confidence measures based on the distribution of votes, making Random Forests particularly valuable in medical diagnostic applications where both accuracy and interpretability are crucial.

A study conducted by Ambale-Venkatesh et al. aimed to assess the ability of random survival forests to predict six cardiovascular outcomes and compare its performance to traditional cardiovascular risk scores [336]. Participants were drawn from the Multi-Ethnic Study of Atherosclerosis (MESA), which followed 6,814 individuals (ages 45 to 84) from four ethnic groups and six centers across the United States over 12 years. MESA participants were initially free of CVD, and baseline measurements were used to predict future cardiovascular events. A total of 735 variables, including imaging, noninvasive tests, questionnaires, and biomarker panels, were analyzed. The random survival forests technique identified the top 20 predictors for each cardiovascular outcome, with imaging, electrocardiography, and serum biomarkers emerging as significant predictors, rather than traditional risk factors. Age was the strongest predictor for all-cause mortality, while fasting glucose levels and carotid ultrasound measures were key for predicting stroke. The coronary artery calcium score was the best predictor for coronary heart disease and overall atherosclerotic CVD, and left ventricular function and cardiac troponin-T were among the top predictors for incident heart failure. Creatinine levels, age, and ankle-brachial index were significant for atrial fibrillation, and inflammatory markers like TNF-α, IL-2 soluble receptors, and NT-proBNP were important across all outcomes. The random survival forests technique outperformed established cardiovascular risk scores, improving prediction accuracy by reducing the Brier score by 10%–25%. This study concluded that machine learning combined with deep phenotyping enhances prediction accuracy for cardiovascular events in an initially asymptomatic population, offering insights into subclinical disease markers without assumptions about causality.

5.11   Adaptive Boosting (AdaBoost)

Adaptive Boosting is an ensemble learning algorithm that synthesizes multiple weak classifiers to form a robust and highly accurate model. By focusing on the misclassified instances from previous iterations and assigning them higher weights, AdaBoost sequentially enhances the performance of weak classifiers, ultimately creating a strong, more reliable predictor. In medical diagnostics, AdaBoost is particularly valuable for improving the performance of simpler models, enabling them to achieve higher accuracy and robustness. Its ability to iteratively refine predictions makes it an effective tool in the classification of complex medical conditions, such as CVDs, where subtle patterns in data are critical for accurate diagnosis.

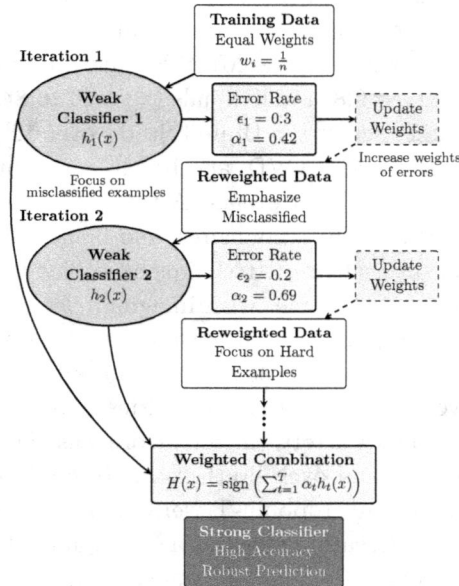

Figure 5.11: Illustration of the Adaptive Boosting (AdaBoost) algorithm: the ensemble method sequentially trains weak classifiers while adaptively adjusting sample weights to focus on previously misclassified examples. Each iteration produces a weak classifier with associated weight α_t based on its error rate ϵ_t. The final strong classifier combines all weak classifiers through weighted majority voting, where classifiers with lower error rates receive higher influence in the final decision.

Adaptive Boosting exemplifies the principle of sequential learning, where each iteration builds upon the knowledge gained from previous mistakes to create increasingly robust predictors. As demonstrated in Figure 5.11, the algorithm initiates with uniformly weighted training examples and proceeds through iterative cycles of classifier training and weight adjustment. At each iteration t, a weak classifier $h_t(x)$ is trained on the current weighted dataset, followed by the calculation of its weighted error rate ϵ_t and corresponding classifier weight $\alpha_t = \frac{1}{2} \ln\left(\frac{1-\epsilon_t}{\epsilon_t}\right)$. The algorithm then increases the weights of misclassified examples while decreasing the weights of correctly classified ones, effectively forcing subsequent classifiers to concentrate on the most challenging cases. This adaptive reweighting mechanism ensures that each new weak classifier complements its predecessors by targeting their weaknesses, leading to a diverse ensemble that captures complex decision boundaries. The final strong classifier $H(x) = \text{sign}\left(\sum_{t=1}^{T} \alpha_t h_t(x)\right)$ combines all weak classifiers through weighted majority voting, where classifiers with superior performance (lower error rates) exert greater influence on the final prediction. This sequential refinement process transforms a collection of marginally better-than-random weak classifiers into a highly accurate ensemble, making AdaBoost particularly effective for medical diagnostic tasks where the distinction between healthy and diseased states may rely on subtle, complex patterns that individual simple classifiers cannot capture alone.

A study conducted by Zhu et al. explored using AdaBoost in assessing the quality of ECG signals. They analyzed 12-lead ECG data provided by PhysioNet, focusing on two time-domain features: the number of R peaks and the amplitude difference [350]. These features were extracted to create a matrix of 24 attributes. Using this feature matrix, the authors trained a classification model, achieving a classification accuracy of 95.80% on the test set. The experimental results demonstrated that the AdaBoost algorithm provided superior accuracy compared to other methods for solving ECG quality assessment problems.

5.12   Extreme Gradient Boosting (XGBoost)

XGBoost, or Extreme Gradient Boosting, is a machine learning algorithm widely employed in medical image classification due to its efficiency and exceptional performance. Based on the principles of gradient boosting, it is capable of addressing both regression and classification tasks. XGBoost is used for various purposes, such as classifying different tissue types, identifying disease markers, or predicting disease progression. Its effectiveness in medical image classification stems from its ability to manage high-dimensional data, handle missing values, and maintain strong performance even when faced with noisy data, which is a common characteristic of medical imaging datasets.

Extreme Gradient Boosting represents a sophisticated advancement in ensemble learning that leverages gradient descent optimization to sequentially construct decision trees for superior predictive accuracy. As illustrated

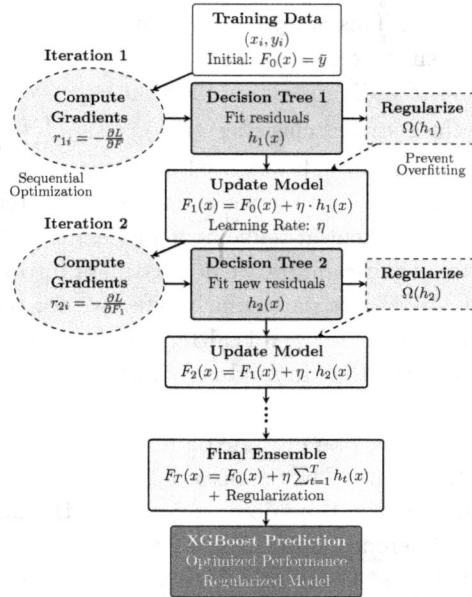

Figure 5.12: Illustration of the Extreme Gradient Boosting (XGBoost) algorithm: the ensemble method sequentially builds decision trees by fitting gradients of the loss function from previous iterations. Each iteration computes negative gradients r_{ti} as pseudo-residuals, trains a new decision tree $h_t(x)$ to fit these residuals, applies regularization $\Omega(h_t)$ to prevent overfitting, and updates the ensemble model $F_t(x) = F_{t-1}(x) + \eta \cdot h_t(x)$ with a learning rate η. The final model combines all trees with regularization to achieve optimal predictive performance.

in Figure 5.12, XGBoost employs a systematic approach where each iteration begins with the computation of negative gradients of the loss function, serving as pseudo-residuals that guide the training of subsequent decision trees. Unlike traditional boosting methods that focus on reweighting misclassified samples, XGBoost directly optimizes the loss function by fitting each new tree $h_t(x)$ to the gradients $r_{ti} = -\frac{\partial L(y_i, F_{t-1}(x_i))}{\partial F_{t-1}(x_i)}$ calculated from the current ensemble's predictions. The algorithm incorporates regularization terms $\Omega(h_t)$ at each iteration to control model complexity and prevent overfitting, a crucial consideration in medical applications where generalization to unseen patient data is paramount. The ensemble model is updated incrementally as $F_t(x) = F_{t-1}(x) + \eta \cdot h_t(x)$, where the learning rate η controls the contribution of each new tree to the overall prediction. This iterative refinement process, combined with XGBoost's built-in capabilities for handling missing values and high-dimensional feature spaces, makes it particularly well-suited for cardiovascular disease prediction tasks where patient data may be incomplete and feature interactions are complex. The final ensemble $F_T(x) = F_0(x) + \eta \sum_{t=1}^{T} h_t(x)$ represents a regularized model that balances predictive accuracy with generalization ability, enabling robust performance on diverse cardiovascular diagnostic challenges ranging from ECG classification to risk stratification in cardiac patients.

A single-center study conducted by Xie et al. included 104 patients with idiopathic dilated cardiomyopathy (DCM) [351]. Left ventricular reverse remodeling (LVRR) was defined as an absolute increase in left ventricular ejection fraction (LVEF) greater than 10%, reaching a final value above 35%, along with a decrease in left ventricular end-diastolic diameter (LVDd) exceeding 10%. The study analyzed various features, including demographic characteristics, comorbidities, physical signs, biochemistry data, echocardiography, electrocardiogram, Holter monitoring, and medication. Logistic regression, random forests, and extreme gradient boosting (XGBoost) were applied using a 10-fold cross-validation model to distinguish between LVRR and non-LVRR, with performance evaluated via receiver operating characteristic (ROC) curves and calibration plots. Results showed that LVRR occurred in 47 patients (45.2%) after optimal medical treatment. Key variables such as cystatin C, right ventricular end-diastolic dimension, high-density lipoprotein cholesterol (HDL-C), left atrial dimension, left ventricular posterior wall dimension, systolic blood pressure, severe mitral regurgitation, eGFR, and NYHA classification were incorporated into the XGBoost model, which demonstrated a higher AU-ROC compared to logistic regression (AU-ROC: 0.8205 vs. 0.5909, $p = 0.0119$). Ablation analysis revealed that cystatin C, right ventricular end-diastolic dimension, and HDL-C made the largest contributions to the model. In conclusion, tree-based models like XGBoost were effective in early differentiating LVRR from non-LVRR in patients with newly diagnosed DCM before drug therapy, aiding in disease management and guiding decisions regarding invasive therapies. Further validation through a multicenter prospective study is warranted.

5.13   RoboFlow 3.0 Object Detection (RF3)

RoboFlow is a comprehensive platform that provides tools and resources for computer vision tasks, including object detection in cardiovascular imaging.

It supports the processing of various cardiology-related medical images, such as echocardiograms, coronary angiograms, cardiac MRIs, CT scans, and X-rays. This versatility allows healthcare professionals to apply object detection models across a broad spectrum of cardiovascular diagnostic modalities, thereby improving the detection and analysis of conditions such as coronary artery disease, heart failure, valve abnormalities, and myocardial infarction. By enhancing the accuracy and efficiency of image analysis, RoboFlow contributes to more precise and timely diagnoses, ultimately leading to improved patient outcomes.

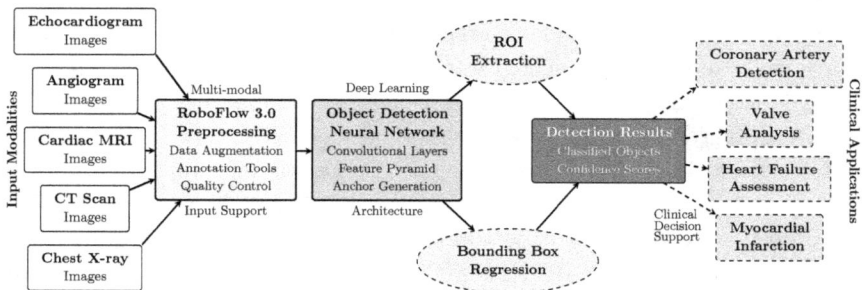

Figure 5.13: Illustration of the RoboFlow 3.0 Object Detection (RF3) workflow for cardiovascular imaging: the system processes multiple imaging modalities including echocardiograms, angiograms, cardiac MRIs, CT scans, and chest X-rays through RoboFlow's comprehensive preprocessing pipeline, which includes data augmentation, annotation tools, and quality control mechanisms. The preprocessed images are fed into a deep learning-based object detection neural network featuring convolutional layers, feature pyramid networks, and anchor generation for precise localization. The model performs simultaneous region of interest (ROI) extraction and bounding box regression to identify and classify cardiovascular structures and pathologies, producing detection results with confidence scores that support various clinical applications including coronary artery detection, valve analysis, heart failure assessment, and myocardial infarction diagnosis.

RoboFlow 3.0 Object Detection represents a state-of-the-art computer vision platform specifically optimized for cardiovascular imaging applications, employing sophisticated deep learning architectures to automatically identify and localize pathological structures across diverse imaging modalities. As depicted in Figure 5.13, the RF3 workflow demonstrates remarkable versatility by accepting input from multiple cardiovascular imaging sources, including echocardiograms for cardiac chamber assessment, coronary angiograms for vessel visualization, cardiac MRIs for tissue characterization, CT scans for anatomical evaluation, and chest X-rays for initial screening. The platform's preprocessing pipeline incorporates advanced data augmentation techniques, comprehensive annotation tools, and rigorous quality control mechanisms that enhance model robustness and ensure consistent performance across varying image acquisition protocols and patient populations. The core object detection neural network utilizes convolutional layers with feature pyramid architectures to extract multi-scale representations, while anchor generation mechanisms enable precise localization of cardiovascular structures ranging from coronary stencses to valvular abnormalities. Through simultaneous region of interest extraction and bounding box regression, RF3 generates detection results with associated confidence scores that directly support clinical decision-making processes. This integrated approach facilitates comprehensive cardiovascular analysis spanning coronary artery disease detection, valve function assessment, heart failure evaluation, and myocardial infarction identification, thereby streamlining diagnostic workflows and potentially improving patient outcomes through enhanced accuracy and reduced interpretation time in cardiovascular imaging.

A study conducted by Ega et al. discusses the development of a Non-Invasive Blood Pressure (NIBP) device reading system using ESP32-CAM and the YOLOv5 (You Only Look Once) algorithm, utilizing Roboflow for NIBP digit recognition [352]. For the development of the model, a dataset consisting of 431 images of NIBP device readings was split for training (392 images) and validation (39 images). Each digit from digit class 0 to digit class 9 was annotated using the Roboflow platform and trained using Python in the Google Colab environment. The results showed that the YOLOv5 model could recognize all the displayed digits in the NIBP device test dataset with a mean average precision of 99.5%, precision of 99.5%, and recall of 99.6% from 39 validation images, consisting of a total of 245 labels for all digits from 0 to 9. Comparison results with the traditional OCR method showed that the trained YOLOv5 model achieved 100% detection accuracy, while the OCR method obtained 73.06% for the same NIBP digit test dataset. This study concluded that the proposed system can be integrated with Internet of Things (IoT) technology to conduct automatic data acquisition and cloud monitoring of blood pressure data with the ThingsBoard IoT platform. An automated alarm system with an IoT setup can also be created to notify the hospital by email, requesting immediate ambulance dispatch to the patient's location if the blood pressure value is critical.

Chapter 6

Standardized Validation Framework

High in-domain accuracy in healthcare machine learning (ML) models does not guarantee reliable clinical performance, especially when training and validation protocols are insufficiently robust. This paper presents a standardized framework for training and validating ML models intended for classifying medical conditions, emphasizing the need for clinically relevant evaluation metrics and external validation. We apply this framework to a case study in knee osteoarthritis grading, demonstrating how overfitting, data leakage, and inadequate validation can lead to deceptively high accuracy that fails to translate into clinical reliability. In addition to conventional metrics, we introduce composite clinical measures that better capture real-world utility. Our findings show that models with strong in-domain performance may underperform on external datasets, and that composite metrics provide a more nuanced assessment of clinical applicability. Standardized training and validation protocols, together with clinically oriented evaluation, are essential for developing ML models that are both statistically robust and clinically reliable across a range of medical classification tasks.

6.1 Introduction

Machine Learning (ML) models have been a topic of interest in medical diagnostics since the late 20th century, primarily due to their potential to assist clinicians in detecting diseases and predicting patient outcomes [353–358]. Over the decades, advancements in computational power and the advent of deep learning architectures, such as convolutional neural networks (CNNs) and transformers [359, 360], have significantly accelerated research in this field [361]. These models promise to transform healthcare, with applications ranging from medical imaging analysis [362, 363], like detecting tumors in X-rays and MRIs [364–366], to predicting patient outcomes based on electronic health records (EHR) [367–371]. Recent frameworks have enhanced this capability through temporal learning with dynamic range features and transfer learning techniques that leverage large observational EHR databases [372]. Many recent studies report exceptional accuracy and precision, boasting metrics that often surpass human-level performance in specific diagnostic tasks. For instance, CNN-based models trained on large datasets have demonstrated specificities and accuracies of over 90% in tasks such as breast cancer detection from mammograms [373], or diabetic retinopathy diagnosis from fundus images [374]. These numbers have garnered attention and optimism within the medical community and beyond. AI implementation in medical imaging is demonstrably linked to enhanced efficiency, with roughly two-thirds of studies reporting improvements [375], yet meta-analyses reveal that its benefits vary widely across different applications [376]. Moreover, while many studies note reduced processing times, a significant number also disclose conflicts of interest that could bias study design or outcome estimation [377]. Moreover, these impressive results can be misleading. In many cases, the reported accuracy and precision do not necessarily reflect a model's clinical utility. A closer look often reveals significant methodological issues.

A critical issue in the development of ML models for medical diagnostics is overfitting to test sets. This occurs when a model becomes excessively tailored to the specific data it was trained and validated on, leading to inflated performance metrics that do not reflect its ability to generalize to new, unseen data. In many studies, models are evaluated on the same datasets used during development or on overly similar validation sets, which results in a performance boost that can create a false sense of accuracy and precision. This practice, known as data leakage, occurs when there is too much overlap between training and testing data, or when the data is not sufficiently diversified to represent real-world variability.

While high accuracy on the training and test datasets may seem promising, it does not guarantee that the model will perform equally well in clinical environments where the data may differ significantly from the training set. Testing the model on entirely unseen datasets, sourced from different hospitals, clinics, or imaging devices, is important for assessing the true generalizability of an ML model. Unfortunately, many studies neglect this critical step, limiting their findings to "in-domain" validation, which only tests the model on data from the same or very similar sources. As a result, performance metrics such as accuracy and precision, may be misleading, failing to capture the true performance of the model in diverse real-world settings.

It is also understandable that obtaining relevant external data can be challenging or even impossible due to ethical, legal, or logistical constraints, as well as the inherent limitations in data availability across institutions. In many practical scenarios, researchers are compelled to work with limited external datasets, making comprehensive out-of-domain validation difficult. Nonetheless, as demonstrated in this article, the absence of adequate external data makes it even more pivotal to establish robust ML training protocols and to scrutinize the underlying learning dynamics. In particular, close examination of learning curves, reflecting the model's behavior during training and validation, can serve as an essential diagnostic tool. When learning curves behave as desired, with a close alignment between training and validation performance, there is greater assurance that the model has captured generalizable patterns; conversely, abnormal or "bad-behaving" learning curves can signal overfitting or data leakage, thus foreshadowing inferior performance on unseen external data. This emphasis on thorough training evaluation underscores the importance of reliable training practices and serves as an effective surrogate for external validation when such data are not readily available.

Recent literature has increasingly emphasized the importance of standardization and trust in the development and validation of AI models for healthcare. For example, Wierzbicki et al. provide a comprehensive review of approaches to standardizing medical descriptions for clinical entity recognition, highlighting the implications for AI implementation [378]. Arora et al. discuss the value of standardized health datasets in enabling robust AI-based applications [379], while Um et al. examine trust management from a standardization perspective [380]. These studies underscore the necessity of adopting standardized frameworks and data practices to ensure the reliability, generalizability, and clinical acceptance of ML models. Our work builds on these insights by proposing a validation methodology that not only aligns with these emerging standards but also addresses the specific challenges of clinical utility and external validation in real-world healthcare settings.

Recent advances in ML have led to a proliferation of studies reporting high accuracy in medical classification tasks; however, many of these models lack standardized validation and do not adequately reflect clinical utility when deployed beyond their development settings. This work addresses the specific challenge of bridging the gap between promising in-domain ML performance and the need for robust, clinically meaningful validation protocols that can ensure generalizability and regulatory alignment for real-world healthcare applications.

The primary goal of this chapter is to present a standardized validation framework for developing clinically actionable healthcare ML models, specifically demonstrated through the case study of knee osteoarthritis grading. Central to our approach is the integration of credibility assessment by analyzing training dynamics (e.g., learning curves and overfitting diagnostics) alongside traditional performance metrics, highlighting the necessity of protocols and evaluation methods that align model performance with true clinical utility and external validity. Our original contributions are threefold: (1) we synthesize and implement a practical, FDA-aligned validation framework applicable to real-world clinical ML workflows; (2) we propose and evaluate composite clinical utility metrics to capture clinically meaningful model performance; and (3) we demonstrate it with a case study on knee osteoarthritis grading, highlighting the importance of robust training assessment and clinically oriented evaluation for improving model generalizability and patient safety. The remainder of this article is organized as follows: Section 2 details the materials and methods, including the proposed validation framework and evaluation protocols; Section 3 presents experimental results, including in-domain and cross-domain validation; Section 4 discusses the clinical implications of our findings; and Section 5 summarizes the key insights and recommendations for future research and clinical practice.

6.2   Materials and Methods

6.2.1   Establishing Clinical Credibility Through Standardized Validation

Establishing clinical credibility in ML models requires following a validation framework that adheres to regulatory standards. The validation process encompasses five interconnected domains as illustrated in Figure 6.1: Model Description, Data Description, Model Training, Model Evaluation, and Life Cycle Maintenance. These components form a structured pathway for ensuring model reliability and clinical applicability in healthcare settings.

The model description phase establishes foundational elements by specifying model inputs, outputs, architecture, and parameter definitions. This transparency enables proper assessment of a model's theoretical underpinnings and computational approach. The framework then progresses to data description, where training datasets undergo rigorous characterization to ensure relevance and reliability. Particular attention must be directed toward data collection methodologies, annotation processes, and potential sources of algorithmic bias that could compromise model performance across diverse patient populations.

Model training represents a critical validation component requiring detailed documentation of learning methodologies, performance metrics, and hyperparameter optimization. This documentation establishes computational reproducibility and enables independent verification of model development processes. As outlined in FDA guidance [312], training procedures should incorporate appropriate strategies to prevent overfitting while maintaining model generalizability across diverse clinical scenarios.

The model evaluation phase introduces stringent requirements for testing with independent datasets that were not utilized during development. This separation between training and testing data constitutes a fundamental validation principle that reveals a model's true clinical utility. Models demonstrating high performance exclusively on development datasets yet failing with independent test data manifest what regulatory frameworks identify as deceptively high accuracy—signaling inadequate clinical validation. The evaluation process must include comprehensive metrics with confidence intervals, uncertainty quantification, and systematic assessment of limitations and potential biases. Additionally, careful consideration of sample size and statistical power is essential for meaningful clinical validation of ML models, as underscored by recent sample size analyses in the field [381].

Life cycle maintenance completes the validation framework by establishing protocols for longitudinal performance monitoring, model updates, and risk-based oversight. This phase acknowledges the dynamic nature of clinical environments and ensures sustained model credibility through structured retraining procedures and regulatory reporting mechanisms. According to FDA guidance, models deployed in clinical settings require ongoing performance verification to maintain credibility as patient populations and clinical practices evolve.

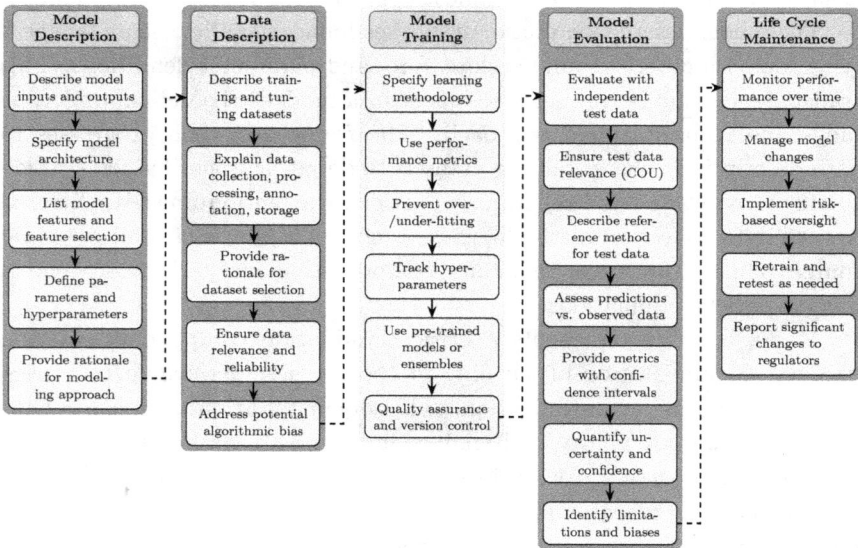

Figure 6.1: Standardized validation framework for establishing and maintaining clinical credibility in healthcare machine learning models. The framework presents five interconnected domains (Model Description, Data Description, Model Training, Model Evaluation, and Life Cycle Maintenance) with sequential validation steps within each domain. Arrows indicate the logical progression within domains (solid lines) and dependencies between domains (dashed lines). This structured approach addresses critical FDA regulatory requirements for AI credibility assessment, ensuring comprehensive documentation of model development, rigorous evaluation with independent test data, and continuous performance monitoring throughout the model lifecycle.

In the context of Figure 6.1, the "Data Description" domain is pivotal for ensuring that the model is developed on datasets that are both representative and reliable for the intended clinical application. This step involves thorough

documentation of the origin and characteristics of all datasets used in
model development, including details about patient demographics, clinical
diversity, acquisition protocols, and annotation standards. Specific attention
is paid to data collection methodologies (e.g., multi-center versus single-
center sourcing), data preprocessing and augmentation techniques, storage
protocols, and the handling of missing or imbalanced data [382]. Annotation
processes are described in terms of both the clinical expertise involved and the
consistency of grading or labeling (for example, the use of standardized scales
such as the Kellgren-Lawrence grading for osteoarthritis). Additionally,
this domain requires a careful evaluation of potential sources of bias, such
as class imbalance, sampling artifacts, or systematic differences between
data sources, and mandates strategies for mitigating such biases to enhance
fairness and generalizability. By systematically addressing these aspects, the
"Data Description" domain provides the foundation for subsequent model
training, evaluation, and regulatory credibility.

Thorough implementation of this standardized validation framework addresses key regulatory concerns regarding model credibility. By establishing
transparent documentation of model development, rigorous testing with independent data, and structured maintenance protocols, healthcare machine
learning applications can progress from promising research tools to clinically
validated decision support systems. The framework systematically mitigates
risks associated with algorithmic bias, overfitting, and performance degradation while providing regulatory authorities with comprehensive evidence
of model reliability for specific clinical contexts of use.

6.2.2   Beyond FDA Guidance

While our validation framework is explicitly aligned with recent FDA draft
guidance on AI for drug and biological product regulation [312], its structure is intentionally designed for broad applicability across regulatory and
best-practice contexts. The FDA's approach, emphasizing transparency,
rigorous evaluation, and continuous monitoring, reflects foundational principles also found in international standards. For example, the International
Council for Harmonisation (ICH) Quality guidelines and the FDA's Office
of Pharmaceutical Quality both stress lifecycle management, risk-based
oversight, and robust model and data control, highlighting the need for clear
standards in areas like adaptive systems, data integrity, and cloud/edge
computing [383, 384]

These principles are echoed in the European Union's Medical Device Regulation (EU MDR) [385], which mandates quality management, systematic risk assessment, clinical evaluation, and ongoing post-market surveillance for medical devices, including AI-based software. The EU MDR's focus on traceability, transparency, and technical documentation closely aligns with our framework, supporting harmonization between US and EU regulatory expectations. The EU's Artificial Intelligence Act [386] further strengthens this alignment by establishing a comprehensive, risk-based legal framework for high-risk AI systems, including those in healthcare. The Act requires strict risk management, data governance, technical documentation, transparency, human oversight, and continuous monitoring, directly mirroring our framework's core domains. By embedding these requirements into law and complementing sectoral regulations like the EU MDR, the AI Act promotes regulatory convergence and cross-border trust.

Finally, the World Health Organization's guidance on AI ethics and governance [387] reinforces the global relevance of these principles, calling for harmonized ethical, legal, and technical standards to ensure safety, equity, and public trust. Hence, our framework is consistent with both US and international regulatory expectations, supporting global adoption of best practices for trustworthy, clinically relevant AI validation in healthcare.

6.2.3   Comparison to Existing Validation Frameworks

Several validation frameworks for ML in healthcare have been proposed in recent years, including those recommended by regulatory bodies such as the FDA and detailed in the broader literature on clinical AI evaluation. These frameworks (such as the FDA's Good Machine Learning Practice (GMLP) and the model reporting guidelines of MI-CLAIM and CONSORT-AI [388–390]) typically emphasize clear documentation of model development, data transparency, rigorous internal and external validation, and ongoing model monitoring. Our proposed framework builds upon these principles but addresses gaps by (i) providing a mathematically formalized approach for validation, (ii) integrating composite clinical utility metrics, and (iii) offering practical, stepwise guidance for model training, evaluation, and life cycle maintenance tailored to real-world clinical needs. Unlike many prior frameworks, which may focus primarily on statistical metrics or narrative reporting, our approach prioritizes clinically actionable assessment and robust mitigation of deceptively high accuracy. As a result, our methodology offers a more comprehensive and practically implementable solution for healthcare ML model validation.

6.2.4   Standardized Validation Framework for Clinical Credibility

In order to address the issue of deceptively high accuracy in healthcare machine learning and to ensure reliable clinical applicability, a standardized model training framework (see Figure 6.1) is established following the recent FDA guidance [312]. The framework is designed to document and verify every aspect of model training and evaluation, thereby guaranteeing that performance metrics reflect true clinical utility rather than artifacts arising from specific data characteristics.

Specify Learning Methodology

The methodology for developing the machine learning (ML) model is explicitly defined, beginning with standardized image preprocessing and extending through the selection of model architecture. The VGG16 model was selected due to its established performance in medical image analysis, particularly in contexts where interpretability and transparency are prioritized. Although more recent architectures such as ResNet or transformer-based models may demonstrate superior performance on large, general image datasets, VGG16 remains a reliable baseline for medical imaging tasks, especially when data availability is limited and model explainability is required. Comparative research in biomedical fields has demonstrated that the choice of ML architecture can significantly influence detection performance, highlighting the importance of benchmarking and selecting models based on the specific clinical context [391]. The methodology and rationale described here are based on a previously published standardized validation framework [392].

The primary objective of this approach is to establish a standardized validation framework and to highlight the risks of overestimating model accuracy in a reproducible and interpretable environment, for which VGG16 is well suited. Standardized normalization procedures are applied to ensure compatibility with the pre-trained VGG16 model, as this is a common practice that supports optimal transfer learning. This approach maintains stable and effective feature extraction from medical images, even when these images differ from those used in the original model training. Full methodological details and justification are provided in the prior work [392].

Use Performance Metrics

A comprehensive set of performance metrics is employed to evaluate the model. These include overall accuracy, as well as class-specific measures such as precision, recall, and the F1 score, which together provide a nuanced understanding of the model's strengths and weaknesses. Additional metrics, such as Cohen's Kappa and the Matthews Correlation Coefficient (MCC), are also calculated to account for chance agreement and to provide robust evaluation in situations where data may be imbalanced across clinical categories. This approach to performance evaluation follows the protocol established in the standardized framework [392].

The overall accuracy is defined as

$$\text{Accuracy} = \frac{1}{N} \sum_{n=1}^{N} \mathbf{1}\{\hat{y}_n = y_n\}, \tag{6.1}$$

where $\mathbf{1}\{\cdot\}$ is the indicator function. In this case, since there are 5 classes $k \in \{1, \ldots, 5\}$. For each class k, the precision and recall are calculated as follows:

$$\text{Precision}_k = \frac{TP_k}{TP_k + FP_k}, \tag{6.2}$$

$$\text{Recall}_k = \frac{TP_k}{TP_k + FN_k}, \tag{6.3}$$

The F1 score for class k is the harmonic mean of precision and recall:

$$\text{F1}_k = 2 \cdot \frac{\text{Precision}_k \cdot \text{Recall}_k}{\text{Precision}_k + \text{Recall}_k}, \tag{6.4}$$

Moreover, Cohen's Kappa is computed to adjust for chance agreement:

$$\kappa = \frac{p_o - p_e}{1 - p_e}, \tag{6.5}$$

where p_o is the observed agreement and p_e is the expected agreement calculated from the marginal probabilities of the classes. Furthermore, the Matthews Correlation Coefficient (MCC) is used as a robust measure even in imbalanced data conditions:

$$\text{MCC} = \frac{TP \cdot TN - FP \cdot FN}{\sqrt{(TP + FP)(TP + FN)(TN + FP)(TN + FN)}}, \tag{6.6}$$

where TP, TN, FP, and FN denote the total true positives, true negatives, false positives, and false negatives, respectively.

Prevent Overfitting and Underfitting

To ensure that the model generalizes well to new data and does not simply memorize the training set, learning curves are generated to monitor performance on both training and validation datasets. Early stopping criteria are implemented to halt training if improvements plateau, thereby reducing the risk of overfitting. Furthermore, a 5-fold cross-validation strategy is used, dividing the dataset into five parts and rotating the validation set, to ensure that the model's performance is consistent and not dependent on a particular subset of data. The choice of resampling and cross-validation methods is particularly important in clinical ML, as it can significantly affect the generalizability of models, especially when data have spatial or domain-specific characteristics [393]. These procedures are detailed in the previously published framework [392].

Track Hyperparameters

All key parameters influencing model training (such as learning rate, dropout rate, number of training cycles, and batch size) are systematically tracked and recorded. This practice supports reproducibility and allows for systematic optimization. A grid search is conducted to explore different combinations of these parameters, with performance averaged across cross-validation folds. All changes and experiments are managed using version control systems to ensure traceability and facilitate iterative improvement, as described in the standardized methodology [392].

Use Pre-trained Models or Ensembles

The training protocol is enhanced by incorporating pre-trained models and ensemble strategies. The pre-trained VGG16 model is used as a feature extractor, allowing the classifier to be trained on high-level image features. Additionally, ensemble methods are employed, combining the outputs of multiple models to reduce variance and improve generalizability. These techniques help mitigate biases that may arise from reliance on a single model architecture. The rationale and implementation of these strategies are outlined in the prior publication [392].

Quality Assurance and Version Control

Quality assurance is integrated throughout the development process via automated testing and continuous integration. Performance changes following code updates are monitored against predefined thresholds to ensure stability. Regular code reviews and systematic audits are conducted in accordance with regulatory standards [312]. All modifications are managed using version control systems, ensuring comprehensive traceability and compliance with clinical validation protocols. Recent studies have highlighted the value of dedicated tools for improving software quality and reproducibility in ML, which further enhances the reliability of clinical ML pipelines [394]. These quality assurance practices are a core component of the standardized framework [392].

By integrating these six methodological components (namely, explicit learning specification, comprehensive performance metrics, measures to prevent overfitting and underfitting, systematic hyperparameter tracking, strategic use of pre-trained and ensemble methods, and robust quality assurance) the framework provides a rigorous approach to developing ML models that are clinically reliable and generalizable. This systematic methodology is essential for translating promising ML prototypes into trusted tools for clinical application, as demonstrated in the previously published work [392].

6.2.5   Datasets

Two distinct datasets were processed using an identical training protocol, employing the same architecture, hyperparameters, and training procedures, with the only difference being the input data. The base neural network architecture and dataset preparation are similar to those described in our prior work [395], but the current study expands upon that work by introducing new composite performance metrics and a standardized evaluation protocol aligned with recent FDA guidance. Specifically, the model was trained on Dataset A and also, separately, on Dataset B, and each model was subsequently cross-tested on the alternate dataset to evaluate their performance on external data. Dataset A was acquired from Kaggle [396] and contains knee X-ray images labeled with Kellgren-Lawrence (KL) grades from 0 (healthy) to 4 (severe osteoarthritis). This dataset provides data for both knee joint detection and KL grading. The images have a balanced distribution across grades and were preprocessed to standardize resolution and orientation. Dataset B was obtained from Mendeley Data [397] and similarly comprises knee X-ray images with KL annotations (grades 0–4) following the same definitions as Dataset A. Including Dataset B allowed us to perform external validation and assess our model's generalizability across different sources.

The selection of Datasets A and B was guided by the need to assess both the in-domain performance and the generalizability of the proposed model for knee osteoarthritis grading. Dataset A (Kaggle) was chosen due to its widespread use in benchmarking ML models for musculoskeletal radiographs and its balanced distribution of KL grades, which enables robust model training. Dataset B (Mendeley Data) was selected as an independent source to enable external validation, as it provides KL-graded knee X-rays collected separately from Dataset A, thus differing in imaging conditions, patient demographics, and potential annotation variability. Including two distinct, publicly available datasets ensures that our evaluation reflects real-world variability and addresses the critical issue of domain shift, thereby supporting a more clinically relevant assessment of model robustness and transferability.

6.2.6 Clinically Oriented Evaluation Protocol

The clinically oriented evaluation protocol is designed to bridge the gap between high statistical performance and the nuanced requirements of patient-centered healthcare. In this protocol, two composite metrics are defined that integrate standard performance measures with clinical priorities. These metrics are central to the clinically oriented evaluation framework and are used to both select and validate models in a manner that aligns with clinical decision-making.

The first composite metric is the overall model score, which is defined as

$$\text{Score}(m_\theta) = \alpha_1 \cdot \text{AUC}(m_\theta) + \alpha_2 \cdot \text{Sensitivity}(m_\theta) \\ + \alpha_3 \cdot \text{Specificity}(m_\theta) \tag{6.7}$$

where:

– $\text{AUC}(m_\theta)$ is the Area Under the Receiver Operating Characteristic (ROC) Curve, computed by

$$\text{AUC} = \int_0^1 \text{TPR}(FPR)\, dFPR, \tag{6.8}$$

with the True Positive Rate (TPR) defined as

$$\text{TPR} = \frac{TP}{TP + FN}, \tag{6.9}$$

and the False Positive Rate (FPR) given by

$$\text{FPR} = 1 - \frac{TN}{TN + FP}. \tag{6.10}$$

– Sensitivity(m_θ), which is equivalent to the TPR, quantifies the model's ability to correctly detect positive cases.

– Specificity(m_θ) is defined as

$$\text{Specificity} = \frac{TN}{TN + FP}, \tag{6.11}$$

and reflects the model's capacity to correctly identify negative cases.

– The weighting coefficients α_1, α_2, and α_3 are selected based on clinical priorities; for instance, in many healthcare applications, a higher weight is assigned to sensitivity to minimize the risk of missing a critical diagnosis.

For example, in cancer screening tasks such as mammography for breast cancer detection, prioritizing sensitivity is important to ensure that cases of malignancy are not missed, as a false negative could result in delayed treatment and adverse outcomes [373]. Similarly, in diabetic retinopathy screening, high sensitivity is often emphasized to minimize the risk of overlooking patients who require urgent ophthalmologic intervention [374]. These examples underscore why, in many healthcare applications, the weighting of sensitivity over other metrics is not only justified but necessary for patient safety.

Equation (6.7) is important in ML for healthcare because it integrates global discriminative performance (via AUC) with more clinically meaningful sensitivities and specificities. This combination ensures that a high overall score is achieved only when the model both discriminates well across classes and meets the clinical requirements for minimizing false negatives and false positives.

The second metric, referred to as the *Clinical Utility* score, is defined as

$$\text{Clinical Utility} = \omega_1 \cdot \text{PPV} + \omega_2 \cdot \text{NPV} + \omega_3 \cdot F1, \tag{6.12}$$

where the components are defined as follows:

$$\text{PPV} = \frac{TP}{TP + FP}, \tag{6.13}$$

$$\text{NPV} = \frac{TN}{TN + FN}, \tag{6.14}$$

$$F1 = 2 \cdot \frac{\text{PPV} \cdot \text{TPR}}{\text{PPV} + \text{TPR}}. \tag{6.15}$$

Here, TPR is as defined in Equation (6.9).

Equation (6.12) is pivotal in healthcare ML because it consolidates three key aspects of clinical performance. By integrating PPV, NPV, and the F1 score, the equation directly correlates the algorithm's predictions with outcomes that are of clinical importance. This is particularly critical in scenarios where the consequences of misclassification are high, and there is a need to balance the trade-offs between over-diagnosis and under-diagnosis.

Together, Equations (6.7) and (6.12) form a dual-layered evaluation framework. The first layer (Equation (6.7)) assesses the inherent discriminative power of the model while accounting for statistical robustness. The second layer (Equation (6.12)) translates statistical performance into clinically actionable insights by emphasizing the predictive values and balanced accuracy. This structured approach ensures that models not only achieve high performance metrics computationally but also translate effectively into real-world clinical environments by addressing the specific risks and rewards associated with medical diagnoses.

In summary, the clinical evaluation protocol leverages these equations to create a quantifiable standard for model assessment relevant to healthcare. By incorporating both statistical and clinical considerations, the protocol mitigates the risk of deceptively high accuracy that lacks clinical relevance and emphasizes the development of models that deliver robust, patient-centered decision support.

6.2.7 Weighted Confusion Matrix Utility Metric

In healthcare applications such as grading knee osteoarthritis severity, where classes range from 0 (healthy) to 4 (severe osteoarthritis), it is pivotal to emphasize accurate prediction of the endpoints, namely the healthy state and the severely affected state. Misclassifications that confuse healthy knees with osteoarthritic states or vice versa may lead to adverse clinical decisions.

To address this concern, a novel metric is introduced, termed the *Weighted Endpoint Accuracy Score (WEAS)*, for evaluating the usefulness of confusion matrices in multi-class classification tasks.

Let $M(i, j)$ denote the (i, j)-th element of the confusion matrix, corresponding to the number of instances with true class i predicted as class j. The per-class accuracy is defined as

$$\text{Acc}_i = \frac{M(i, i)}{\sum_j M(i, j)}, \quad i = 0, 1, \ldots, n, \tag{6.16}$$

where n is the highest classification index (i.e., $n = 4$ in this study's knee osteoarthritis example).

To reflect clinical priorities, a heavier weight w is assigned to the endpoint classes (i.e., classes 0 and n) and a weight of 1 to all intermediate classes ($1 \leq i \leq n - 1$). The overall metric is computed as:

$$\text{WEAS} = \frac{w \cdot \text{Acc}_0 + \sum_{i=1}^{n-1} \text{Acc}_i + w \cdot \text{Acc}_n}{2w + (n - 1)}. \tag{6.17}$$

For instance, in the case of grading knee osteoarthritis (with $n = 4$), choosing $w = 2$ (or another clinically-motivated value) ensures that high accuracy in classifying a healthy knee (class 0) and a severely affected knee (class 4) substantially influences the overall metric. This metric is designed to capture the clinical utility of the model by highlighting performance in the most critical classification regions.

Furthermore, the metric can be extended to incorporate a misclassification penalty based on the distance between true and predicted classes. Let a penalty function be defined as

$$d(i, j) = |i - j|, \tag{6.18}$$

which imposes larger penalties for misclassifications that deviate further from the true class. A composite utility function can then be formulated as

$$U = \lambda \cdot \text{WEAS} - (1 - \lambda) \cdot \text{Penalty}, \tag{6.19}$$

with $\lambda \in [0, 1]$ balancing the trade-off between the weighted endpoint accuracy and the overall misclassification cost.

By adopting the WEAS and its extensions, the proposed metric enhances the evaluation of machine learning models in healthcare settings, ensuring that models which excel in distinguishing clinically essential endpoints are favored, thereby better aligning performance measures with clinical decision-making requirements.

Summary of Notation

For clarity, we summarize below the notation and symbols used in Equations (6.16) – (6.19) and throughout the manuscript:

- $M(i,j)$: Element in the i-th row and j-th column of the confusion matrix, indicating the number of samples with true class i predicted as class j.

- n: Highest class index (e.g., $n = 4$ for five classes labeled 0 to 4).

- Acc_i: Per-class accuracy for class i.

- w: Weight assigned to endpoint classes ($i = 0$ and $i = n$) to emphasize their clinical importance; all other classes have weight 1.

- WEAS: Weighted Endpoint Accuracy Score, as defined in Eq. (6.17).

- $d(i,j)$: Penalty function, defined as the absolute difference $|i - j|$ between true and predicted class.

- U: Composite utility function, combining WEAS and the misclassification penalty, as defined in Eq. (6.19).

- $\lambda \in [0,1]$: Trade-off parameter that balances the emphasis between WEAS and the misclassification penalty.

- $\sum$: All summations are taken over the specified class indices as indicated in the equations.

6.3   Results

As a reminder, a concise description of the model and training protocol utilized in this study are as follows. The model is a CNN implemented in Keras, based on a VGG16 backbone pre-trained on ImageNet. Input images were resized to 224×224 pixels and normalized using ImageNet statistics. The classification head consists of two dense layers (1024 and 512 units, respectively, each followed by ReLU activation and dropout at $p = 0.5$), ending with a five-unit softmax output corresponding to the KL grades.

Training was performed for 20 epochs with a batch size of 32 and learning rate of 0.001, using sparse categorical cross-entropy loss and Adam optimizer. Stratified 80/20 splits ensured class balance, and all key hyperparameters were tracked and are available upon request. The model's performance was evaluated using accuracy, Cohen's Kappa, Matthews Correlation Coefficient, precision, recall, F1 score, and clinically oriented composite metrics as described above.

The following subsection examines a case study in which an ML model was independently trained on two distinct datasets using the same methodology. Although both training processes yielded confusion matrices with similar overall patterns of class distribution, the learning curves exhibited markedly different behaviors. One training instance produced learning curves that deviated from the expected pattern, suggesting issues such as potential overfitting or ineffective regularization. In contrast, the other instance displayed learning curves that progressed in a more stable and predictable manner. This discrepancy ultimately manifested in the model's external performance, where the training exhibiting unfavorable learning dynamics corresponded to inferior results when evaluated on an external dataset. The subsections that follow detail the performance metrics from the within-dataset evaluations, the outcomes of the cross-dataset external testing, and an analysis of the learning curves, thereby linking training behavior to generalizability outcomes.

6.3.1   ML model trained on two datasets

The performance of CNN based on the Keras framework when it is trained and evaluated on two separate datasets (Dataset A and Dataset B) is presented as follows. Figure 6.2 shows two confusion matrices that detail the classification outcomes for each dataset. In these matrices the rows denote the true class labels while the columns represent the predicted labels for a 5-class problem. This visualization helps to pinpoint where misclassifications occur and highlights which classes are most often confused by the model.

Complementing the visual analysis, Table 6.1 summarizes a set of quantitative performance metrics including Overall Accuracy, Cohen's Kappa, MCC, Precision, Recall, and F1 score. By comparing the metrics between Dataset A and Dataset B, one can observe that the model achieves improved performance on Dataset B, indicated by higher accuracy and better inter-class agreement, suggesting potential differences in data quality or inherent

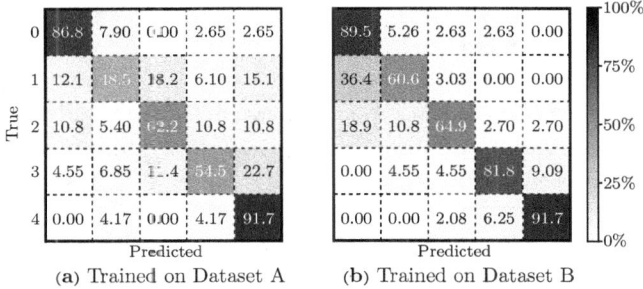

(a) Trained on Dataset A   (b) Trained on Dataset B

Figure 6.2: Two confusion matrices, evaluated on (a) Dataset A, and (b) Dataset B, illustrating the performance of Keras Framework in classifying knee X-ray images. Each matrix shows the true classifications (rows) versus the predicted classifications (columns). Adapted from [395].

Metric	Dataset A	Dataset B
Overall Accuracy	70.00%	79.00%
Cohen's Kappa	62.19%	73.60%
Matthews CC	62.57%	73.90%
Precision	69.48%	79.19%
Recall	68.74%	77.69%
F1	69.14%	77.70%

Table 6.1: Performance Metrics of the ML model trained and (in-domain) tested on Datasets A and B.

feature distinctiveness between the two datasets.

6.3.2 Cross-dataset external testing

To further evaluate the generalizability of this model, cross-dataset (i.e., external) testing was performed. In this scenario, the model trained on one dataset was tested on the other to expose its resilience against domain shifts. Figure 6.3 presents the confusion matrices obtained under these conditions. Subfigure (a) displays the confusion matrix when the model trained on Dataset A is tested on Dataset B, while subfigure (b) shows the matrix for the case where the model trained on Dataset B is evaluated using data from Dataset A. These cross-dataset comparisons help to understand how variations in data distributions can affect model predictions.

Table 6.2 details the corresponding performance metrics for the cross-dataset experiments. The metrics demonstrate a notable performance drop compared to the within-dataset evaluations. Particularly, the model trained on Dataset A suffers a more significant decrease in accuracy when tested on Dataset B. In contrast, the model trained on Dataset B shows a comparatively better generalization on Dataset A. These results underscore the importance of rigorous external validation to ensure that models remain reliable when exposed to data from different sources.

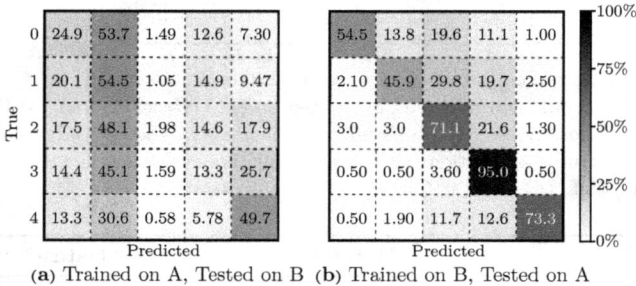

(a) Trained on A, Tested on B (b) Trained on B, Tested on A

Figure 6.3: Confusion matrices illustrating the cross-dataset evaluation of the deep learning model for a 5-class classification problem using the Keras framework. (a) Model trained on Dataset A and tested on Dataset B; (b) Model trained on Dataset B and tested on Dataset A. Adapted from [395].

Metric	Dataset A (Tested on B)	Dataset B (Tested on A)
Overall Accuracy	49.94%	68.36%
Cohen's Kappa	24.92%	60.45%
Matthews CC	26.15%	61.12%
Precision	38.92%	69.14%
Recall	49.94%	68.36%
F1	43.79%	68.74%

Table 6.2: Performance Metrics for ML model trained on Datasets A and B and (externally) tested on Datasets B and A, respectively.

6.3.3   Learning Curves

The anomalous learning curves for the model trained on Dataset A (Figure 6.4(a)), where the validation accuracy is higher than the training accuracy, are an immediate red flag. The ideal scenario is to see a small gap between the training and validation curves with the validation accuracy slightly lower than the training accuracy (as seen in Figure 6.4(b)). This gap reflects that the model is learning useful patterns from the training data while still being somewhat regularized, ensuring it can generalize well.

When the two curves are nearly overlapping or, worse, when the validation accuracy exceeds the training accuracy, it is a red flag. It often that the validation procedure is contaminated or that the model suffers from improper regularization or data leakage. In this case, the validation set from Dataset A may have been overly "friendly" or unrepresentative of the true complexity present in the training examples, leading the model to appear as if it were generalizing better than it really was.

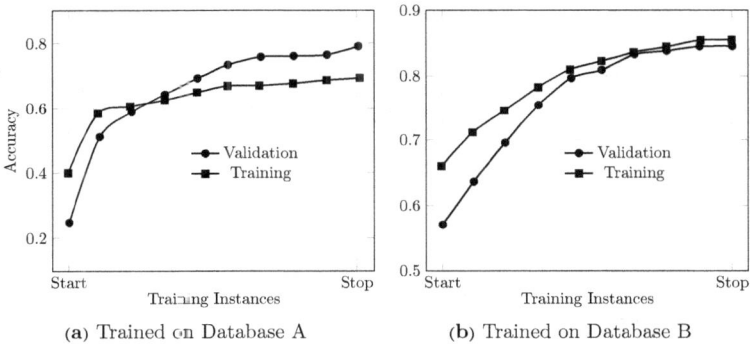

(a) Trained on Database A   (b) Trained on Database B

Figure 6.4: Learning curves for accuracy returned by the Deep Learning model using the Keras Framework trained on the Dataset A (a) and Dataset B (b).

This deceptive behavior means that the model's apparent in-domain performance (70% overall accuracy on Dataset A during training) is not a reliable indicator of its true generalization ability. When the model is later tested on an external dataset (Dataset B), the mismatch in data characteristics is exposed and the performance deteriorates significantly; dropping to 49.94% overall accuracy with similarly reduced Cohen's Kappa and Matthews CC values. Essentially, the inflated validation accuracy masked underlying issues such as overfitting to Dataset A's spurious patterns or artifacts. As a result, the model failed to adapt to the new data distribution in Dataset B.

In contrast, the model trained on Dataset B, which did not suffer from such deceptive learning curves, maintained higher performance even when tested on Dataset A (68.36% accuracy). This comparison underscores that a reliable validation strategy, reflected by proper learning curves where training accuracy at least matches or exceeds validation accuracy, is critical to developing models that generalize well across datasets. Thus, the "bad-behaving" learning curves for the model from Dataset A are directly linked to its poor cross-dataset performance: they reveal that the validation metrics were misleading, and that the model had not truly learned robust features but rather had adapted to quirks in its in-domain data.

6.3.4   Composite Clinical Score Analysis

To bridge the quantitative performance evaluation with clinical applicability, two composite metrics are computed as defined above: the overall model score (Equation 6.7) and the clinical utility score (Equation 6.12). These scores integrate standard statistical measures with clinically relevant priorities, providing a single performance index that reflects both the model's discriminative power and its potential impact in a clinical setting.

As reported in Table 6.1, the macro-averaged sensitivity (i.e., recall), PPV, and F1 score for Dataset B are 0.7769, 0.7919, and 0.7770, respectively. The remaining metrics required for the composite scores were computed directly from the confusion matrix. Specifically, a macro-averaged specificity is of approximately 0.9478 and a macro-averaged negative predictive value (NPV) of about 0.9487.

Using these values, and an independently computed AUC of 0.87, the overall model score is calculated by equally weighting AUC, sensitivity, and specificity:

$$\text{Score}(m_\theta) \approx \frac{0.87 + 0.7769 + 0.9478}{3} \approx 0.8649 \quad (86.5\%).$$

Similarly, the clinical utility score is computed by equally weighting the PPV, NPV, and F1 score:

$$\text{Clinical Utility} \approx \frac{0.7919 + 0.9487 + 0.7770}{3} \approx 0.8392 \quad (83.9\%).$$

These composite scores, an overall model score of approximately 86.5% and a clinical utility score of roughly 83.9%, demonstrate that the model not only achieves strong statistical performance but also meets key clinical requirements. In other words, the model's high global discriminative ability is well aligned with its capability to provide clinically actionable insights, thereby supporting its potential as a reliable decision support tool.

In the context of knee osteoarthritis grading, concrete clinical requirements refer to criteria that ensure the model's outputs are directly useful for patient care and decision-making. These include: (1) high sensitivity for detecting severe and healthy cases to minimize missed diagnoses and unnecessary interventions, (2) high specificity to avoid over-diagnosis, (3) strong positive and negative predictive values to support reliable clinical triage, and (4) robust performance in distinguishing clinically actionable endpoints (such as differentiating between grades that mandate intervention versus those that do not). The weighting schemes and composite scores used in this study are explicitly designed to align with these requirements, prioritizing the accurate identification of cases with significant clinical implications.

6.3.5 Evaluation of Weighted Endpoint Accuracy Score

The utility of the proposed WEAS is evaluated using the confusion matrix derived from the test set after the ML model was trained on Dataset B (see Figure6.2(b)). It is important to note that the confusion matrix reflects the model's performance on the independent test (or validation) data, not on the training data itself. Thus, the total number of instances reported in the confusion matrix corresponds to the size of the test set used for evaluation, rather than the dataset used for model training. This distinction is relevant, as the confusion matrix and associated metrics (such as WEAS) provide an assessment of how well the trained model generalizes to unseen data, rather than its performance on the data it was trained on.

For this 5-class problem (with class labels 0–4, where class 0 signifies healthy patients and class 4 represents severe pathology), the per-class accuracies, as reported in Figure 6.2(b), are as follows:

$$\text{Acc}_0 \approx 89.47\%, \quad \text{Acc}_1 \approx 60.61\%, \quad \text{Acc}_2 \approx 64.86\%,$$
$$\text{Acc}_3 \approx 81.82\%, \quad \text{Acc}_4 \approx 91.67\%.$$

Recognizing the higher clinical importance of correctly predicting the endpoints (classes 0 and 4), we assign them a weight $w = 2$, while the intermediate classes (1, 2, and 3) remain unweighted (i.e., weight $= 1$). The overall WEAS (Equation 6.17) is defined as

$$\text{WEAS} = \frac{w \cdot \text{Acc}_0 + \sum_{i=1}^{3} \text{Acc}_i + w \cdot \text{Acc}_4}{2w + 3}.$$

Substituting the computed accuracies with $w = 2$, we obtain:

$$\text{WEAS} = \frac{2(0.8947) + 0.6061 + 0.6486 + 0.8182 + 2(0.9167)}{7} \approx \frac{5.6956}{7}$$

$$\approx 0.8137.$$

This metric indicates an overall utility of approximately 81.4%, underscoring the model's strong performance on the clinically critical endpoints.

An extension to the WEAS incorporates a misclassification penalty that accounts for the severity of off-diagonal errors. With a distance penalty defined as $d(i,j) = |i - j|$, the cumulative penalty for misclassifications is given by

$$\text{Penalty} = \frac{\sum_{i \neq j} |i - j| \, M(i,j)}{\text{Total Instances}}.$$

For ML model trained on Dataset B, yielding the following confusion matrix

$$\mathbf{M} = \begin{bmatrix} 34 & 2 & 1 & 1 & 0 \\ 12 & 20 & 1 & 0 & 0 \\ 7 & 4 & 24 & 1 & 1 \\ 0 & 2 & 2 & 36 & 4 \\ 0 & 0 & 1 & 3 & 44 \end{bmatrix}.$$

the penalty per row is computed as follows:

- Row 0 $(i = 0)$: $2 \times 1 + 1 \times 2 + 1 \times 3 = 7$.

- Row 1 $(i = 1)$: $12 \times 1 + 1 \times 1 = 13$.

- Row 2 $(i = 2)$: $7 \times 2 + 4 \times 1 + 1 \times 1 + 1 \times 2 = 21$.

- Row 3 $(i = 3)$: $2 \times 2 + 2 \times 1 + 4 \times 1 = 10$.

- Row 4 $(i = 4)$: $1 \times 2 + 3 \times 1 = 5$.

Summing these penalties yields a total penalty of $7 + 13 + 21 + 10 + 5 = 56$. Dividing by the total number of instances ($38 + 33 + 37 + 44 + 48 = 200$), we obtain

$$\text{Penalty} = \frac{56}{200} = 0.28.$$

This penalty is then integrated into a composite utility function (Equation 6.19: $U = \lambda \cdot \text{WEAS} - (1 - \lambda) \cdot \text{Penalty}$), where $\lambda \in [0, 1]$ is a parameter that balances the importance of endpoint accuracy against the cost of misclassification. For example, with $\lambda = 0.5$, the utility becomes

$$U \approx 0.5(0.8137) - 0.5(0.28) \approx 0.4069 - 0.14 = 0.2669.$$

These findings indicate that, while the elevated WEAS (81.4%) demonstrates robust discrimination between healthy and severely ill patients, the composite utility metric U provides a more comprehensive evaluation by also accounting for the cost of misclassifications. Such an assessment aligns the model's evaluation with clinical priorities, ensuring that both endpoint accuracy and the severity of errors are appropriately reflected.

6.4   Discussion

Ensuring robust and well-documented training of ML models in healthcare is pivotal for their clinical utility, as described in Figure 6.1 (especially the middle square highlighted in red). The model training phase, which encompasses proper learning methodologies, prevention of overfitting or underfitting, and use of appropriate performance metrics, is foundational to achieving clinically actionable outcomes. Without rigorous training protocols, high accuracy metrics may be deceptive, creating a false sense of reliability in a model's clinical applicability.

A model trained inadequately or with methodological flaws, such as overfitting to training data or insufficient validation, can yield inflated accuracy metrics that fail to generalize to real-world scenarios [398]. For instance, as demonstrated in the case study, a model achieving 70% accuracy on its training dataset catastrophically failed during cross-dataset evaluation, with accuracy plummeting to under 2% for a critical grade 2 osteoarthritis classification. This highlights a systemic issue where models validated solely on in-domain data appear promising but ultimately lack the robustness necessary for diverse clinical environments. Robust training ensures that the model learns meaningful patterns from data rather than memorizing noise or artifacts. Overfitting, characterized by exceptional performance on training data but poor generalization to unseen data, can render a model clinically useless. Similarly, underfitting, where a model fails to capture the underlying data structure, results in subpar performance across all datasets. Both scenarios undermine the validity of reported performance metrics, making them clinically irrelevant.

Learning Curve Behavior	Potential Cause	Clinical Implication
Training and validation curves converge and plateau, but the validation curve is higher than the training curve.	Data leakage or overly simplistic training data. Improper regularization.	Indicates that the validation set is not representative of real-world data. Clinically, this could lead to overconfidence in the model's performance, resulting in poor generalization to unseen patient data.
Training and validation curves never converge.	Model underfitting due to insufficient complexity, poor feature representation, or inadequate training.	Suggests that the model fails to learn meaningful patterns. Clinically, this results in low diagnostic accuracy and unreliable predictions.
Training curve plateaus, but the validation curve continues to improve.	Validation set may be easier or less diverse than the training set.	Indicates a mismatch between training and validation data. Clinically, this could lead to overestimation of the model's generalizability.
Training and validation curves converge but never plateau.	Model is overfitting to noise or artifacts in the data.	Suggests that the model is learning spurious patterns. Clinically, this could lead to unreliable predictions and increased false positives or negatives.
Large gap between training and validation curves.	Overfitting due to excessive model complexity or insufficient regularization.	Indicates poor generalization. Clinically, this could result in high accuracy on training data but poor performance in real-world scenarios.
Training and validation curves oscillate significantly.	High learning rate or unstable optimization process.	Suggests instability in training. Clinically, this could lead to unpredictable model behavior and unreliable predictions.
Validation curve improves initially but then deteriorates.	Overfitting due to prolonged training or lack of early stopping.	Indicates that the model is memorizing the training data. Clinically, this could result in poor generalization and unreliable diagnostic outcomes.

Table 6.3: Problematic learning (accuracy) curve behaviors, their potential causes, and clinical implications.

Properly trained models are better equipped to handle variability in patient data, imaging protocols, and disease presentations, ensuring they are reliable tools for clinical decision-making. Incorporating standardized training methodologies, as outlined in regulatory frameworks like the FDA's guidance on AI credibility, bridges the gap between research prototypes and bedside applications. By adhering to these practices, healthcare ML models can transition from deceptively high accuracy metrics to robust, actionable tools that prioritize patient safety and ethical deployment.

6.4.1 Clinical Implications of Learning Curve Behaviors in ML Models

In ML model training, learning curves, i.e., plots of training and validation performance over time or epochs, serve as critical diagnostic tools for assessing the health of the training process. A well-trained ML model typically exhibits learning curves where the training and validation curves converge and plateau together, with the training curve slightly above the validation curve (see Figure 6.4(b)). This behavior indicates that the model has learned meaningful patterns from the data without overfitting or underfitting. However, deviations from this ideal behavior can signal significant issues in the training process, which, if unaddressed, can lead to clinically unreliable models. Table 6.3 summarizes various problematic learning curve behaviors, their potential causes, and their clinical implications.

Analysis of Problematic Learning Curve Behaviors

The analysis of problematic learning curve behaviors reveals several key patterns that can indicate issues in ML model training, each with distinct causes and clinical implications (summarized in Table 6.3). When the validation curve is higher than the training curve, it often points to data leakage, where information from the validation set inadvertently influences the training process. This can also occur if the training data is overly simplistic or lacks diversity. Clinically, such a model may appear to perform well during validation but fail catastrophically when exposed to real-world data, leading to misdiagnoses or inappropriate treatment recommendations.

Non-converging curves, where the training and validation curves fail to converge, indicate underfitting. This issue arises from insufficient model complexity, poor feature engineering, or inadequate training data. Clinically, an underfitted model is incapable of capturing the underlying patterns in the data, resulting in low diagnostic accuracy and unreliable predictions. On the other hand, non-plateauing curves, where the curves converge but fail to plateau, suggest overfitting to noise or artifacts in the data. This behavior implies that the model is learning spurious patterns rather than clinically relevant features, which could lead to unreliable predictions, particularly in edge cases or less common conditions.

A large gap between the training and validation curves is a hallmark of overfitting. This occurs when the model is too complex relative to the amount of training data, allowing it to memorize the training data rather than generalize. Clinically, this results in a model that performs well on training data but poorly on unseen data, undermining its utility in real-world settings. Oscillating curves, characterized by significant fluctuations in performance, often indicate an unstable optimization process, potentially due to a high learning rate or poor initialization. Clinically, this instability translates to unpredictable model behavior, making it unsuitable for deployment in critical healthcare applications.

Another problematic behavior is validation curve deterioration, where the validation curve initially improves but later deteriorates. This is a clear sign of overfitting, typically occurring when training continues beyond the point of optimal generalization. Clinically, this could lead to a model that performs well during initial testing but fails to maintain accuracy over time, especially as patient populations or data distributions evolve.

The clinical implications of these poor learning curve behaviors are significant. Overfitting can lead to false positives, resulting in unnecessary treatments or interventions, while underfitting can result in missed diagnoses, delaying critical care for patients. Data leakage can create a false sense of confidence in the model's performance, leading to its premature deployment in clinical settings. To mitigate these risks, it is essential to monitor learning curves during training and address any anomalies promptly. Techniques such as cross-validation, early stopping, regularization, and robust data preprocessing can help ensure that the model learns meaningful patterns and generalizes well to unseen data. By understanding and addressing problematic learning curve behaviors, researchers and clinicians can develop ML models that are not only statistically robust but also clinically reliable. This ensures that the models are capable of improving patient outcomes and advancing the field of healthcare AI.

Assessing Learning Dynamics Beyond Learning Curves

While this study demonstrates the value of analyzing learning curves to diagnose overfitting, data leakage, and generalization issues, it is important to recognize that other forms of training dynamics analysis can further strengthen model validation. In particular, recent work in AI-based glaucoma detection [399] has highlighted the importance of reporting and interpreting model performance metrics (such as accuracy, precision, recall, and F1-score) across each data subset: training, validation, test, and external (cross-dataset) evaluation. As shown in that study, a properly trained and generalizable ML model should exhibit a slight and continuous decrease in performance metrics as evaluation moves from the training set to the validation set, to the test set, and finally to external data. This expected trend reflects the model's ability to generalize, with only modest declines in performance as the data becomes less similar to the training distribution. In contrast, large drops or erratic changes in these metrics across subsets are indicative of overfitting, data leakage, or poor generalization.

Although this current work focuses on learning curve analysis as a primary tool for diagnosing training issues, incorporating subset-wise performance metric analysis (following the approach demonstrated in [399]) would provide an additional layer of insight into the model's learning dynamics and generalizability. It is recommended that future studies routinely include such analyses to complement learning curve evaluation, thereby ensuring a more comprehensive assessment of model robustness and clinical applicability.

6.4.2   Clinical Implications of the Composite Utility Metric

In order to bridge the gap between traditional performance metrics and the nuanced requirements of clinical decision-making, a series of composite measures have been proposed to evaluate ML models in healthcare. Table 6.4 summarizes four key metrics—the Overall Model Score (Eq. 6.7), Clinical Utility Score (Eq. 6.12), Weighted Endpoint Accuracy Score (WEAS; Eq. 6.17), and the Composite Utility Metric (Eq. 6.19). These metrics not only capture a model's global discriminative capacity (via AUC, sensitivity, and specificity) but also incorporate predictive values and a misclassification penalty, thereby aligning model evaluation with clinical priorities. Such an integrated approach is essential to ensure that the models are both statistically robust and clinically actionable.

The resulting composite utility U is of significant clinical relevance as it combines the model's performance on critical endpoints with an explicit penalty for misclassification errors. While the WEAS of approximately 81.4% demonstrates that the model reliably distinguishes between the healthy (class 0) and severely pathological cases (class 4), the composite metric U further addresses the impact of misclassifications across all classes.

Metric	Equation	Clinical Relevance
Overall Model Score (Eq. 6.7)	$\text{Score}(m_\theta) = \alpha_1 \cdot \text{AUC}(m_\theta) + \alpha_2 \cdot \text{Sensitivity}(m_\theta) + \alpha_3 \cdot \text{Specificity}(m_\theta)$	Integrates global discriminative performance with sensitivity and specificity to ensure that both the ability to detect true positive cases and to correctly identify negatives are balanced, reflecting the dual clinical need to avoid missed diagnoses and false alarms.
Clinical Utility Score (Eq. 6.12)	$\text{Clinical Utility} = \omega_1 \cdot \text{PPV} + \omega_2 \cdot \text{NPV} + \omega_3 \cdot \text{F1}$	Consolidates predictive positive value, negative predictive value, and the F1 score to directly connect model performance with patient management outcomes, thereby mitigating diagnostic ambiguity in clinical practice.
Weighted Endpoint Accuracy Score (WEAS) (Eq. 6.17)	$\text{WEAS} = \dfrac{w \cdot \text{Acc}_0 + \sum_{i=1}^{n-1} \text{Acc}_i + w \cdot \text{Acc}_n}{2w + (n-1)}$	Emphasizes the accurate classification of critical endpoints (e.g., healthy vs. severely pathological cases) by assigning extra weight to these classes, which is relevant when prioritizing patient safety in high-stakes clinical decisions.
Composite Utility Metric (Eq. 6.19)	$U = \lambda \cdot \text{WEAS} - (1 - \lambda) \cdot \text{Penalty}$	Combines the weighted endpoint accuracy (WEAS) with a penalty for misclassifications, thereby quantifying not only the model's success in critical classifications but also the clinical cost of errors—a balance central to safe and effective patient care.

Table 6.4: Suggested Clinical Evaluation Metrics for ML in Healthcare.

Specifically, the penalty component in U quantifies the cost of errors based on their distance from the true class, reflecting the clinical intuition that misclassifying a healthy patient as severely ill (or vice versa) is more consequential than errors involving intermediate classes. For example, with a balancing parameter $\lambda = 0.5$, the computed utility $U \approx 0.2669$ indicates that, despite robust performance at the endpoints, the model incurs a non-negligible cost when it strays from accurate classification in a clinically meaningful way.

This approach aligns with clinical decision protocols where endpoint accuracy remains paramount but intermediate class errors still require mitigation. The integration of macro-averaged sensitivity (77.69%) and specificity (94.78%) in the composite model score provides critical insights into real-world functionality. These metrics reveal how well models balance the detection of positive cases (minimizing false negatives) against the ability to correctly identify negative cases (minimizing false positives); both fundamental requirements for clinical adoption. Similarly, the clinical utility score (83.9%) emphasizes predictive values that directly correlate with patient management outcomes, as clinicians prioritize minimizing diagnostic ambiguity through high positive and negative predictive values.

In a healthcare setting, such as grading knee osteoarthritis severity [395, 400], this composite measure provides a more holistic evaluation of the model's clinical usefulness. It ensures that models selected for clinical use not only exhibit high accuracy in discriminating between the most critical cases but also maintain an acceptable level of performance across intermediate stages. Consequently, U serves as a relevant tool for clinicians and stakeholders by aligning the performance evaluation with clinical priorities, thus supporting safer and more effective patient management decisions.

The clinical prioritization of endpoint accuracy through weighting ($w = 2$ for classes 0 and 4 vs. intermediate classes) mirrors established medical protocols where clear differentiation between normal and severely affected states drives treatment pathways. However, the additional penalty mechanism acknowledges that even smaller misclassifications between adjacent grades (e.g., class 2 mislabeled as class 3) accumulate operational costs through unnecessary referrals, repeated imaging, or delayed interventions. This dual focus, prioritizing critical distinctions while disincentivizing all errors proportionally, creates performance benchmarks that better reflect clinical workflows compared to conventional accuracy metrics.

Ultimately, composite scoring methodologies address a fundamental disconnect between ML evaluation and medical practice. By translating statistical performance into risk-adjusted utility measures, they provide frameworks for model assessment that account for both diagnostic priorities and the asymmetric consequences of different error types. This alignment is essential for validating AI systems in healthcare, where computational metrics must be subordinated to patient safety considerations and clinical decision-making realities. A critical consideration in the clinical deployment of ML models is the selection and justification of weighting coefficients for composite evaluation metrics. The optimal balance between sensitivity and specificity is not universal, but rather context-dependent and should be tailored to the intended clinical application. For example, in population-level screening programs (e.g., national mammography campaigns or infectious disease surveillance) the primary objective is to identify as many true positive cases as possible, even at the expense of increased false positives. In these scenarios, maximizing sensitivity is paramount to ensure that no cases are missed, as the public health consequences of undetected disease can be severe. Conversely, when managing the care of an individual patient, the clinical focus often shifts toward specificity. Here, the goal is to minimize false positives to avoid unnecessary anxiety, invasive follow-up procedures, or unwarranted treatments. For instance, a highly specific confirmatory test is essential before initiating a potentially harmful therapy. Thus, the weighting coefficients in composite metrics must be carefully chosen to reflect whether the model is intended for broad screening or for guiding individual patient management, ensuring that the evaluation framework aligns with real-world clinical priorities.

6.4.3   Limitations and Future Research Directions

While this work has addressed core issues in the standardized validation of ML models for medical classification, several avenues for future research remain. First, the development and evaluation of advanced model architectures that further mitigate overfitting and improve domain generalization should be explored, particularly in more heterogeneous and multi-center clinical datasets. Second, the real-world deployment of such validated models (integrating them into clinical workflows and assessing their ongoing impact on patient outcomes and care efficiency) warrants thorough investigation. Third, the creation of standardized benchmarks and open challenges for external validation in diverse clinical settings would further advance the field. Finally, additional work is needed to align composite utility metrics with evolving clinical guidelines and regulatory standards, ensuring models remain relevant and actionable as healthcare practices progress.

Additionally, while the composite evaluation metrics and their associated formulas (including weighting schemes, penalty functions, and aggregation strategies) were designed to be consistent with established clinical reasoning and to reflect priorities commonly recognized in medical decision-making, we acknowledge that these formulas were not formally validated through direct physician input or structured expert consensus in this study. Future work could incorporate expert clinician feedback or employ a formal Delphi consensus process [401] to systematically refine and validate these formulas and weighting strategies, thereby ensuring that all aspects of the evaluation framework are optimally aligned with real-world clinical priorities and expert judgment.

Furthermore, benchmarking composite clinical scores against baseline models (such as random or majority-class classifiers) and, when available, against human expert performance would provide valuable context and further strengthen the clinical relevance of these findings. Incorporating such comparisons represents an important direction for future work and would help to more clearly position the utility of the evaluation framework within real-world clinical practice.

6.5   Conclusions

While robust assessment of an ML model's training process is an important precursor to interpreting its reported performance, we emphasize that learning dynamics (such as the analysis of learning curves and detection of overfitting or data leakage) should be considered as a valuable complement to, rather than a replacement for, established performance metrics. Insights into training dynamics can help identify potential pitfalls that may not be immediately evident from final accuracy or F1 scores alone, particularly in situations where external validation data is limited. However, it is important to recognize that no single evaluation approach is universally sufficient; both the trajectory of model learning and the ultimate performance metrics provide distinct, meaningful information about model reliability and generalizability. Accordingly, we recommend integrating the assessment of learning dynamics alongside comprehensive performance evaluation, in order to build a more holistic and reliable understanding of model readiness for clinical deployment.

Our results demonstrate that even models with strong in-domain performance, such as the 79% accuracy and 0.78 F1 score obtained on Dataset

B, may exhibit substantial drops in external validity (e.g., to 68% accuracy when cross-tested) if robust training and validation protocols are not rigorously enforced. The observed discrepancies between in-domain and out-of-domain performance, as well as the analysis of learning curve behaviors, directly highlight the risks of overfitting and data leakage. Importantly, the application of composite clinical utility metrics provided a more nuanced assessment of the model's clinical relevance than conventional accuracy alone. For instance, a WEAS of 81.4% for Dataset B emphasizes the model's strength in predicting clinically critical endpoints, while the composite utility metric additionally penalizes misclassifications in a manner reflective of clinical risk. These findings underscore that standardized protocols and clinically oriented evaluation are essential for ensuring that ML models for medical classification deliver reliable, generalizable, and patient-centered results in real-world settings.

Chapter 7

Data Leakage and Feature Selection

If we do not urgently educate current and future medical professionals to critically evaluate and distinguish credible AI-assisted diagnostic tools from those whose performance is artificially inflated by data leakage or improper validation, we risk undermining clinician trust in all AI diagnostics and jeopardizing future advances in patient care. For instance, machine learning models have shown high accuracy in diagnosing Parkinson's Disease when trained on clinical features that are themselves diagnostic, such as tremor and rigidity. This study systematically investigates the impact of data leakage and feature selection on the true clinical utility of machine learning models for early Parkinson's Disease detection. We constructed two experimental pipelines: one excluding all overt motor symptoms to simulate a subclinical scenario, and a control including these features. Nine machine learning algorithms were evaluated using a robust three-way data split and comprehensive metric analysis. Results revealed that, without overt features, all models exhibited superficially acceptable F1 scores but failed catastrophically in specificity, misclassifying most healthy controls as Parkinson's Disease. Inclusion of overt features dramatically improved performance, confirming that high accuracy was due to data leakage rather than genuine predictive power. These findings underscore the necessity of rigorous experimental design, transparent reporting, and critical evaluation of machine learning models in clinically realistic settings. Our work highlights the risks of overestimating model utility due to data leakage and provides guidance for developing robust, clinically meaningful machine learning tools for early disease detection.

7.1   Introduction

Machine learning (ML) has rapidly emerged as a promising tool for the early detection and diagnosis of neurodegenerative diseases [402, 403], including Parkinson's Disease (PD) [404, 405]. Numerous studies have reported high diagnostic accuracy for ML models trained on clinical and paraclinical data, often exceeding 90% when leveraging features such as tremor, rigidity, bradykinesia, and other overt motor symptoms [406]. These results have fueled optimism about the potential for ML to augment or even surpass traditional clinical assessment, particularly in resource-limited or high-throughput screening settings.

However, a critical methodological challenge in the development and evaluation of ML models for clinical diagnosis is the risk of *data leakage*, i.e., the inadvertent use of information during model training that would not be available at the time of prediction in real-world scenarios [407]. Data leakage can arise from improper data splitting, inclusion of post-diagnostic features, or subtle correlations that artificially inflate model performance [408]. When present, leakage leads to overestimation of a model's true predictive utility, undermining both scientific validity and clinical safety [409].

In the context of PD, most published ML models derive their predictive power from features that are themselves diagnostic criteria, such as motor symptoms or scores from clinical rating scales [410, 411]. While this approach can yield impressive accuracy, it does not address the more challenging and clinically relevant question: can ML models detect PD *before* the emergence of overt symptoms, using only subtle or prodromal indicators? This distinction is crucial, as early detection could enable timely intervention and improved patient outcomes, whereas models that simply recapitulate existing diagnostic criteria offer little added value [404, 412].

Recent literature has begun to recognize this gap. For example, studies that exclude obvious motor features or focus on prodromal PD consistently report a dramatic drop in model performance, with high rates of false positives and poor specificity [413]. Moreover, many studies rely on aggregate metrics such as accuracy or F1 score, which can mask pathological model behaviors, such as defaulting to predicting all patients as diseased, that render the models clinically unusable. Confusion matrix analysis, though rarely reported, often reveals these underlying failures [414, 415].

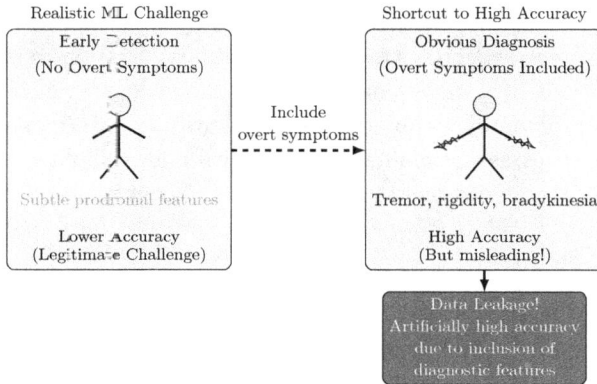

Figure 7.1: Illustration of the impact of feature selection on ML model accuracy for PD diagnosis. Left: Excluding overt motor symptoms simulates early detection, resulting in low accuracy. Right: Including overt symptoms (e.g., tremor, rigidity) yields high accuracy, but this is misleading due to data leakage; these features are themselves diagnostic and not available for true early detection. The temptation to include such features leads to artificially inflated performance metrics.

The present study was designed to systematically investigate the impact of data leakage and feature selection on the apparent and actual performance of ML models for PD diagnosis. Specifically, we constructed two experimental pipelines: one in which all overt motor symptoms and clinically obvious features were excluded to simulate a subclinical diagnostic scenario, and a control in which these features were included (Figure 7.1). By training and evaluating nine distinct ML models (including logistic regression, LASSO, SVM, gradient boosting, XGBoost, KNN, AdaBoost, random forest, and deep neural networks) on both feature sets, we aimed to disentangle the contributions of algorithmic complexity, feature signal, and evaluation methodology to observed performance.

Our results demonstrate that, in the absence of overt features, all models exhibited superficially acceptable F1 scores but failed catastrophically in terms of specificity, misclassifying the vast majority of healthy controls as PD. This pattern was consistent across model types and persisted despite hyperparameter tuning and regularization. When overt features were reintroduced, model performance improved dramatically, confirming that the observed diagnostic failures were not due to algorithmic limitations but to the absence of strong diagnostic signals. These findings underscore the necessity of rigorous experimental design, transparent reporting of confusion matrices, and critical evaluation of model utility in clinically realistic scenarios. They also highlight the dangers of data leakage and the importance of aligning ML evaluation with real-world clinical decision-making.

This work provides a cautionary example of how data leakage and feature selection can profoundly distort the perceived utility of ML models in clinical diagnosis. By contrasting model behavior with and without access to overt diagnostic features, we reveal the limitations of current approaches and offer guidance for the development of more robust, clinically meaningful ML tools for early PD detection.

7.2   Materials and Methods

This section outlines each stage of the experimental workflow, including data preprocessing, model development, and evaluation. All procedures related to data handling, such as feature selection and exclusion criteria, are described in detail to minimize the risk of inadvertent data leakage and to reflect clinically realistic scenarios. Strategies for data partitioning, model training, and hyperparameter optimization are specified to facilitate reproducibility. Evaluation metrics and visualization approaches are reported to ensure an unbiased assessment of model performance. Where relevant, methodological choices are clarified [416].

7.2.1   Dataset and Preprocessing

A structured dataset comprising $N = 2,105$ patients was utilized, with each individual labeled as either having Parkinson's disease (PD) or as a healthy control [417]. To emulate a subclinical diagnostic context, all features directly corresponding to overt motor symptoms (such as tremor, rigidity, bradykinesia, postural instability, speech problems, sleep disorders, and constipation) and other clinically obvious indicators were systematically excluded prior to analysis. The following variables were removed: PatientID, DoctorInCharge, UPDRS, MoCA, FunctionalAssessment, Tremor, Rigidity, Bradykinesia, PosturalInstability, SpeechProblems, SleepDisorders, and Constipation. The original dataset is then denoted as $\mathcal{D}$, and the dataset after column removal as $\mathcal{D}'$.

Feature selection was guided by established clinical knowledge and expert consensus, rather than by automated feature selection or importance ranking algorithms [418]. This approach was adopted to ensure that only features plausibly available and relevant in a true subclinical context were retained, thereby aligning the analysis with real-world diagnostic challenges. By prioritizing clinical input over purely data-driven selection, the inclusion of variables that, while statistically informative, would not be accessible or meaningful in early-stage patient assessment was avoided.

During data preprocessing, categorical variables were systematically converted into a format suitable for analysis alongside numerical variables. This ensured that all patient characteristics, regardless of their original format, could be incorporated into the modeling process. The dataset was then organized so that the relevant patient features were separated from the diagnostic labels, allowing for subsequent model development and evaluation.

No explicit normalization or standardization of features was performed. Most variables retained after preprocessing were either binary indicators or clinical scores with similar numeric ranges, which are generally well-handled by the types of models used in this study. It is acknowledged, however, that some modeling approaches may be sensitive to differences in feature scale; this is recognized as a limitation, and future work will assess whether additional data scaling could influence model performance.

To further minimize the risk that subtle proxies for overt motor symptoms remained in the dataset, a manual review of all retained features was conducted. This review aimed to exclude any variables that might indirectly reflect the presence of overt symptoms, such as those related to downstream clinical consequences, medication use, or subjective assessments of motor function. Demographic and categorical variables were also examined to ensure they did not inadvertently serve as proxies through imbalanced representation or encoding patterns. Although no automated methods for detecting hidden correlations were applied, this conservative approach was intended to closely simulate the information available in a real-world subclinical diagnostic scenario [416].

7.2.2   Data Splitting

To ensure that the evaluation of model performance reflected real-world clinical scenarios, the dataset was divided into three distinct subsets: a training set, a validation set, and a test set. The majority of the data was allocated to the training set, which was used to develop the models and perform internal validation. A smaller portion was set aside as a validation set, which served to optimize model parameters and prevent overfitting during development. The remaining data formed a test set, which was held out entirely from the model development process and used only for the final, unbiased assessment of model performance. Stratified random sampling was employed throughout this process to maintain the original balance between patients with Parkinson's disease and healthy controls, thereby ensuring that each subset was representative of the overall population. This approach was chosen to rigorously assess the generalizability of the models and to avoid the risk of data leakage, which can occur if information from the test set inadvertently influences model development [416].

7.2.3 Machine Learning Models

A range of machine learning models was evaluated to determine their ability to distinguish between patients with Parkinson's disease and healthy controls under clinically realistic conditions. The models included both traditional statistical approaches and more complex algorithms, such as logistic regression, regularized regression, support vector machines, tree-based ensemble methods, and deep neural networks. All models were developed using the same data pipeline to ensure comparability. Model parameters were systematically optimized using the validation set, with the aim of maximizing predictive performance while minimizing overfitting. For each model, a range of parameter values was explored to identify the optimal configuration. This thorough approach allowed for a robust comparison of different modeling strategies and provided insights into the strengths and limitations of each method in the context of early disease detection [416].

7.2.4 Learning Curve Analysis

To better understand how the amount of available training data influenced model performance, learning curve analysis was conducted. This involved training each model on progressively larger subsets of the training data and evaluating performance on both the training and validation sets. By examining how accuracy changed as more data became available, it was possible to assess whether the models were able to generalize from the training data to new, unseen cases, or whether they were prone to overfitting.

This analysis provided valuable information about the data requirements for reliable model development and highlighted the challenges associated with early detection of Parkinson's disease when only subtle or non-specific features are available [416].

7.2.5   Prediction and Evaluation Metrics

Model performance was assessed using a range of standard metrics, including accuracy, precision, recall, and the F1 score. These metrics were calculated for each of the three data subsets (training, validation, and test) to provide a comprehensive view of model behavior. In addition, confusion matrices were generated to offer a more detailed understanding of the types of errors made by each model, such as the rates of false positives and false negatives. This granular analysis was particularly important in the context of early disease detection, where the clinical consequences of misclassification can be significant. The use of multiple metrics and confusion matrix analysis ensured that the evaluation captured both overall performance and specific patterns of diagnostic error [416].

Although techniques such as synthetic data augmentation or class weighting are sometimes used to address imbalances between disease and control groups [382], these approaches were deliberately not applied in this study. The rationale was to maintain the natural class distribution present in the dataset, thereby reflecting the true prevalence of Parkinson's disease in a screening population. This decision was made to avoid artificially enhancing model performance in ways that may not translate to real-world clinical settings. Instead, the focus was placed on evaluating how well the models performed under authentic conditions, with particular attention to the rates of false positives and negatives as revealed by confusion matrix analysis. This approach allowed for a transparent assessment of the limitations and potential of current machine learning methods for early disease detection [416].

7.2.6   Visualization and Model Diagnostics

To facilitate interpretation and diagnostic insight, model performance was visualized using learning curves and comparative plots of key metrics across the different data subsets. Confusion matrices were also visualized to highlight patterns of misclassification and to identify systematic errors.

These visual tools provided an accessible means for clinicians and researchers to assess model reliability, detect overfitting, and understand the practical implications of model predictions in a clinical context [416].

7.2.7 Comparative Experiments with and Without Overt Features

To determine whether the observed limitations in model performance were due to the absence of strong diagnostic signals or to inherent algorithmic constraints, all models were also retrained and evaluated using the full set of clinical features, including those directly indicative of Parkinson's disease. This comparison served as a control, demonstrating that the same models could achieve high accuracy when provided with overtly diagnostic information. The dramatic improvement in performance under these conditions highlighted the risk of data leakage and underscored the importance of excluding such features when evaluating models intended for early detection [416].

7.2.8 Visualization and Model Diagnostics

To support clinical interpretation and diagnostic insight, model performance was visualized using several complementary approaches. Learning curves were generated to illustrate how model accuracy changed as the amount of training data increased, providing a means to identify whether models were underfitting or overfitting. For each model, key performance metrics (including accuracy, precision, recall, and F1-score) were compared across the training, validation, and test sets. This allowed for a clear assessment of how well each model generalized to new, unseen data. Special attention was given to the F1-score, as it reflects the balance between correctly identifying patients with Parkinson's disease and avoiding false positives. Confusion matrices were also visualized for each model and data split, offering a detailed view of the types of errors made, such as misclassifying healthy controls as patients or vice versa. These visual tools enabled clinicians and researchers to better understand model reliability, detect patterns of systematic error, and appreciate the practical implications of model predictions in a clinical context [416].

7.2.9 Comparative Experiments with and Without Overt Features

To clarify whether the observed limitations in model performance were due to the absence of strong diagnostic signals or to inherent constraints of the algorithms themselves, all models were also retrained and evaluated using the full set of clinical features, including those directly indicative of Parkinson's disease such as tremor, rigidity, and bradykinesia. This comparison served as a control, demonstrating that the same models could achieve high accuracy when provided with overtly diagnostic information. The marked improvement in performance under these conditions highlighted the risk of data leakage and underscored the importance of excluding such features when evaluating models intended for early detection [416].

7.2.10 Summary of Workflow

The overall workflow was designed to evaluate the clinical utility of machine learning models for early detection of Parkinson's disease. This included careful data preprocessing to exclude overtly diagnostic features, stratified splitting of the dataset into training, validation, and test sets, and the development and comparison of multiple machine learning models. Learning curve analysis was performed to assess the impact of training set size, and model performance was evaluated using a comprehensive set of metrics and visualizations. Finally, all analyses were repeated with the full feature set to provide a direct comparison and to highlight the effects of including overt clinical indicators. This approach ensured that the study's conclusions were grounded in clinically realistic scenarios and avoided artificial enhancements to model performance [416].

7.3 Results

To assess the ability of ML models to detect PD in the absence of overt clinical symptoms, we constructed two experimental pipelines. In the first, all features corresponding to classical motor symptoms (e.g., tremor, rigidity, bradykinesia) and other clinically obvious indicators were excluded, simulating a subclinical diagnostic scenario. In the second, these features were included, representing a control condition that allows for potential data leakage. Nine ML models were trained and evaluated using a three-way split (train/validation/test), and performance was assessed using accuracy, F1 score, and confusion matrix analysis.

7.3.1 Superficial Performance Masks Diagnostic Failure in the Absence of Overt Features

At first glance, several models appeared to perform reasonably well when overt features were excluded. For example, logistic regression and LASSO achieved test F1 scores of 0.74 and 0.76, respectively, while SVM and Gradient Boosting hovered around 0.73. However, as shown in Table 7.1, a closer examination revealed that all models exhibited substantial false positive rates when classifying healthy controls. Notably, LASSO and logistic regression misclassified over 90% of controls as having PD, while DNN and KNN also showed false positive rates exceeding 60%. These findings underscore a consistent diagnostic failure pattern: models achieved seemingly strong metrics by over-predicting PD in the absence of overt motor symptom features.

Model	F1 Score	Accuracy	% Falsely Predicted PD
Logistic Regression	0.7381	0.5968	92.5%
LASSO	0.7555	0.6095	98.3%
DNN	0.6209	0.5270	63.3%
Random Forest	0.7222	0.5873	86.7%
SVM	0.7261	0.5905	87.5%
Gradient Boosting	0.7253	0.5937	85.0%
KNN	0.6450	0.5143	80.8%
AdaBoost	0.6339	0.5270	69.2%
XGBoost	0.7253	0.5937	85.0%

Table 7.1: Performance of ML models on the held-out test set. While F1 scores and overall accuracies varied across models, all exhibited substantial false positive rates when attempting to classify healthy controls. Notably, LASSO and logistic regression misclassified over 90% of controls as having PD, while DNN and KNN also showed false positive rates exceeding 60%. These findings underscore a consistent diagnostic failure pattern: models achieving seemingly strong metrics did so by over-predicting PD in the absence of overt motor symptom features, reinforcing the need to evaluate clinical utility beyond accuracy or F1 score.

Although overt motor symptoms were excluded to simulate a subclinical scenario, the retained features included demographic and general health variables such as age, gender, BMI, and education level. While some of these features have been loosely associated with PD risk in prior epidemiological studies, their inclusion did not yield clinically meaningful predictive performance in our analysis. This suggests that, although subtle correlations may exist, they are insufficient in isolation to support early-stage PD classification using standard ML algorithms. These findings further emphasize the limitations of relying solely on non-diagnostic features and reinforce the clinical relevance of our negative results.

7.3.2 Overfitting and Model Collapse Across Complexity Levels

Overfitting was most pronounced in high-capacity models such as Random Forest, DNN, and AdaBoost, which achieved nearly perfect training scores but suffered test set F1 drops of 25–40%. Figure 7.2 illustrates the accuracy of all nine ML models across training, validation, and test splits. High-capacity models showed marked performance drops on unseen test data, indicative of memorization rather than learning. In contrast, simpler models like logistic regression maintained lower, but more stable, performance across splits.

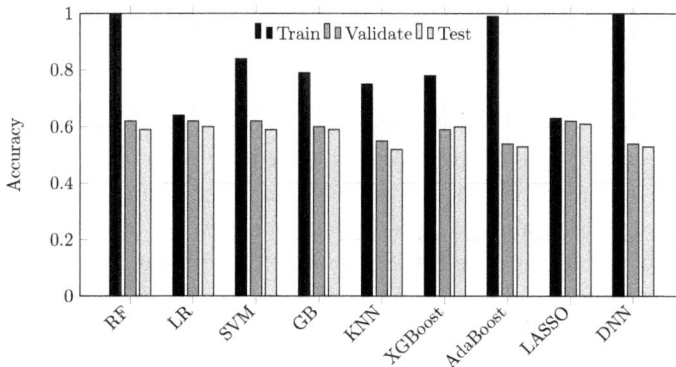

Figure 7.2: Bar graph illustrating training, validation, and test accuracy for each ML model. High-capacity models such as Random Forest, DNN, and AdaBoost achieve near-perfect training accuracy but show marked drops on the test set, indicating overfitting. Simpler models like logistic regression maintain lower but more consistent performance across splits.

Figure 7.3 further highlights this phenomenon by comparing F1 scores across splits. Large discrepancies between training and test F1 scores in models like DNN, Random Forest, and AdaBoost reveal significant generalization failures, while logistic regression and LASSO show more consistent but modest F1 scores.

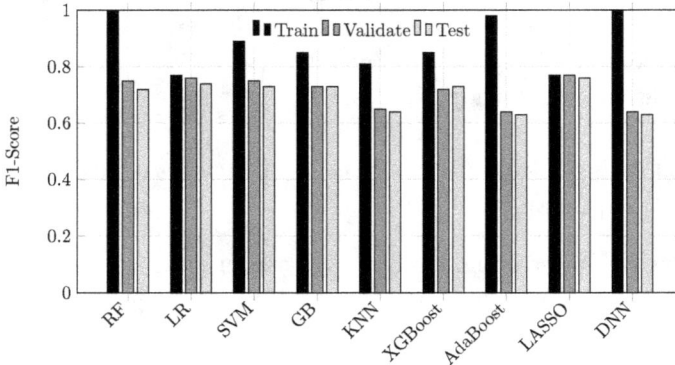

Figure 7.3: Bar graph of training, validation, and test F1 scores for each ML model. Large discrepancies between training and test F1 scores in complex models highlight generalization failure. More consistent but modest F1 scores are seen in logistic regression and LASSO.

7.3.3 Confusion Matrices Reveal the True Clinical Utility

Aggregate metrics such as F1 score and accuracy failed to capture the near-complete collapse of specificity exhibited by every model. As shown in Figure 7.4, confusion matrices for DNN and LASSO on the test set reveal that most models defaulted to predicting nearly every subject as having PD, regardless of true class. The LASSO model, for example, misclassified 118 of 120 healthy controls as having PD, despite a high F1 score. In contrast, the DNN model, while exhibiting lower F1 and accuracy scores overall, achieved the lowest false positive rate among all models. These contrasting confusion matrices emphasize the limitations of relying solely on aggregate metrics.

In addition to the high false positive rates (Type I errors), we also evaluated false negatives (Type II errors) across all models. While many models defaulted to predicting most subjects as having PD (resulting in high false positives) the impact on false negatives varied. For example, the DNN model misclassified 44 actual PD cases as healthy controls (Figure 7.4), representing a substantial Type II error rate despite its lower false positive rate. This pattern suggests a trade-off between overprediction and sensitivity

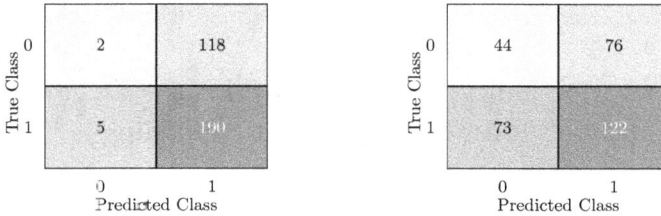

Figure 7.4: Confusion matrices highlighting diagnostic behavior of LASSO (left) and DNN (right) on the test set, with overt features excluded. The LASSO model demonstrates extreme overprediction of PD, misclassifying 111 of 120 healthy controls as having PD. The DNN model, while less accurate overall, achieves the lowest false positive rate among all models. These results illustrate how confusion matrices can reveal pathological model behavior that is hidden by summary metrics.

loss, reinforcing the limitations of relying solely on metrics like F1 score. Including overt features, as seen in the following sections, reduced both false positives and false negatives substantially, highlighting how access to diagnostically informative features artificially improves both types of error rates.

Notably, while the DNN model demonstrated lower overall F1 and accuracy scores compared to simpler models, it achieved the lowest false positive rate among all models evaluated without overt features (Figure 7.4). This paradoxical pattern (relatively better specificity despite poorer aggregate metrics) was also observed in models such as AdaBoost and KNN, both of which reported modest F1 scores but demonstrated improved ability to correctly identify healthy controls compared to models like LASSO or logistic regression. This phenomenon may be partially explained by differences in model architecture and regularization behavior. For instance, the DNN's use of dropout and weight decay likely encouraged a more conservative decision boundary, reducing overconfident misclassification. Similarly, KNN's instance-based learning approach is sensitive to local density, which may yield cautious predictions in sparsely populated control regions. AdaBoost, by emphasizing misclassified instances through iterative weighting, may have inadvertently focused on recovering specificity at the expense of recall. These findings suggest that certain model types, particularly those with non-linear representation capacity or adaptive weighting mechanisms, may be better suited to managing class imbalance in subclinical scenarios where overt signals are absent. However, this increased specificity does not necessarily equate to superior clinical utility, as most of these models still exhibited substantial false positive rates overall.

7.3.4   Model Behavior with Obvious PD Features Included: The Effect of Data Leakage

To determine whether the observed diagnostic failures were due to algorithmic limitations or the absence of strong diagnostic signals, all models were retrained on the full dataset, including classical Parkinsonian symptoms. As shown in Table 7.2, performance improved dramatically across all metrics. Random Forest and Gradient Boosting achieved test accuracies exceeding 92%, with false positive rates as low as 8.3%. This sharp contrast to the >90% false positive rates observed without obvious clinical symptoms demonstrates that the same models, when given access to overtly diagnostic features, achieve artificially high performance, i.e., an effect attributable to data leakage.

Model	F1 Score	Accuracy	% Falsely Predicted PD
Logistic Regression	0.8440	0.8063	25.8%
LASSO	0.8550	0.8190	25.0%
DNN	0.8342	0.7968	25.0%
Random Forest	0.9487	0.9365	8.3%
SVM	0.8483	0.8127	24.2%
Gradient Boosting	0.9361	0.9206	10.8%
KNN	0.7712	0.7175	36.7%
AdaBoost	0.9207	0.9016	13.3%
XGBoost	0.9361	0.9206	10.8%

Table 7.2: F1 scores, accuracy, and false positive rates on the test set reported for each model after retraining to include overt motor symptoms of PD. All models demonstrated substansial performance gains compared to runs excluding these features. Notably, Random Forest and Gradient Boosting achieved the highest accuracies (93.7% and 92.1%, respectively) and the lowest false positive rates (8.3% and 10.8%, respectively), indicating that clinical feature richness substantially enhances model precision and reliability.

Figure 7.5 presents confusion matrices for Random Forest and KNN on the test set when overt features were included. The Random Forest model demonstrates superior specificity, with only 29 false positives, while KNN exhibits the highest false positive count (44) among the models analyzed.

To preserve readability and avoid redundancy, we do not present confusion matrices for all nine models across the three data partitions. Visual inspection shows that the misclassification patterns are highly concordant

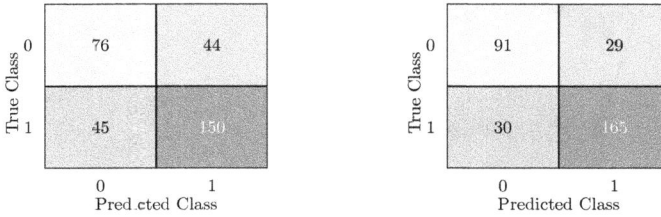

Figure 7.5: Confusion matrices for KNN (left) and Random Forest (right) on the test dataset when overt Parkinsonian motor features were included. The Random Forest model demonstrates superior specificity, with only 29 false positives, while KNN exhibits the highest false positive count (44) among the models analyzed.

(e.g., elevated false-positive rates when overt clinical features are omitted), and these trends are already captured by the reported specificity and "percent falsely predicted PD" metrics in Tables 7.1–7.2. Accordingly, we display only representative matrices that illustrate the two dominant behaviors (specificity collapse vs. more balanced errors).

7.3.5 Learning Curves Reveal the Impact of Overt Feature Inclusion

To directly illustrate the effect of including overt clinical features on model learning dynamics, we compared learning curves for LASSO logistic regression (trained without overt features) and KNN (trained with overt features). Figure 7.6 shows training and validation accuracy as a function of training set size for both scenarios.

In well-behaved learning scenarios, training and validation curves should gradually converge toward each other as the training set size increases, eventually plateauing at similar performance levels with only a small, stable gap between them This convergence pattern suggests that the model is learning genuine patterns rather than memorizing noise, and that additional training data helps reduce overfitting while improving generalization.

These results highlight the dramatic difference in achievable accuracy and generalization when overt clinical features are included. The LASSO model, trained without overt features, shows limited learning capacity and converges to moderate accuracy, reflecting the true difficulty of early PD detection. In contrast, the KNN model, trained with overt features, achieves much higher accuracy, but this performance is largely attributable to the inclusion of features that are themselves diagnostic, thus inflating apparent

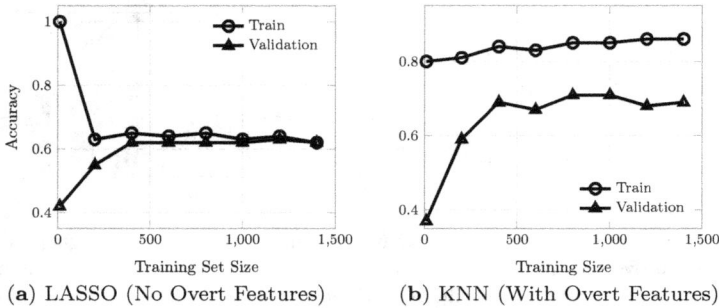

(a) LASSO (No Overt Features)   **(b)** KNN (With Overt Features)

Figure 7.6: Learning curves for (a) LASSO logistic regression trained without overt features and (b) KNN trained with overt features. Excluding overt features (left) results in modest and plateauing accuracy, with minimal gap between training and validation curves. Including overt features (right) yields substantially higher accuracy, but a persistent gap between training and validation curves, indicating potential overfitting and the artificial boost in performance due to data leakage.

model utility.

Figure 7.7 presents learning curves for two representative high-capacity machine learning models (i.e., Random Forest (a) and AdaBoost (b)) trained on a set that explicitly excludes overtly diagnostic indicators of PD, such as tremor, rigidity, and other classical motor symptoms. In both models, the training accuracy remains at or near 1.0 (100%) across all training set sizes, indicating that the models are able to perfectly memorize the training data regardless of how much data is provided. This is a hallmark of overfitting, especially in high-capacity models with sufficient flexibility to capture even random noise in the absence of strong predictive signals.

In stark contrast, the validation accuracy for both Random Forest and AdaBoost plateaus at substantially lower levels, i.e., approximately 0.5 to 0.6, regardless of the amount of training data. Notably, increasing the training set size does not close the gap between training and validation accuracy; the two curves remain widely separated, with a persistent gap of 0.4–0.5. This persistent discrepancy demonstrates that the models are not learning generalizable patterns from the data, but are instead memorizing idiosyncrasies of the training set that do not translate to improved performance on unseen cases.

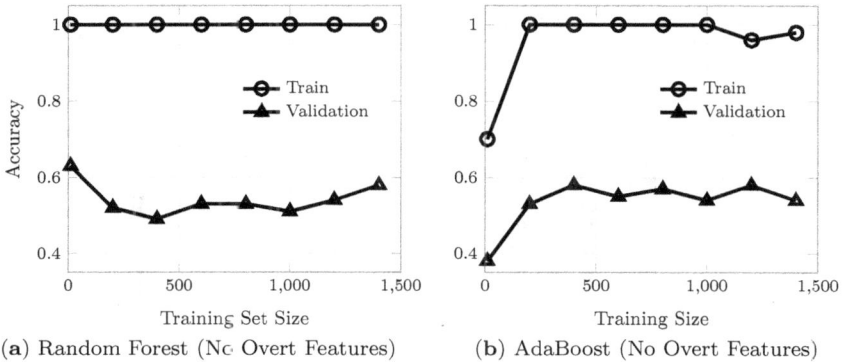

(a) Random Forest (No Overt Features)   (b) AdaBoost (No Overt Features)

Figure 7.7: Learning curves for (a) Random Forest and (b) AdaBoost, both trained without overtly diagnostic features (i.e., features directly indicative of Parkinson's Disease such as tremor or rigidity). Both models exhibit persistent overfitting: training accuracy remains near-perfect across all data sizes, while validation accuracy plateaus at substantially lower levels (approximately 0.5–0.6), with a large and stable gap between the two curves. This pattern indicates that, in the absence of strongly predictive features, high-capacity models such as Random Forest and AdaBoost are unable to generalize and instead memorize the training data.

7.3.6   Direct Comparison and Clinical Implications

The stark contrast between model performance with and without overt features is summarized in Figure 7.8. This graph illustrates how excluding overt features simulates a realistic early detection scenario, resulting in low accuracy, while including overt features (data leakage) yields high but misleading accuracy. The temptation to include such features leads to artificially inflated performance metrics that do not translate to real-world clinical utility.

Hence, these results provide a cautionary example of how data leakage and feature selection can profoundly distort the perceived utility of ML models in clinical diagnosis. Only by rigorously excluding diagnostic features and critically evaluating model behavior using confusion matrices can the true limitations and potential of ML for early PD detection be revealed.

While statistical comparisons between ML algorithms (e.g., McNemar's test or bootstrap-based confidence intervals) are common in model benchmarking studies, such analyses were intentionally omitted here. Our primary aim was not to identify statistically superior models but to evaluate whether any model could demonstrate clinically meaningful performance in the absence of overt motor features. Given that all models exhibited unacceptably

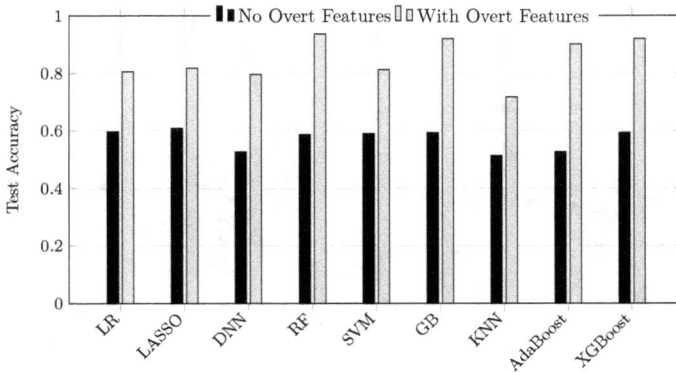

Figure 7.8: Direct comparison of test accuracy for nine ML models with and without overt features. Including overt features (orange) yields dramatically higher accuracy across all models, highlighting the risk of data leakage and the misleading nature of such results for early detection scenarios.

high false positive rates under realistic conditions, comparative statistical testing between them would offer limited practical value. Instead, we emphasize clinical thresholds of utility (such as false positive and negative rates) over small statistical differences between algorithms, as even the "best" model under these conditions failed to reach a level of diagnostic performance that would justify clinical deployment.

7.4   Discussion

In designing and interpreting this study, our perspective was consistently guided by the realities and priorities of clinical medicine. As a research group rooted in clinical science, our priorities differ from those of purely computational or engineering teams: rather than approaching the work solely from a computational or algorithmic vantage point, we maintained a focus on clinical translation, ensuring that our experimental decisions (such as the choice of features, validation methods, and performance metrics) were all selected to mirror the constraints and needs of real-world healthcare environments. This clinical orientation shaped our entire workflow, motivating us to move beyond technical performance and instead interrogate whether the specific ML models we evaluated in this study can genuinely contribute to earlier and more accurate diagnosis in practical, patient-facing settings.

ML holds a promise for advancing medical diagnostics, but its true predictive power can only be demonstrated when models are trained on data that do not include features directly indicative of the target pathology [407, 419]. If input data contain variables that are themselves diagnostic (such as overt clinical signs or test results that would immediately reveal the disease to a clinician) the resulting model may appear highly accurate, but this performance is misleading and does not reflect genuine predictive capability [420, 421]. Instead, such models risk simply replicating existing diagnostic criteria rather than uncovering novel patterns or providing early detection [422, 423]. As ML-based solutions become increasingly available for clinical use, it is essential for medical professionals to critically evaluate these tools and understand the nature of the data used in their development [424]. This requires learning to ask the right questions about which features were included, how the models were validated, and whether the reported performance truly reflects real-world predictive utility rather than artificial inflation due to data leakage or circular reasoning [425, 426].

7.4.1 Analysis of Learning Curve Patterns

The two learning curves in Figure 7.6 reveal dramatically different behaviors that illuminate the impact of feature selection on model learning dynamics. The LASSO model (Figure 7.6a) demonstrates healthy learning curve characteristics. Both training and validation curves converge and plateau together at approximately 0.62-0.64 accuracy, with a minimal gap between them (typically less than 0.02). This convergence pattern indicates that the model has reached its true learning capacity given the available features and is not overfitting to the training data [427]. The small, stable gap between curves suggests good generalization, i.e., the model performs similarly on both seen and unseen data. However, the modest plateau level (around 62-64% accuracy) reflects the inherent difficulty of early PD detection when relying solely on legitimate, non-diagnostic features [428].

In stark contrast, the KNN model (Figure 7.6b) exhibits problematic learning curve behavior that violates the principles of healthy model learning [429]. The training and validation curves fail to converge, maintaining a persistent, large gap of approximately 0.15-0.17 (15-17 percentage points) even as training set size increases to 1,400 samples. This behavior is characteristic of overfitting and suggests that the model is memorizing training-specific patterns rather than learning generalizable relationships [430]. The consistently high training accuracy (85-86%) combined with substantially lower validation accuracy (68-71%) indicates that the model's apparent performance is artificially inflated by its ability to exploit the overt clinical features that directly encode the diagnostic outcome.

The failure of curves to converge in the KNN model is particularly concerning because it suggests that even with substantial increases in training data, the model cannot achieve the generalization performance that its training accuracy would suggest [431]. This persistent gap is a hallmark of data leakage, where the model has access to information that would not be available in real-world deployment scenarios [432]. The overt features essentially provide "shortcuts" to the diagnosis, allowing the model to achieve high training performance without learning the subtle, early indicators that would be clinically valuable [433].

A similar pattern is observed in high-capacity models such as Random Forest and AdaBoost (Figure 7.7), both trained without overtly diagnostic features. These models consistently achieve near-perfect performance on the training data, regardless of how much data is provided, reflecting their ability to memorize even subtle or irrelevant patterns. However, this apparent success does not translate to improved performance on new, unseen cases: their validation results remain substantially lower, and the gap between training and validation performance persists even as the training set grows. This persistent discrepancy is a classic indicator of overfitting, underscoring that, in the absence of strong predictive signals, such models are prone to capturing noise rather than learning generalizable patterns. These findings reinforce the importance of careful feature selection and robust validation [434], as high-capacity models can easily give a false impression of effectiveness if evaluated solely on their training performance.

These findings reinforce the central message of the study: high apparent accuracy in ML models for clinical diagnosis is often an artifact of data leakage or the inclusion of features that are themselves diagnostic. When such features are removed to reflect a true early detection challenge, model performance collapses, and overfitting becomes pervasive. This highlights the critical importance of proper feature selection and experimental design to avoid misleading conclusions about model utility in real-world clinical settings.

7.4.2   Strengths of the Study

This study provides a systematic investigation into the impact of feature selection and data leakage on the apparent and actual performance of ML models for PD diagnosis. By explicitly constructing parallel pipelines (with and without overtly diagnostic features) and evaluating nine distinct ML algorithms using a robust three-way data split, we offer a transparent, reproducible framework for assessing true model generalizability. The inclusion of learning curve analysis, confusion matrix visualization, and detailed metric reporting goes beyond conventional aggregate metrics, revealing subtle but clinically critical model behaviors that would otherwise remain hidden. This approach aligns with recent recommendations for standardized validation and transparent reporting in clinical AI research, and serves as a practical template for future studies seeking to avoid common methodological pitfalls [392, 398].

7.4.3   Limitations and Weaknesses

As always, several limitations must be acknowledged. First, while the exclusion of overt clinical features simulates a subclinical diagnostic scenario, the remaining feature set may still contain subtle proxies for disease status, potentially introducing residual bias. Second, the dataset, though relatively large and balanced, is derived from a single source and may not capture the full heterogeneity of real-world patient populations, limiting external generalizability. Although the original dataset used in this study was relatively balanced between PD cases and controls, we recognize that real-world clinical datasets are often imbalanced. In such cases, resampling techniques (e.g., SMOTE) or class weighting may be necessary to mitigate bias in model evaluation metrics, particularly regarding false positive and false negative rates. In this study, the high false positive rates observed in the early detection scenario were due primarily to the lack of predictive signal in the available features, rather than class imbalance. Future work should systematically evaluate the impact of resampling and cost-sensitive methods, especially for deployment in settings with unbalanced prevalence. Third, the study does not include external validation on independent datasets from other institutions or geographic regions; a step increasingly recognized as essential for establishing clinical robustness [392, 398]. Additionally, while multiple ML algorithms were compared, the study did not exhaustively explore all possible model architectures or ensemble strategies, nor did it incorporate advanced techniques for model interpretability or explainability. Finally, the weighting of performance metrics and the clinical relevance of specific thresholds were not formally established through expert consensus, which could further refine the evaluation of clinical utility [392].

However, it is important to note that additional regularization techniques, such as more aggressive dropout or early stopping, would not have materially altered these findings. The persistent gap between training and validation accuracy in high-capacity models reflects the intrinsic limitations of the available feature set, rather than insufficient regularization or premature stopping. This underscores that the primary barrier to improved generalization is the lack of predictive signal in the features, not the choice of model or training protocol.

A key limitation of the present study is the use of a dataset derived from a single source. While the controlled and standardized nature of this dataset allows for consistent feature collection and preprocessing, it may limit the generalizability of findings across more heterogeneous clinical populations. Differences in demographics, comorbidities, recording equipment, and diagnostic protocols could all influence model performance when applied outside the original context. As a potential next step (if suitable external data become available) we would seek to validate our models on datasets from multiple clinical sites or community-based cohorts. Such external validation would enable a more comprehensive assessment of generalizability and may reveal population- or site-specific adjustments needed for optimal model performance. Furthermore, future work could explore domain adaptation techniques and federated learning to address inter-site variability while preserving data privacy.

While recent studies have increasingly leveraged multimodal or longitudinal data (such as sensor-derived gait metrics [435], voice recordings [436–438], or handwriting samples [439, 440]) for prodromal PD detection, our study intentionally focused on purely tabular clinical and demographic data. This design choice was driven by the desire to evaluate whether subclinical PD could be identified using low-cost, routinely collected variables that would be accessible in typical primary care or screening settings. In contrast, multimodal approaches often require specialized equipment, extensive preprocessing pipelines, or repeated longitudinal measurements that may not be feasible in all clinical environments. By deliberately restricting our feature set, we aimed to highlight the limitations and risks of overestimating model utility in early-stage PD when only minimal, non-diagnostic data are available. We acknowledge that this approach trades off sensitivity for broader accessibility and have clarified this design rationale accordingly.

7.4.4   Ensuring Clinical Value

A key lesson from this study is that the development of clinically actionable ML models requires genuine collaboration between computer science experts and medical professionals at every stage of the process. For example, in this work, rather than relying solely on automated feature selection algorithms, we deliberately used clinical expertise to determine which features should be included for early detection. This approach ensured that the retained variables were not only statistically relevant, but also plausible and meaningful in a real-world subclinical context. When ML developers work in isolation and depend exclusively on algorithmic feature selection, there is a significant risk of producing models that are technically impressive but clinically irrelevant; either by including variables unavailable at the point of care, or by missing subtle but important clinical cues. Only by integrating domain knowledge with technical innovation can we create ML tools that address real diagnostic challenges and support actionable decision-making in healthcare. This underscores the importance of interdisciplinary teamwork to bridge the gap between algorithmic performance and true clinical utility.

7.4.5   Future Directions

Building on these findings, several avenues for future research are warranted. First, future studies should prioritize external validation using datasets from diverse clinical settings to rigorously assess model generalizability and mitigate the risk of overfitting to local data idiosyncrasies [392,398]. Second, the development and adoption of standardized, clinically oriented composite metrics (such as those that integrate sensitivity, specificity, predictive values, and misclassification penalties) would provide a more nuanced assessment of model utility in real-world scenarios [392]. Third, collaboration with clinical experts to define clinically meaningful endpoints and thresholds, as well as to guide feature selection, will help ensure that ML models address genuine unmet needs rather than merely replicating existing diagnostic criteria. Fourth, future work should explore the integration of explainable AI (XAI) techniques to enhance model transparency and foster clinician trust [441], as recommended in recent reviews [398,442]. Finally, as regulatory frameworks for clinical AI continue to evolve [312,388], adherence to emerging standards for documentation, validation, and post-deployment monitoring will be critical for translating research advances into safe and effective clinical tools [392, 442].

Furthermore, recent advances in deep learning for industrial fault diagnosis offer useful lessons for the challenges of early disease detection discussed in this study. For example, recent work has shown that combining time-frequency analysis methods, such as wavelet transforms, with deep learning models that can focus on important patterns in complex sensor data can greatly improve the detection of subtle faults in machinery, even when signals are noisy or variable [443]. Other research has demonstrated that integrating information from multiple types of sensors (such as vibration and acoustic emission) using specialized neural network architectures can further enhance the reliability of fault classification, especially in real-world industrial environments where any single signal may be ambiguous or affected by interference [444]. These trends highlight the value of using richer data representations and combining complementary sources of information to improve model robustness. While our current approach does not yet incorporate these advanced signal processing or multimodal strategies, such methods may represent promising directions for future work; particularly as wearable sensors and other non-invasive technologies continue to expand the range of physiological data available for early detection of conditions like PD.

7.5   Conclusions

This study highlights the critical importance of rigorous experimental design, transparent reporting, and critical evaluation of machine learning models for early disease detection. By demonstrating how data leakage and feature selection can profoundly distort perceived model utility, we underscore the need for the medical AI community to move beyond superficial performance metrics and toward robust, clinically meaningful validation. Only through such efforts can the promise of ML in advancing early diagnosis and improving patient outcomes be fully realized.

If we do not begin educating our current and future medical professionals right now on how to critically evaluate and distinguish credible AI-assisted diagnostic tools from those that simply inflate their performance metrics through practices like data leakage or improper validation, we risk a future where well-intentioned clinicians adopt unreliable AI solutions in hopes of improving patient care. When these tools inevitably fail on real-world, unseen data, the resulting disappointment could foster widespread distrust of all AI-assisted diagnostics throughout the healthcare sector. Once that trust is lost, it will be difficult and time-consuming to regain. This is why it is imperative that we act now to equip medical professionals with the knowledge and skills to ask the right questions about AI validation, learning dynamics, feature selection, data leakage, and generalizability, so they can reliably identify robust, clinically meaningful AI solutions and prevent a future defined by skepticism and missed opportunities for patient care improvement.

Chapter 8

Practical Integration of AI in Clinical Practice

8.1 Questions Every Clinician Should Ask

As AI transforms medical practice, clinicians face an unprecedented challenge: evaluating complex algorithmic tools that may fundamentally alter patient care decisions. The rapid proliferation of AI-powered diagnostic aids, risk prediction models, and clinical decision support systems has outpaced the development of standardized evaluation frameworks, leaving many healthcare providers ill-equipped to distinguish between robust, clinically validated tools and potentially harmful applications built on flawed methodologies.

The stakes of this evaluation challenge cannot be overstated. Unlike traditional medical devices with well-established regulatory pathways and clinical testing protocols, many AI tools operate in regulatory gray areas with performance claims based on retrospective analyses that may not reflect real-world clinical scenarios. The complexity of machine learning algorithms, combined with the technical expertise gap between developers and clinicians, creates a dangerous asymmetry of information that can lead to the adoption of tools that appear sophisticated but harbor fundamental flaws.

This section provides a detailed framework for clinicians to systematically evaluate AI tools through structured questioning that probes beyond marketing claims and surface-level performance metrics. The framework is organized into two complementary domains: validation concerns that address the scientific rigor of model development (Table 8.1), and operational concerns that examine real-world deployment considerations (Table 8.2). Together, these questions enable clinicians to identify critical weaknesses, demand appropriate transparency, and make informed decisions about AI adoption that prioritize patient safety and clinical effectiveness.

8.1.1 Validation Concerns

The validation questions outlined in Table 8.1 address the most common and dangerous methodological flaws that plague AI tools in healthcare. Data splitting practices represent perhaps the most fundamental concern, as improper splitting can lead to catastrophic overestimation of model performance. When developers report that they "split randomly" without specifying the unit of splitting, this often indicates image-level or observation-level splitting rather than the patient-level or site-level splitting required to prevent data leakage. For imaging applications, this distinction is critical: if multiple images from the same patient appear in both training and test sets, the model may simply learn to recognize individual patients rather than generalizable diagnostic patterns.

Performance evaluation requires scrutiny beyond headline accuracy numbers. Large gaps between training and test performance (>10-15 percentage points) suggest overfitting, while the absence of external validation studies indicates that the tool may only work in the specific environment where it was developed. Clinicians should insist on seeing comprehensive metrics including sensitivity, specificity, positive and negative predictive values, and area under the receiver operating characteristic curve, stratified by relevant clinical subgroups.

Feature engineering questions expose whether the AI tool can actually function in real clinical workflows. Tools that use post-diagnosis information as predictive features, include outcomes data as inputs, or incorporate "future" information not available at the time of prediction represent fundamental design flaws that render the tool unusable in practice. The temporal sequence of clinical events must be carefully respected, with features limited to information genuinely available at the point of clinical decision-making.

External validation serves as the ultimate test of model generalizability. Tools that have only been tested internally, show dramatic performance drops across different patient populations, or cannot provide references from other institutions using the system should be viewed with extreme skepticism.

True external validation requires testing on completely independent datasets from different clinical sites, ideally with different patient demographics and practice patterns.

Category	Critical Question	Good Response
Data Splitting	How was your dataset split into training, validation, and test sets?	Clear patient- or site-level splitting
Data Splitting	For imaging, was splitting done at patient or image level?	"Patient-level splitting ensures no leakage"
Data Splitting	Were preprocessing steps performed before splitting?	"All preprocessing done after splitting"
Data Splitting	Was temporal order considered in splitting?	"Splitting respects clinical timelines"
Performance	What are your training, validation, and test accuracy metrics?	Realistic, similar performance across splits
Performance	How large is the performance gap between training and test sets?	Small gap (5–10 points)
Performance	Can you show performance on independent, external datasets?	External validation from multiple sites
Performance	Are all relevant metrics (e.g., sensitivity, specificity, F1) reported?	Full set of clinically relevant metrics
Feature Engineering	What features does your model use for prediction?	Clear, clinically justified feature list
Feature Engineering	Are all features available at prediction time?	Only uses pre-decision information
Feature Engineering	Do any features include info only known after diagnosis?	Features match clinical workflow
Feature Engineering	How were features selected?	"Features selected for clinical relevance"
External Validation	Has your model been validated at other hospitals/sites?	Multiple external validation studies
External Validation	How does performance vary across patient populations?	Consistent across demographics
External Validation	Can you provide references from institutions using your tool?	Provides references and contacts
Temporal Validity	What is the realistic timeline for using your tool in workflow?	Matches current clinical workflow
Temporal Validity	Do you use any "future" information not available at prediction time?	Only uses info available at prediction time
Temporal Validity	How do you handle the temporal sequence of clinical events?	Clear understanding of clinical sequence

Table 8.1: Critical questions for evaluating AI tool development and validation methodologies.

8.1.2 Operational Concerns

The operational questions in Table 8.2 address the practical realities of deploying AI tools in clinical practice. Explainability and transparency have evolved from nice-to-have features to clinical necessities, as clinicians must be able to understand and communicate the basis for AI-driven recommendations. Tools that operate as "black boxes" without interpretable outputs or comprehensive documentation of model updates create liability concerns and undermine clinical decision-making.

Bias and fairness considerations have gained prominence as studies reveal systematic disparities in AI tool performance across racial, ethnic, gender, and socioeconomic groups. Developers who have not conducted bias audits or cannot provide stratified performance metrics may be deploying tools that exacerbate healthcare disparities. The absence of ongoing bias monitoring represents a particularly serious concern, as model performance can drift over time as patient populations and clinical practices evolve.

Deployment and support infrastructure often receives insufficient attention during the evaluation process, yet inadequate support can render even well-designed tools clinically useless. Tools backed by minimal technical support, unclear update processes, or vendors who disclaim responsibility for model failures represent poor investments that may ultimately compromise patient care.

Category	Critical Question	Good Response
Explainability	Can you explain how the model makes predictions?	"We provide explainable outputs"
Transparency	Is there documentation for model updates?	Full version history and change logs
Bias	How do you assess and mitigate bias?	"We audit for bias and report subgroups"
Fairness	Are metrics stratified by race, sex, age, etc.?	"Yes, we provide subgroup analyses"
Support	What support is available for integration and troubleshooting?	"Dedicated support team & resources"
Support	How is the model updated and maintained post-deployment?	"Regular updates with user notification"
Support	What happens if the model fails or gives unexpected results?	"Clear escalation and remediation"

Table 8.2: Critical questions for evaluating AI tool deployment, transparency, and operational support.

8.1.3   Red Flag Responses to Avoid

When evaluating AI tools for clinical use, several types of responses should raise immediate concerns. Vague or evasive answers about fundamental methodology, such as "we split randomly" without specifying patient-level versus image-level splitting, indicate poor understanding of data leakage risks. Performance red flags include large gaps between training and test accuracy (>10-15 percentage points), inability to provide external validation results, or reporting only overall accuracy without clinically relevant metrics like sensitivity and specificity. Feature engineering concerns arise when developers cannot clearly articulate their feature list, admit to using post-diagnosis information as predictors, or claim to use all available data without clinical justification. Temporal validity issues emerge when tools require future information for supposedly real-time predictions or when developers show vague understanding of clinical workflows and event sequences. Transparency red flags include absence of version control or update documentation, inability to explain model decisions ("it's a black box"), and failure to assess bias across patient subgroups. Finally, deployment concerns include minimal technical support, unclear model maintenance processes, and disclaimers of responsibility when models fail or produce unexpected results.

8.1.4   The Need for Developer-Clinician Collaboration

The evaluation framework presented in Tables 8.1 and 8.2 highlights a fundamental truth about AI in healthcare: successful implementation requires unprecedented collaboration between technical developers and clinical practitioners. Unlike previous generations of medical technology, where clinicians could evaluate devices based primarily on clinical outcomes, AI tools require assessment of complex statistical methodologies, data handling practices, and algorithmic design choices that may not be immediately apparent from clinical performance alone.

This collaboration must begin during the development phase, not after deployment. Clinicians must actively participate in defining clinically relevant outcomes, establishing appropriate validation protocols, and ensuring that model features align with real-world clinical workflows. Conversely, developers must embrace transparency, provide comprehensive documentation [193, 445], and design tools that enhance rather than replace clinical judgment.

The asymmetry of expertise between developers and clinicians creates particular challenges. While developers may excel at optimizing algorithmic performance, they often lack deep understanding of clinical contexts, temporal workflows, and the practical constraints of healthcare delivery. Clinicians, meanwhile, may struggle to evaluate complex statistical methodologies or identify subtle forms of data leakage that can invalidate model performance claims.

8.1.5   Addressing the Urgency of the Current Moment

The rapid expansion of machine learning in diagnostic applications has created a critical window where the standards and practices established today will shape the future of AI in healthcare. The current regulatory environment, while evolving, has not kept pace with technological innovation, leaving clinicians as the primary gatekeepers responsible for distinguishing between beneficial and harmful applications.

Several factors contribute to the urgency of establishing robust evaluation practices. First, the scale of AI deployment is accelerating rapidly, with hundreds of AI tools receiving regulatory clearance and thousands more operating in clinical settings without formal oversight. Second, the complexity of modern AI systems makes traditional clinical evaluation methods insufficient, requiring new frameworks that address algorithmic bias, data leakage, and generalizability concerns. Third, the potential for widespread harm from poorly validated tools means that individual adoption decisions can have population-level consequences.

The healthcare industry stands at a crossroads. The path forward requires clinicians to develop new competencies in AI evaluation while demanding unprecedented transparency from developers. The questions and frameworks presented here represent essential tools for navigating this transition, but they require widespread adoption and continuous refinement as the technology evolves.

Ultimately, the goal is not to slow AI adoption but to ensure that it proceeds safely and effectively. By establishing rigorous evaluation standards and fostering meaningful collaboration between developers and clinicians, the healthcare community can harness the transformative potential of artificial intelligence while maintaining the highest standards of patient care and safety.

8.2 Reporting Guidelines for Clinical AI

The TRIPOD+AI statement marks a significant milestone in the standardization of reporting for clinical prediction models that employ AI and ML techniques. Developed through an international, multi-expert consensus process, TRIPOD+AI updates and supersedes the original TRIPOD 2015 checklist, offering harmonized guidance for transparent reporting, regardless of whether regression modeling or machine learning methods are used [445]. This detailed framework aims to foster complete, accurate, and transparent reporting, thereby facilitating critical appraisal, model evaluation, and eventual implementation in clinical practice [445].

The TRIPOD+AI statement introduces a robust 27-item checklist that covers all critical aspects of AI-powered clinical research. These include:

- Model description: Detailed characterization of the model, including inputs, outputs, and rationale for its use.

- Data handling: Clear documentation of data sources, preparation, and representativeness.

- Training procedures: Explicit reporting of model development steps, including data splitting and hyperparameter tuning.

- Performance evaluation: Comprehensive reporting of metrics such as discrimination, calibration, and clinical utility, including subgroup analyses for fairness.

- Lifecycle maintenance: Guidance on model updating and monitoring post-deployment.

- Open science practices: Requirements for sharing protocols, data, and code.

- Patient and public involvement: Encouragement for incorporating diverse stakeholder perspectives.

A particularly notable innovation is the embedding of fairness considerations throughout the checklist, addressing algorithmic bias, data representativeness, and subgroup performance [445]. The guidelines also address open science, transparency, reproducibility, and equity in healthcare AI.

Despite its strengths, it is crucial to recognize that assessing training dynamics is not the primary focus of the TRIPOD+AI framework. TRI-POD+AI provides guidance on 'what' to report in AI studies, but it does not delve into the methodological details required to evaluate whether the AI models have been properly trained, whether overfitting or data leakage has occurred, or how learning curve behaviors should be interpreted. While the checklist includes items related to overfitting and underfitting, it stops short of offering clinicians and researchers the technical depth necessary for a critical evaluation of model development and training quality [445].

This distinction is of critical importance. A study can fully comply with TRIPOD+AI reporting guidelines and still present a fundamentally flawed model that suffers from overfitting, data leakage, or other training pathologies. Conversely, a study with modest documentation may contain a technically robust and clinically valuable model. In other words, excellent documentation cannot compensate for poor training dynamics, but proper evaluation of training dynamics can reveal the true clinical utility of AI tools, irrespective of how well the study is written.

8.2.1   The Critical Gap

For a comprehensive assessment of training dynamics, which is arguably 'more important' than ensuring polished documentation, readers should consult specialized resources. In this context, Chapter 3 of this book provides the necessary technical guidance for:

- Recognizing problematic learning curves and distinguishing healthy convergence from overfitting or underfitting.

- Detecting data leakage, both temporal and patient-level, through careful examination of workflow and data splitting.

- Understanding the implications of class imbalance and how it distorts standard metrics like accuracy.

- Interpreting performance metrics across training, validation, test, and external cohorts to assess generalization and real-world applicability.

Chapter 3 emphasizes that learning curves, subset-wise performance analysis, and rigorous reporting of training dynamics are indispensable for credible and clinically useful AI models. This technical evaluation is the only way to distinguish between models that truly generalize and those that merely memorize training data or exploit methodological shortcuts.

The optimal strategy for evaluating clinical AI research combines the comprehensive reporting requirements of TRIPOD+AI with the technical depth and practical diagnostics described in Chapter 3. TRIPOD+AI should be used for ensuring transparency and reproducibility, while the assessment of training dynamics ensures that the underlying machine learning methodology is robust, free from overfitting or leakage, and genuinely generalizable. This dual approach is essential for meeting the standards required for safe, effective, and equitable clinical implementation [445].

Hence, TRIPOD+AI represents a significant advance in the reporting standards for clinical AI, but it is not sufficient on its own. True model reliability, clinical safety, and trustworthiness require detailed assessment of training dynamics; an area covered in greater depth in Chapter 3 of this book. Only by mastering both transparent reporting and technical evaluation can the medical community ensure that AI models deliver on their promise without compromising patient safety or equity.

8.3 Becoming a Future-Ready Physician

The integration of ML and AI into medicine heralds a new era of diagnostic and therapeutic possibilities. However, the safe and effective use of these technologies requires clinicians to move beyond passive acceptance and become critical, informed evaluators of AI tools. As AI systems become increasingly embedded in clinical workflows, the role of the physician is evolving: from sole decision-maker to collaborative partner with digital systems. This transformation demands new competencies, a commitment to lifelong learning, and a willingness to engage with the ethical, technical, and practical challenges that AI introduces.

8.3.1 From Passive User to Critical Evaluator

To ensure that AI serves as a tool for enhancing, rather than undermining, patient care, clinicians must develop a foundational understanding of how these systems work, their limitations, and the potential risks they pose. This includes:

- Understanding Model Evaluation: Clinicians should be familiar with the basics of model validation, including the importance of external validation, the dangers of data leakage, and the interpretation of key performance metrics beyond simple accuracy (such as sensitivity, specificity, and F1 score).

- Recognizing Limitations and Bias: AI models are only as good as the data they are trained on. Clinicians must be vigilant for sources of bias, class imbalance, and lack of representativeness, and should demand transparency regarding how models were developed and validated.

- Demanding Transparency and Explainability: The ability to interpret and explain AI-driven recommendations is not a luxury but a necessity. Clinicians should advocate for tools that provide interpretable outputs and clear documentation of model updates and limitations.

- Identifying Red Flags: Vague or evasive answers from developers, lack of external validation, absence of subgroup performance metrics, or reliance on features unavailable at the time of prediction should all raise immediate concerns about the reliability of an AI tool.

The future-ready physician is not one who blindly trusts algorithms, but one who leverages them judiciously, always prioritizing patient safety, equity, and clinical judgment. This requires a commitment to ongoing education in digital health and AI, as well as active participation in interdisciplinary teams that include data scientists, engineers, and ethicists. By fostering a culture of collaboration and continuous learning, clinicians can help shape the responsible integration of AI into healthcare.

8.3.2 Actionable Steps for Clinicians

To become critically engaged and future-ready, clinicians should:

- Seek Education and Training: Participate in workshops, courses, and continuing medical education (CME) activities focused on AI, ML, and digital health.

- Engage with Developers: Collaborate with AI developers early in the design process to ensure that clinical workflows, relevant outcomes, and real-world constraints are incorporated into model development.

- Advocate for Standards: Support the adoption of standardized reporting guidelines (such as TRIPOD+AI) and demand adherence to best practices in model validation and transparency.

- Participate in Evaluation: Take an active role in the evaluation and selection of AI tools for clinical use, using structured frameworks and checklists to assess methodological rigor and operational readiness.

- Promote Equity and Fairness: Insist on the reporting of subgroup performance metrics and ongoing bias monitoring to ensure that AI tools do not exacerbate healthcare disparities.

- Maintain Clinical Judgment: Remember that AI is a tool to augment, not replace, clinical expertise. Final decisions should always be grounded in the clinician's knowledge of the patient and the broader clinical context

8.3.3 Shaping the Future of AI in Healthcare

The healthcare industry stands at a crossroads. The rapid expansion of AI in diagnostic and therapeutic applications has created a critical window where the standards and practices established today will shape the future of medicine. Clinicians are uniquely positioned to serve as gatekeepers, ensuring that only robust, validated, and equitable AI tools are integrated into patient care. By developing new competencies in AI evaluation, demanding transparency from developers, and fostering meaningful collaboration across disciplines, clinicians can help harness the transformative potential of artificial intelligence while maintaining the highest standards of patient care and safety.

Ultimately, the goal is not to slow AI adoption but to ensure that it proceeds safely, ethically, and effectively. The future-ready, critically engaged physician will be a leader in this transformation, leveraging AI to enhance patient outcomes, reduce disparities, and uphold the core values of medicine. Through ongoing education, critical engagement, and a steadfast commitment to patient-centered care, clinicians can help shape the responsible integration of AI into healthcare for generations to come.

Chapter 9

Practical Tools for Clinical AI Evaluation

This chapter provides practical, clinician-friendly tools to appraise AI and ML systems in healthcare. It complements the earlier chapters by translating concepts such as data leakage, generalization, external validation, fairness, calibration, and clinical utility into actionable checklists you can apply when reviewing papers, vendor materials, or internal development reports.

Practical steps for use:

– Define the clinical question and decision point (screening vs. confirmatory vs. monitoring).

– Gather the evidence packet: a methods section, data flow schematic, model documentation, performance tables, learning curves, and confusion matrices for test/external sets.

– Work through the two checklists in order. For each item, mark pass/fail/NA and add a short note.

– Triage outcomes: Green (most items pass, no critical red flags), Yellow (several gaps but remediable with additional evidence/analyses), Red (critical red flags such as leakage, no external validation, or missing confusion matrices).

– Where evidence is missing, request it explicitly from the developer or research team; document the response for governance and procurement.

9.1 Evaluation Checklists for Clinical ML

#	Training Feature	What to Look For	✓
Critical: Any single failure = Do not deploy			
1	Patient-level data splitting	For imaging: splitting done at patient level, not image level. Multiple images from same patient stay together	☐
2	Preprocessing after splitting	All normalization, feature selection, imputation, etc., performed after train/test split using only training data parameters; applied identically to validation/test sets	☐
3	Features available at prediction time	All input features must be available before the clinical decision point	☐
4	No post-diagnosis features used	Model doesn't use treatment codes, discharge summaries, or other post-decision information	☐
5	No label-derived features used	Features that are direct or indirect proxies for the outcome (e.g., discharge summary, treatment codes) are excluded; feature importance reviewed by clinical experts	☐
6	Temporal validity	Future information not used to predict past events	☐
Important: 1 failure = caution; >1 failures = Do not deploy			
7	Class imbalance properly addressed	If classes are imbalanced, appropriate techniques used and reported (not just overall accuracy)	☐
8	Cross-validation appropriately used	If used, k-fold CV respects patient boundaries and temporal ordering	☐
9	No data leakage indicators	Validation accuracy never exceeds training accuracy; no suspicious performance patterns	☐
Transparency: Missing evidence = request, but do not block deployment			
10	Multiple institutions involved	Training and/or validation performed across different clinical sites when possible	☐
11	External validation performed	Model tested on completely independent dataset from different institution/time period	☐
12	Class prevalence and distribution reported	Explicit reporting of class proportions in all splits (train, validation, test, external); confusion matrices provided for each	☐
13	Subgroup performance and fairness reported	Performance metrics stratified by demographics (age, race, gender, etc.) and fairness metrics (e.g., equal opportunity) to assess equity	☐
14	Explicit data leakage audit performed	Authors describe steps taken to check for and prevent all forms of data leakage (temporal, patient-level, preprocessing, label)	☐

Table 9.1: Checklist for Data Handling and Experimental Design in Clinical ML Studies, grouped by deployment criticality.

#	ML Training Feature	What to Look For	✓
Critical: Any single failure = Do not deploy			
15	Learning curves converge and plateau	Both training and validation curves should rise together and plateau at similar levels with a small, stable gap ($<10\%$)	☐
16	Proper curve order maintained	Training accuracy should be consistently above validation accuracy throughout training	☐
17	Performance trends are monotonic	Metrics should decrease gradually: Train > Validate > Test > External (no erratic jumps)	☐
18	Small generalization gap	Difference between training and test performance is modest ($<15\%$ points)	☐
Important: 1 failure = caution; >1 failures = Do not deploy			
19	Comprehensive metrics reported	Beyond accuracy: sensitivity, specificity, precision, recall, F1-score, and AUC all reported	☐
20	Confusion matrices provided	Full confusion matrices shown for test/external sets, revealing true positive/negative patterns	☐
21	Learning dynamics transparent	Full learning curves (not just final values) shown for both training and validation sets; convergence behavior discussed	☐
Transparency: Missing evidence = request, but do not block deployment			
22	Model architecture justified	Choice of algorithm explained based on data type and clinical context	☐
23	Hyperparameter tuning documented	Process for model optimization transparent, done only on training/validation sets	☐
24	Model calibration assessed	Calibration plots (e.g., reliability diagrams) provided; calibration metrics (e.g., Brier score) reported	☐
25	Decision threshold and clinical utility analysis	Threshold selection justified (e.g., maximizing F1, clinical utility, or cost-benefit); decision/utility curves provided if relevant	☐

Table 9.2: Checklist for Model Training and Reporting in Clinical ML Studies, grouped by deployment criticality.

The checklist in Table 9.1 is designed to help you rapidly assess whether a study's data pipeline and experimental design are fit for clinical use. Items are grouped by deployment criticality to make triage straightforward:

– Critical: any single failure means do not deploy.

– Important: one failure warrants caution; more than one failure means do not deploy.

– Transparency: missing evidence should be requested, but gaps alone should not block deployment if all critical and important items are sound.

How to use Table 9.1: Work through each row and mark the box ($\square$) as pass/fail/NA, adding a short note if needed.

- Pay special attention to rows 1–6 (patient-level splitting; preprocessing after splitting; features available at the decision time; no post-diagnosis or label-derived features; temporal validity). Any single failure here is a hard stop.

- For rows 7–9, verify that class imbalance is addressed beyond accuracy, cross-validation respects patient/time boundaries, and there are no leakage indicators (e.g., validation outperforming training).

- For rows 10–14, request the missing artifacts if not provided: multi-site involvement, external validation, class prevalence per split with confusion matrices, subgroup/fairness metrics, and an explicit leakage audit.

Document your findings and escalation steps (e.g., "Provide external-site confusion matrices and subgroup performance by age/sex/race before further consideration").

Similarly, Table 9.2 focuses on whether the model actually learned generalizable patterns and whether reporting enables clinical interpretation. As with Table 9.1, items are grouped by deployment criticality. How to use Table 9.2:

- Confirm healthy learning dynamics (rows 15–18): training and validation curves rising and plateauing together with a small, stable gap; training above validation throughout; performance that degrades gradually from Train $\rightarrow$ Validate $\rightarrow$ Test $\rightarrow$ External; and a modest generalization gap (<10-15 percentage points).

- Verify complete, clinically relevant reporting (rows 19–21): beyond accuracy (sensitivity, specificity, precision, recall, F1, AUC), confusion matrices for test/external sets, and the actual learning curves; not just final point estimates.

- Ensure transparency about the modeling choices and bedside use (rows 22–25): architecture justified for the data and task; hyperparameter tuning confined to training/validation; calibration assessed (plots and a metrics); decision thresholds justified for the clinical context, with utility/decision curves where appropriate.

– Record pass/fail/NA and request missing artifacts (e.g., "Share learning curves and reliability diagrams; provide external-set confusion matrices; explain threshold selection for screening vs. confirmatory use").

Typical red flags:
– Missing or inverted learning-curve order (validation above training), large or unstable gaps, or erratic subset-wise trends.

– Reporting only accuracy without confusion matrices and class-wise metrics.

– No calibration despite probability outputs guiding care pathways.

– Thresholds set to maximize a single metric without regard to clinical trade-offs.

9.2   Quick Triage for Busy Clinicians

Five-minute screen

Ask for: (1) dataflow diagram; (2) patient-level split confirmation; (3) test/external confusion matrices; (4) learning curves; (5) list of features available at prediction time only. If any are missing or problematic, pause adoption.

Deep dive

Walk through both checklists. Note failure points and send a consolidated query to the developer/researcher (e.g., "Please provide external-set confusion matrices and calibration plots; confirm temporal ordering; share subgroup metrics by age, sex, race, site.")

9.3   Discussion

Checklists increase consistency, transparency, and speed of evaluation, but they do not replace clinical judgment. Some high-value tools will initially lack ideal evidence (e.g., early external validation) yet may be piloted under governance, while others with impressive in-domain accuracy will fail due to leakage, poor calibration, or misaligned thresholds. Considerations:

- Context of use matters: Screening vs. diagnosis vs. monitoring require different thresholds and tolerance for false positives/negatives.

- Generalizability and equity: External validation across sites and demographics is essential to avoid performance cliffs and disparities in care.

- Lifecycle management: Commit to post-deployment monitoring, periodic revalidation, and change control; models and populations drift.

- Documentation and reproducibility: Insist on sufficient detail to reproduce training, splitting, preprocessing, and evaluation.

The safest and most clinically useful AI systems are built on sound data handling and transparent training dynamics. Learning curves, confusion matrices, calibration, and external validation together provide a realistic picture of performance. The two checklists in this chapter distill best practices into a repeatable evaluation process that clinicians, data scientists, and decision-makers can share. Use them to triage tools rapidly, focus requests on missing evidence, and guide responsible adoption.

Practical tips for physicians

- Always request: dataflow diagram, feature list limited to information available at prediction time, learning curves, test/external confusion matrices, calibration, subgroup metrics.

- Match thresholds to clinical intent (screening vs. diagnosis); one-size-fits-all thresholds are rarely appropriate.

- Prefer tools with prospective or external validation; pilot with governance if evidence is incomplete.

- Document every assumption and evidence gap; build a revalidation plan before deployment.

- Keep humans in the loop: Use AI to augment (not replace) clinical judgment, and align use with patient values and safety.

Bottom line: If the data pipeline is clean and the learning dynamics are healthy, the model is far likelier to help your patients. Use these checklists to make that determination clear, consistent, and defensible.

Bibliography

[1] Michael Matheny Sonoo Thadaney Israni, Mahnoor Ahmed, and Danielle Whicher. *Artificial Intelligence in Health Care: The Hope, the Hype, the Promise, the Peril.* NAM Special Publication. National Academy of Medicine, Washington, DC, 2019.

[2] Sali Abubaker Bagabir, Nahla Khamis Ibrahim, Hala Abubaker Bagabir, and Raghdah Hashem Ateeq. Covid-19 and artificial intelligence: Genome sequencing, drug development and vaccine discovery. *Journal of Infection and Public Health*, 15(2):289–296, February 2022. doi:10.1016/j.jiph.2022.01.011.

[3] Chris Giordano, Meghan Brennan, Basma Mohamed, Parisa Rashidi, François Modave, and Patrick Tighe. Accessing artificial intelligence for clinical decision-making. *Frontiers in Digital Health*, 3, June 2021. doi:10.3389/fdgth.2021.645232.

[4] Camillo Lamanna and Lauren Byrne. Should artificial intelligence augment medical decision making? the case for an autonomy algorithm. *AMA Journal of Ethics*, 20(9):E902–910, September 2018. doi:10.1001/amajethics.2018.902.

[5] Silvana Secinaro, Davide Calandra, Aurelio Secinaro, Vivek Muthurangu, and Paolo Biancone. The role of artificial intelligence in healthcare: a structured literature review. *BMC Medical Informatics and Decision Making*, 21(1), April 2021. doi:10.1186/s12911-021-01488-9.

[6] Mohammad Mohammad Amini, Marcia Jesus, Davood Fanaei Sheikholeslami, Paulo Alves, Aliakbar Hassanzadeh Benam, and Fatemeh Hariri. Artificial intelligence ethics and challenges in healthcare applications: A comprehensive review in the context of the european GDPR mandate. *Machine Learning and Knowledge Extraction*, 5(3):1023–1035, August 2023. doi:10.3390/make5030053.

[7] Lena Petersson, Ingrid Larsson, Jens M. Nygren, Per Nilsen, Margit Neher, Julie E. Reed, Daniel Tyskbo, and Petra Svedberg. Challenges to implementing artificial intelligence in healthcare: a qualitative interview study with healthcare leaders in sweden. *BMC Health Services Research*, 22(1), July 2022. doi:10.1186/s12913-022-08215-8.

[8] Shuroug A. Alowais, Sahar S. Alghamdi, Nada Alsuhebany, Tariq Alqahtani, Abdulrahman I. Alshaya, Sumaya N. Almohareb, Atheer Aldairem, Mohammed Alrashed, Khalid Bin Saleh, Hisham A. Badreldin, Majed S. Al Yami, Shmeylan Al Harbi, and Abdulkareem M. Albekairy. Revolutionizing healthcare: the role of

artificial intelligence in clinical practice. *BMC Medical Education*, 23(1), September 2023. doi:10.1186/s12909-023-04698-z.

[9] Vangelis D. Karalis. The integration of artificial intelligence into clinical practice. *Applied Biosciences*, 3(1):14–44, January 2024. doi:10.3390/applbiosci3010002.

[10] Alfonso Maria Ponsiglione, Paolo Zaffino, Carlo Ricciardi, Danilo Di Laura, Maria Francesca Spadea, Gianmaria De Tommasi, Giovanni Improta, Maria Romano, and Francesco Amato. Combining simulation models and machine learning in healthcare management: strategies and applications. *Progress in Biomedical Engineering*, 6(2):022001, February 2024. doi:10.1088/2516-1091/ad225a.

[11] Kathleen Murphy, Erica Di Ruggiero, Ross Upshur, Donald J. Willison, Neha Malhotra, Jia Ce Cai, Nakul Malhotra, Vincci Lui, and Jennifer Gibson. Artificial intelligence for good health: a scoping review of the ethics literature. *BMC Medical Ethics*, 22(1), February 2021. doi:10.1186/s12910-021-00577-8.

[12] Christina Silcox, Eyal Zimlichmann, Katie Huber, Neil Rowen, Robert Saunders, Mark McClellan, Charles N. Kahn, Claudia A. Salzberg, and David W. Bates. The potential for artificial intelligence to transform healthcare: perspectives from international health leaders. *npj Digital Medicine*, 7(1), April 2024. doi:10.1038/s41746-024-01097-6.

[13] Dezhi Mi, Yong Li, Kangying Zhang, Chaoni Huang, Wenjia Shan, and Jiangbo Zhang. Exploring intelligent hospital management mode based on artificial intelligence. *Frontiers in Public Health*, 11, August 2023. doi:10.3389/fpubh.2023.1182329.

[14] Irene Dankwa-Mullan. Health equity and ethical considerations in using artificial intelligence in public health and medicine. *Preventing Chronic Disease*, 21, August 2024. doi:10.5888/pcd21.240245.

[15] Stephanie B. Shamir, Arielle L. Sasson, Laurie R. Margolies, and David S. Mendelson. New frontiers in breast cancer imaging: The rise of AI. *Bioengineering*, 11(5):451, May 2024. doi:10.3390/bioengineering11050451.

[16] Nour Kenaan, George Hanna, Moustafa Sardini, Mhd Omar Iyoun, Khedr Layka, Zein Alabdin Hannouneh, and Zuheir Alshehabi. Advances in early detection of non-small cell lung cancer: A comprehensive review. *Cancer Medicine*, 13(18), September 2024. doi:10.1002/cam4.70156.

[17] Dan Zhao, Wei Wang, Tian Tang, Ying-Ying Zhang, and Chen Yu. Current progress in artificial intelligence-assisted medical image analysis for chronic kidney disease: A literature review. *Computational and Structural Biotechnology Journal*, 21:3315–3326, 2023. doi:10.1016/j.csbj.2023.05.029.

[18] Kit-Kay Mak, Yi-Hang Wong, and Mallikarjuna Rao Pichika. *Artificial Intelligence in Drug Discovery and Development*, pages 1–38. Springer International Publishing, 2023. doi:10.1007/978-3-030-73317-9_92-1.

[19] M. K. G. Abbas, Abrar Rassam, Fatima Karamshahi, Rehab Abunora, and Maha Abouseada. The role of AI in drug discovery. *ChemBioChem*, 25(14), June 2024. doi:10.1002/cbic.202300816.

[20] Amit Gangwal and Antonio Lavecchia. Unleashing the power of generative AI in drug discovery. *Drug Discovery Today*, 29(6):103992, June 2024. doi:10.1016/j.drudis.2024.103992.

[21] Catrin Hasselgren and Tudor I. Oprea. Artificial intelligence for drug discovery: Are we there yet? *Annual Review of Pharmacology and Toxicology*, 64(1):527–550, January 2024. doi:10.1146/annurev-pharmtox-040323-040828.

[22] Anita Ioana Visan and Irina Negut. Integrating artificial intelligence for drug discovery in the context of revolutionizing drug delivery. *Life*, 14(2):233, February 2024. doi:10.3390/life14020233.

[23] Ifra Saifi, Basharat Ahmad Bhat, Syed Suhail Hamdani, Umar Yousuf Bhat, Carlos Alberto Lobato-Tapia, Mushtaq Ahmad Mir, Tanvir Ul Hasan Dar, and Showkat Ahmad Ganie. Artificial intelligence and cheminformatics tools: a contribution to the drug development and chemical science. *Journal of Biomolecular Structure and Dynamics*, 42(12):6523–6541, July 2023. doi:10.1080/07391102.2023.2234039.

[24] Seoin Back, Alan Aspuru-Guzik, Michele Ceriotti, Ganna Gryn'ova, Bartosz Grzybowski, Geun Ho Gu, Jason Hein, Kedar Hippalgaonkar, Rodrigo Hormazabal, Yousung Jung, Seonah Kim, Woo Youn Kim, Seyed Mohamad Moosavi, Juhwan Noh, Changyoung Park, Joshua Schrier, Philippe Schwaller, Koji Tsuda, Tejs Vegge, O. Anatole von Lilienfeld, and Aron Walsh. Accelerated chemical science with AI. *Digital Discovery*, 3(1):23–33, 2024. doi:10.1039/d3dd00213f.

[25] Anna Cichonska, Balaguru Ravikumar, and Rayees Rahman. Ai for targeted polypharmacology The next frontier in drug discovery. *Current Opinion in Structural Biology*, 84:102771, February 2024. doi:10.1016/j.sbi.2023.102771.

[26] Anthony K. Cheetham and Ram Seshadri. Artificial intelligence driving materials discovery? perspective on the article: Scaling deep learning for materials discovery. *Chemistry of Materials*, 36(8):3490–3495, April 2024. doi:10.1021/acs.chemmater.4c00643.

[27] Renan Gonçalves Leonel da Silva. The advancement of artificial intelligence in biomedical research and health innovation: challenges and opportunities in emerging economies. *Globalization and Health*, 20(1), May 2024. doi:10.1186/s12992-024-01049-5.

[28] Gary Tom, Stefan P. Schmid, Sterling G. Baird, Yang Cao, Kourosh Darvish, Han Hao, Stanley Lo, Sergio Pablo-Garcia, Ella M. Rajaonson, Marta Skreta, Naruki Yoshikawa, Samantha Corapi, Gun Deniz Akkoc, Felix Strieth-Kalthoff, Martin Seifrid, and Alán Aspuru-Guzik. Self-driving laboratories for chemistry and materials science. *Chemical Reviews*, 124(16):9633–9732, August 2024. doi:10.1021/acs.chemrev.4c00055.

[29] Jia-Min Lu, Jian-Zhang Pan, Yi-Ming Mo, and Qun Fang. Automated intelligent platforms for high-throughput chemical synthesis. *Artificial Intelligence Chemistry*, 2(1):100057, June 2024. doi:10.1016/j.aichem.2024.100057.

[30] Feng Ren, Alex Aliper, Jian Chen, Heng Zhao, Sujata Rao, Christoph Kuppe, Ivan V. Ozerov, Man Zhang, Klaus Witte, Chris Kruse, Vladimir Aladinskiy, Yan Ivanenkov, Daniil Polykovskiy, Yanyun Fu, Eugene Babin, Junwen Qiao, Xing Liang, Zhenzhen Mou, Hui Wang, Frank W. Pun, Pedro Torres Ayuso, Alexander Veviorskiy, Dandan Song, Sang Liu, Bei Zhang, Vladimir Naumov, Xiaoqiang Ding, Andrey Kukharenko, Evgeny Izumchenko, and Alex Zhavoronkov. A small-molecule TNIK inhibitor targets fibrosis in preclinical and clinical models. *Nature Biotechnology*, March 2024. doi:10.1038/s41587-024-02143-0.

[31] Yi Shi. Drug development in the ai era: Alphafold 3 is coming! *The Innovation*, 5(5):100685, September 2024. `doi:10.1016/j.xinn.2024.100685`.

[32] Shiho Ohno, Noriyoshi Manabe, and Yoshiki Yamaguchi. Prediction of protein structure and ai. *Journal of Human Genetics*, 69(10):477–480, January 2024. `doi:10.1038/s10038-023-01215-4`.

[33] Miles McGibbon, Steven Shave, Jie Dong, Yumiao Gao, Douglas R Houston, Jiancong Xie, Yuedong Yang, Philippe Schwaller, and Vincent Blay. From intuition to ai: evolution of small molecule representations in drug discovery. *Briefings in Bioinformatics*, 25(1), November 2023. `doi:10.1093/bib/bbad422`.

[34] Xiangru Tang, Howard Dai, Elizabeth Knight, Fang Wu, Yunyang Li, Tianxiao Li, and Mark Gerstein. A survey of generative ai for de novo drug design: new frontiers in molecule and protein generation. *Briefings in Bioinformatics*, 25(4), May 2024. `doi:10.1093/bib/bbae338`.

[35] Mohamed Khalifa and Mona Albadawy. Artificial intelligence for clinical prediction: Exploring key domains and essential functions. *Computer Methods and Programs in Biomedicine Update*, 5:100148, 2024. `doi:10.1016/j.cmpbup.2024.100148`.

[36] Isabelle Ruchonnet-Metrailler, Johan N Siebert, Mary-Anne Hartley, and Laurence Lacroix. Automated interpretation of lung sounds by deep learning in children with asthma: Scoping review and strengths, weaknesses, opportunities, and threats analysis. *Journal of Medical Internet Research*, 26:e53662, August 2024. `doi:10.2196/53662`.

[37] Rejath Jose, Faiz Syed, Anvin Thomas, and Milan Toma. Cardiovascular health management in diabetic patients with machine-learning-driven predictions and interventions. *Applied Sciences*, 14(5):2132, March 2024. `doi:10.3390/app14052132`.

[38] Jung Sun Cho and Jae-Hyeong Park. Application of artificial intelligence in hypertension. *Clinical Hypertension*, 30(1), May 2024. `doi:10.1186/s40885-024-00266-9`.

[39] Shiva Maleki Varnosfaderani and Mohamad Forouzanfar. The role of ai in hospitals and clinics: Transforming healthcare in the 21st century. *Bioengineering*, 11(4):337, March 2024. `doi:10.3390/bioengineering11040337`.

[40] Valentina Bellini, Michele Russo, Tania Domenichetti, Matteo Panizzi, Simone Allai, and Elena Giovanna Bignami. Artificial intelligence in operating room management. *Journal of Medical Systems*, 48(1), February 2024. `doi:10.1007/s10916-024-02038-2`.

[41] Christina Zhu, Pradeep K. Attaluri, Peter J. Wirth, Ellen C. Shaffrey, Jeffrey B. Friedrich, and Venkat K. Rao. Current applications of artificial intelligence in billing practices and clinical plastic surgery. *Plastic and Reconstructive Surgery - Global Open*, 12(7):e5939, July 2024. `doi:10.1097/gox.0000000000005939`.

[42] Ali Ahmadi. Artificial intelligence revolution: A comprehensive review of its transformative impact on hospital data management in the future. *International Journal of BioLife Sciences (IJBLS)*, 3(3), October 2024. `doi:10.22034/ijbls.2024.199024`.

[43] Hans-Christoph Pape, Adam J. Starr, Boyko Gueorguiev, and Guido A. Wanner. The role of big data management, data registries, and machine learning algorithms

for optimizing safe definitive surgery in trauma: a review. *Patient Safety in Surgery,* 18(1), June 2024. doi:10.1186/s13037-024-00404-0.

[44] Nishita Kalra, Prachi Verma, and Surajpal Verma. Advancements in ai based healthcare techniques with focus on diagnostic techniques. *Computers in Biology and Medicine*, 179:108917, September 2024. doi:10.1016/j.compbiomed.2024. 108917.

[45] Esteban Zavaleta-Monestel, Ricardo Quesada-Villasenor, Sebastian Arguedas-Chacon, Jonathan Garcia-Montero, Monserrat Barrantes-Lopez, Juliana Salas-Segura, Adriana Anchia-Alfaro, Daniel Nieto-Bernal, and Daniel E Diaz-Juan. Revolutionizing healthcare: Qure.ai's innovations in medical diagnosis and treatment. *Cureus*, June 2024. doi:10.7759/cureus.61585.

[46] Shefali V Bhagat and Deepika Kanyal. Navigating the future: The transformative impact of artificial intelligence on hospital management- a comprehensive review. *Cureus*, February 2024. doi:10.7759/cureus.54518.

[47] Rawan Eskandarani, Ahmed Almuhainy, and Abdulrahman Alzahrani. Creating a master training rotation schedule for emergency medicine residents and challenges in using artificial intelligence. *International Journal of Emergency Medicine*, 17(1), July 2024. doi:10.1186/s12245-024-00657-7.

[48] Ciro Mennella, Umberto Maniscalco, Giuseppe De Pietro, and Massimo Esposito. Ethical and regulatory challenges of AI technologies in healthcare: A narrative review. *Heliyon*, 10(4):e26297, February 2024. doi:10.1016/j.heliyon.2024. e26297.

[49] Marie Geny, Emmanuel Andres, Samy Talha, and Bernard Geny. Liability of health professionals using sensors, telemedicine and artificial intelligence for remote healthcare. *Sensors*, 24(11):3491, May 2024. doi:10.3390/s24113491.

[50] Harish Padmanaban. Revolutionizing regulatory reporting through ai/ml: Approaches for enhanced compliance and efficiency. *Journal of Artificial Intelligence General science (JAIGS) ISSN:3006-4023*, 2(1):71–90, February 2024. doi:10.60087/jaigs.v2i1.98.

[51] Roy Snell. Meeting present and future challenges - how to build a more effective compliance department. *Journal of Health Care Compliance*, 26(4):17–22, Jul/Aug 2024.

[52] Abeer Malik and Barry Solaiman. *AI in hospital administration and management: ethical and legal implications*, pages 21–40. Edward Elgar Publishing, July 2024. doi:10.4337/9781802205657.00008.

[53] Vusumuzi Maphosa and Brighton Mpofu. An artificial intelligence-based random forest model for reducing prescription errors and improving patient safety. *SSRN Electronic Journal*, 2024. doi:10.2139/ssrn.4842105.

[54] Eun-Sung Kim. Can data science achieve the ideal of evidence-based decision-making in environmental regulation? *Technology in Society*, 78:102615, September 2024. doi:10.1016/j.techsoc.2024.102615.

[55] Mohit Lakkimsetti, Swati G Devella, Keval B Patel, Sarvani Dhandibhotla, Jasleen Kaur, Midhun Mathew, Janvi Kataria, Manisha Nallani, Umm E Farwa, Tirath Patel, Uzoamaka C Egbujo, Dakshin Meenashi Sundaram, Samar Kenawy, Mehak

Roy, and Saniyal Farheen Khan. Optimizing the clinical direction of artificial intelligence with health policy: A narrative review of the literature. *Cureus*, April 2024. doi:10.7759/cureus.58400.

[56] Francesco Chirico and Jaime A Teixeira da Silva. Evidence-based policies in public health to address COVID-19 vaccine hesitancy. *Future Virology*, 18(4):261–273, March 2023. doi:10.2217/fvl-2022-0028.

[57] Richard J. Chen, Judy J. Wang, Drew F. K. Williamson, Tiffany Y. Chen, Jana Lipkova, Ming Y. Lu, Sharifa Sahai, and Faisal Mahmood. Algorithmic fairness in artificial intelligence for medicine and healthcare. *Nature Biomedical Engineering*, 7(6):719–742, June 2023. doi:10.1038/s41551-023-01056-8.

[58] Margaret A. Goralski and Tay Keong Tan. *Artificial Intelligence: Poverty Alleviation, Healthcare, Education, and Reduced Inequalities in a Post-COVID World*, pages 97–113. Springer International Publishing, 2023. doi:10.1007/978-3-031-21147-8_6.

[59] E.-H. Kluge. The ethics of artificial intelligence in healthcare: From hands-on care to policy-making. *Healthcare Management Forum*, 37(5):406–408, May 2024. doi:10.1177/08404704241253985.

[60] Kavitha Palaniappan, Elaine Yan Ting Lin, and Silke Vogel. Global regulatory frameworks for the use of artificial intelligence (AI) in the healthcare services sector. *Healthcare*, 12(5):562, February 2024. doi:10.3390/healthcare12050562.

[61] Mohamed Khalifa and Mona Albadawy. Ai in diagnostic imaging: Revolutionising accuracy and efficiency. *Computer Methods and Programs in Biomedicine Update*, 5:100146, 2024. doi:10.1016/j.cmpbup.2024.100146.

[62] Heidi Lindroth, Keivan Nalaie, Roshini Raghu, Ivan N. Ayala, Charles Busch, Anirban Bhattacharyya, Pablo Moreno Franco, Daniel A. Diedrich, Brian W. Pickering, and Vitaly Herasevich. Applied artificial intelligence in healthcare: A review of computer vision technology application in hospital settings. *Journal of Imaging*, 10(4):81, March 2024. doi:10.3390/jimaging10040081.

[63] Francisca Chibugo Udegbe, Ogochukwu Roseline Ebulue, Charles Chukwudalu Ebulue, and Chukwunonso Sylvester Ekesiobi. AI's impact on personalized medicine: tailoring treatments for improved health outcomes. *Engineering Science & Technology Journal*, 5(4):1386–1394, April 2024. doi:10.51594/estj.v5i4.1040.

[64] Yu-Hao Li, Yu-Lin Li, Mu-Yang Wei, and Guang-Yu Li. Innovation and challenges of artificial intelligence technology in personalized healthcare. *Scientific Reports*, 14(1), August 2024. doi:10.1038/s41598-024-70073-7.

[65] Michela Ferrara, Giuseppe Bertozzi, Nicola Di Fazio, Isabella Aquila, Aldo Di Fazio, Aniello Maiese, Gianpietro Volonnino, Paola Frati, and Raffaele La Russa. Risk management and patient safety in the artificial intelligence era: A systematic review. *Healthcare*, 12(5):549, February 2024. doi:10.3390/healthcare12050549.

[66] Fatemeh Arjmandnia and Ehsan Alimohammadi. The value of machine learning technology and artificial intelligence to enhance patient safety in spine surgery: a review. *Patient Safety in Surgery*, 18(1), March 2024. doi:10.1186/s13037-024-00393-0.

[67] Rakibul Islam, Azrin Sultana, and Mohammad Rashedul Islam. A comprehensive review for chronic disease prediction using machine learning algorithms. *Journal of Electrical Systems and Information Technology*, 11(1), July 2024. doi:10.1186/s43067-024-00150-4.

[68] Yanzhen Liu, Xinbao Wu, Yudi Sang, Chunpeng Zhao, Yu Wang, Bojing Shi, and Yubo Fan. Evolution of surgical robot systems enhanced by artificial intelligence: A review. *Advanced Intelligent Systems*, 6(5), April 2024. doi:10.1002/aisy.202300268.

[69] Chi Zhang, M. Susan Hallbeck, Hojjat Salehinejad, and Cornelius Thiels. The integration of artificial intelligence in robotic surgery: A narrative review. *Surgery*, 176(3):552–557, September 2024. doi:10.1016/j.surg.2024.02.005.

[70] J. Everett Knudsen, Umar Ghaffar, Runzhuo Ma, and Andrew J. Hung. Clinical applications of artificial intelligence in robotic surgery. *Journal of Robotic Surgery*, 18(1), March 2024. doi:10.1007/s11701-024-01867-0.

[71] Tran Van Duong, Vu Pham Thao Vy, and Truong Nguyen Khanh Hung. Artificial intelligence in plastic surgery: Advancements, applications, and future. *Cosmetics*, 11(4):109, June 2024. doi:10.3390/cosmetics11040109.

[72] Ben Barris, Avrohom Karp, Menachem Jacobs, and William H. Frishman. Harnessing the power of AI: A comprehensive review of left ventricular ejection fraction assessment with echocardiography. *Cardiology in Review*, March 2024. doi:10.1097/crd.0000000000000691.

[73] Muhammad Ali Muzammil, Saman Javid, Azra Khan Afridi, Rupini Siddineni, Mariam Shahabi, Muhammad Haseeb, F.N.U. Fariha, Satesh Kumar, Sahil Zaveri, and Abdulqadir J. Nashwan. Artificial intelligence-enhanced electrocardiography for accurate diagnosis and management of cardiovascular diseases. *Journal of Electrocardiology*, 83:30–40, March 2024. doi:10.1016/j.jelectrocard.2024.01.006.

[74] Alexis Pengfei Zhao, Shuangqi Li, Zhidong Cao, Paul Jen-Hwa Hu, Jiaojiao Wang, Yue Xiang, Da Xie, and Xi Lu. Ai for science: Predicting infectious diseases. *Journal of Safety Science and Resilience*, 5(2):130–146, June 2024. doi:10.1016/j.jnlssr.2024.02.002.

[75] Chunhui Li, Guogio Ye, Yinghan Jiang, Zhiming Wang, Haiyang Yu, and Minghui Yang. Artificial intelligence in battling infectious diseases: A transformative role. *Journal of Medical Virology*, 96(1), January 2024. doi:10.1002/jmv.29355.

[76] Bradley J Langford, Westyn Branch-Elliman, Priya Nori, Alexandre R Marra, and Gonzalo Bearman. Confronting the disruption of the infectious diseases workforce by artificial intelligence: What this means for us and what we can do about it. *Open Forum Infectious Diseases*, 11(3), January 2024. doi:10.1093/ofid/ofae053.

[77] Md. Moradul Siddique, Md. Masrafi Bin Seraj, Md. Nasim Adnan, and Syed Md. Galib. *Artificial Intelligence for Infectious Disease Detection: Prospects and Challenges*, pages 1–22. Springer Nature Switzerland, 2024. doi:10.1007/978-3-031-59967-5_1.

[78] Amna Zar, Lubna Zar, Sara Mohsen, Yosra Magdi, and Susu M. Zughaier. *A Comprehensive Review of Algorithms Developed for Rapid Pathogen Detection and*

Surveillance, pages 23–49. Springer Nature Switzerland, 2024. `doi:10.1007/978-3-031-59967-5_2`.

[79] Geraldine A. Lynch, Nick A. Maskell, and Anna Bibby. Recent advances in mesothelioma. *Current Pulmonology Reports*, 13(3):256–265, May 2024. `doi:10.1007/s13665-024-00357-w`.

[80] Hyun Jae Kim, Nasim Parsa, and Michael F. Byrne. The role of artificial intelligence in colonoscopy. *Seminars in Colon and Rectal Surgery*, 35(1):101007, March 2024. `doi:10.1016/j.scrs.2024.101007`.

[81] Adriel Abraham, Rejath Jose, Jawad Ahmad, Jai Joshi, Thomas Jacob, Aziz-ur-rahman Khalid, Hassam Ali, Pratik Patel, Jaspreet Singh, and Milan Toma. Comparative analysis of machine learning models for image detection of colonic polyps vs. resected polyps. *Journal of Imaging*, 9(10):215, October 2023. `doi:10.3390/jimaging9100215`.

[82] Adarsh Mishra and Saima Aleem. Integration of artificial intelligence in hospital management systems: An overview. *SSRN Electronic Journal*, 2024. `doi:10.2139/ssrn.4838066`.

[83] Pouyan Esmaeilzadeh. Challenges and strategies for wide-scale artificial intelligence (AI) deployment in healthcare practices: A perspective for healthcare organizations. *Artificial Intelligence in Medicine*, 151:102861, May 2024. `doi:10.1016/j.artmed.2024.102861`.

[84] Sushant Kumar, Sumit Datta, Vishakha Singh, Sanjay Kumar Singh, and Ritesh Sharma. Opportunities and challenges in data-centric AI. *IEEE Access*, 12:33173–33189, 2024. `doi:10.1109/access.2024.3369417`.

[85] Ruth P. Evans, Louise D. Bryant, Gregor Russell, and Kate Absolom. Trust and acceptability of data-driven clinical recommendations in everyday practice: A scoping review. *International Journal of Medical Informatics*, 183:105342, March 2024. `doi:10.1016/j.ijmedinf.2024.105342`.

[86] Argyrios Perivolaris, Chris Adams-McGavin, Yasmine Madan, Teruko Kishibe, Tony Antoniou, Muhammad Mamdani, and James J. Jung. Quality of interaction between clinicians and artificial intelligence systems. a systematic review. *Future Healthcare Journal*, 11(3):100172, September 2024. `doi:10.1016/j.fhj.2024.100172`.

[87] Mary Nankya, Allan Mugisa, Yusuf Usman, Aadesh Upadhyay, and Robin Chataut. Security and privacy in e-health systems: A review of AI and machine learning techniques. *IEEE Access*, 2024. `doi:10.1109/access.2024.3469215`.

[88] Sandra Camacho Clavijo. AI assessment tools for decision-making on telemedicine: liability in case of mistakes. *Discover Artificial Intelligence*, 4(1), March 2024. `doi:10.1007/s44163-024-00117-4`.

[89] David B. Olawade, Aanuoluwapo C. David-Olawade, Ojima Z. Wada, Akinsola J. Asaolu, Temitope Adereni, and Jonathan Ling. Artificial intelligence in healthcare delivery: Prospects and pitfalls. *Journal of Medicine, Surgery, and Public Health*, 3:100108, August 2024. `doi:10.1016/j.glmedi.2024.100108`.

[90] Luis B. Elvas, Miguel Nunes, Joao C. Ferreira, and Berit Irene Helgheim. Hospital remote care assistance ai to reduce workload. *International Journal of Computer Information Systems and Industrial Management Applications*, 16(2):197–209, 2024.

[91] Sung Hyun Yoon, Sunyoung Park, Sowon Jang, Junghoon Kim, Kyung Won Lee, Woojoo Lee, Seungjae Lee, Gabin Yun, and Kyung Hee Lee. Use of artificial intelligence in triaging of chest radiographs to reduce radiologists' workload. *European Radiology*, 34(2):1094–1103, August 2023. doi:10.1007/s00330-023-10124-1.

[92] Dirk Hunstein, Lena Frischen, and Madlen Fiebig. *Development of a Data Model to Predict Nursing Workload Using Routine Clinical Data*. IOS Press, August 2024. doi:10.3233/shti240588.

[93] Nasrullah Abbasi and Hafiz Khawar Hussain. Integration of artificial intelligence and smart technology: AI-driven robotics in surgery: Precision and efficiency. *Journal of Artificial Intelligence General science (JAIGS) ISSN:3006-4023*, 5(1):381–390, August 2024. doi:10.60087/jaigs.v5i1.207.

[94] Phuoc Pham, Huilan Zhang, Wenlian Gao, and Xiaowei Zhu. Determinants and performance outcomes of artificial intelligence adoption: Evidence from U.S. hospitals. *Journal of Business Research*, 172:114402, February 2024. doi:10.1016/j.jbusres.2023.114402.

[95] Sabyasachi Pramanik. *AI-Powered Hospital Accounting: Towards Sound Financial Management*, pages 121–142. IGI Global, February 2024. doi:10.4018/979-8-3693-1561-3.ch005.

[96] Chun-You Chen, Ya-Lin Chen, Jeremiah Scholl, Hsuan-Chia Yang, and Yu-Chuan (Jack) Li. Ability of machine-learning based clinical decision support system to reduce alert fatigue, wrong-drug errors, and alert users about look alike, sound alike medication. *Computer Methods and Programs in Biomedicine*, 243:107869, January 2024. doi:10.1016/j.cmpb.2023.107869.

[97] Elizabeth A. Johnson, Katherine M. Dudding, and Jane M. Carrington. When to err is inhuman: An examination of the influence of artificial intelligence-driven nursing care on patient safety. *Nursing Inquiry*, 31(1), July 2023. doi:10.1111/nin.12583.

[98] Md Abu Sayem, Nazifa Taslima, Gursahildeep Singh Sidhu, and Dr. Jerry W. Ferry. A quantitative analysis of healthcare fraud and utilization of AI for mitigation. *International journal of business and management sciences*, 04(07):13–36, July 2024. doi:10.55640/ijbms-04-07-03.

[99] Zarif Bin Akhtar. The design approach of an artificial intelligent (ai) medical system based on electronical health records (ehr) and priority segmentations. *The Journal of Engineering*, 2024(4), April 2024. doi:10.1049/tje2.12381.

[100] Xu-Hui Li, Jian-Peng Liao, Mu-Kun Chen, Kuang Gao, Yong-Bo Wang, Si-Yu Yan, Qiao Huang, Yun-Yun Wang, Yue-Xian Shi, Wen-Bin Hu, and Ying-Hui Jin. The application of computer technology to clinical practice guideline implementation: A scoping review. *Journal of Medical Systems*, 48(1), December 2023. doi:10.1007/s10916-023-02007-1.

[101] N Rajesh Pandian and Meena Krishna. Real-time diagnostics with ai/ml: An assessment of its usefulness in smart health care. In *2023 2nd International Conference on Futuristic Technologies (INCOFT)*, pages 1–6. IEEE, November 2023. doi:10.1109/incoft60753.2023.10425316.

[102] Sahib Singh and Susheela Hooda. A study of challenges and limitations to applying machine learning to highly unstructured data. In *2023 7th International Conference*

On Computing, Communication, Control And Automation (ICCUBEA), volume 7, pages 1–6. IEEE, August 2023. doi:10.1109/iccubea58933.2023.10392115.

[103] Yanshan Wang, Shyam Visweswaran, Sumit Kapoor, Shravan Kooragayalu, and Xizhi Wu. ChatGPT-CARE: a superior decision support tool enhancing chatgpt with clinical practice guidelines. *medRxiv*, August 2023. doi:10.1101/2023.08.09.23293890.

[104] A.M. Arun Mohan, S. Senthil Kumar, Vamseedhar Annam, Mohit Yadav, and P Vishnu Prasanth. Role of AI (artificial intelligence) and machine learning in transforming operations in healthcare industry: An empirical study. *International Journal of Membrane Science and Technology*, 10(2):2069–2076, October 2023. doi:10.15379/ijmst.v10i2.2774.

[105] Sarah Jabbour, David Fouhey, Stephanie Shepard, Thomas S. Valley, Ella A. Kazerooni, Nikola Banovic, Jenna Wiens, and Michael W. Sjoding. Measuring the impact of AI in the diagnosis of hospitalized patients: A randomized clinical vignette survey study. *JAMA*, 330(23):2275, December 2023. doi:10.1001/jama.2023.22295.

[106] Nafiseh Ghaffar Nia, Erkan Kaplanoglu, and Ahad Nasab. Evaluation of artificial intelligence techniques in disease diagnosis and prediction. *Discover Artificial Intelligence*, 3(1), January 2023. doi:10.1007/s44163-023-00049-5.

[107] Jun Zhang, Jingyue Wu, Yiyi Qiu, Aiguo Song, Weifeng Li, Xin Li, and Yecheng Liu. Intelligent speech technologies for transcription, disease diagnosis, and medical equipment interactive control in smart hospitals: A review. *Computers in Biology and Medicine*, 153:106517, February 2023. doi:10.1016/j.compbiomed.2022.106517.

[108] Huda M. Alshanbari, Hasnain Iftikhar, Faridoon Khan, Moeeba Rind, Zubair Ahmad, and Abd Al-Aziz Hosni El-Bagoury. On the implementation of the artificial neural network approach for forecasting different healthcare events. *Diagnostics*, 13(7):1310, March 2023. doi:10.3390/diagnostics13071310.

[109] Amine En-Naaoui, Mohammed Kaicer, and Aicha Aguezzoul. A novel decision support system for proactive risk management in healthcare based on fuzzy inference, neural network and support vector machine. *International Journal of Medical Informatics*, 186:105442, June 2024. doi:10.1016/j.ijmedinf.2024.105442.

[110] Yagmur Yigit, Kubra Duran, Naghmeh Moradpoor, Leandros Maglaras, Nguyen Van Huynh, and Berk Canberk. *Machine Learning for Smart Healthcare Management Using IoT*, pages 135–166. Springer Nature Singapore, 2024. doi:10.1007/978-981-97-5624-7_4.

[111] Demet Topal Koç and Yeliz Mercan. *Artificial Intelligence and Digital Transformation in Healthcare Management*, pages 87–100. Emerald Publishing Limited, July 2023. doi:10.1108/978-1-83753-096-020231007.

[112] Alina Zhukovska, Tetiana Zheliuk, Dmytro Shushpanov, Vasyl Brych, Oleksandr Brechko, and Nataliia Kryvokulska. Management of the development of artificial intelligence in healthcare. In *2023 13th International Conference on Advanced Computer Information Technologies (ACIT)*, volume 2, pages 241–247. IEEE, September 2023. doi:10.1109/acit58437.2023.10275435.

[113] Michael Barnett, Dongang Wang, Heidi Beadnall, Antje Bischof, David Brunacci, Helmut Butzkueven, J. William L. Brown, Mariano Cabezas, Tilak Das, Tej Dugal, Daniel Guilfoyle, Alexander Klistorner, Stephen Krieger, Kain Kyle, Linda Ly, Lynette Masters, Andy Shieh, Zihao Tang, Anneke van der Walt, Kayla Ward, Heinz Wiendl, Gerg Zhan, Robert Zivadinov, Yael Barnett, and Chenyu Wang. A real-world clinical validation for AI-based MRI monitoring in multiple sclerosis. *npj Digital Medicine*, 6(1), October 2023. doi:10.1038/s41746-023-00940-6.

[114] Jonas Asgaard Bojsen, Mohammad Talal Elhakim, Ole Graumann, David Gaist, Mads Nielsen, Frederik Severin Gråe Harbo, Christian Hedeager Krag, Malini Verdela Sagar, Christina Kruuse, Mikael Ploug Boesen, and Benjamin Schnack Brandt Rasmussen. Artificial intelligence for MRI stroke detection: a systematic review and meta-analysis. *Insights into Imaging*, 15(1), June 2024. doi:10.1186/s13244-024-01723-7.

[115] Manuel A. Morales, Warren J. Manning, and Reza Nezafat. Present and future innovations in AI and cardiac MRI. *Radiology*, 310(1), January 2024. doi:10.1148/radiol.231269.

[116] Kain Kim, Samir C. Faruque, Shivani Lam, David Kulp, Xinwei He, Laurence S. Sperling and Danny J. Eapen. Implications of diagnosis through a machine learning algorithm on management of people with familial hypercholesterolemia. *JACC: Advances*, 3(9):101184, September 2024. doi:10.1016/j.jacadv.2024.101184.

[117] Md. Afroz, Emmanuel Nyakwende, and Birendra Goswami. Predictive analytics in oncology: A comprehensive study on lung cancer risk factors and machine learning model performance. In *2024 IEEE International Conference on Contemporary Computing and Communications (InC4)*, pages 1–7. IEEE, March 2024. doi:10.1109/inc460750.2024.10649176.

[118] Karuna Wongtangman, Boudewijn Aasman, Shweta Garg, Annika S. Witt, Arshia A. Harandi Omid Azimaraghi, Parsa Mirhaji, Selvin Soby, Preeti Anand, Carina P. Himes, Richard V. Smith, Peter Santer, Jeffrey Freda, Matthias Eikermann, and Priya Ramaswamy. Development and validation of a machine learning asa-score to identify candidates for comprehensive preoperative screening and risk stratification. *Journal of Clinical Anesthesia*, 87:111103, August 2023. doi:10.1016/j.jclinane.2023.111103.

[119] Michael D. Abramoff, Noelle Whitestone, Jennifer L. Patnaik, Emily Rich, Munir Ahmed, Lutful Husain, Mohammad Yeadul Hassan, Md. Sajidul Huq Tanjil, Dena Weitzman, Tinglong Dai, Brandie D. Wagner, David H. Cherwek, Nathan Congdon, and Khairul Islam. Autonomous artificial intelligence increases real-world specialist clinic productivity in a cluster-randomized trial. *npj Digital Medicine*, 6(1), October 2023. doi:10.1038/s41746-023-00931-7.

[120] Humaid Al Naqbi, Zied Bahroun, and Vian Ahmed. Enhancing work productivity through generative artificial intelligence: A comprehensive literature review. *Sustainability*, 16(3):1166, January 2024. doi:10.3390/su16031166.

[121] Anand E. Rajesh, Oliver Q. Davidson, Cecilia S. Lee, and Aaron Y. Lee. Artificial intelligence and diabetic retinopathy: Ai framework, prospective studies, head-to-head validation, and cost-effectiveness. *Diabetes Care*, 46(10):1728–1739, September 2023. doi:10.2337/dci23-0032.

[122] Kevin Zhai, Mohammad S. Yousef, Sawsan Mohammed, Nader I. Al-Dewik, and M. Walid Qoronfleh. Optimizing clinical workflow using precision medicine and advanced data analytics. *Processes*, 11(3):939, March 2023. doi:10.3390/pr11030939.

[123] Tesfamariam M Abuhay, Stewart Robinson, Adane Mamuye, and Sergey V Kovalchuk. Machine learning integrated patient flow simulation: why and how? *Journal of Simulation*, 17(5):580–593, May 2023. doi:10.1080/17477778.2023.2217334.

[124] Miguel Ortiz-Barrios, Sebastian Arias-Fonseca, Alessio Ishizaka, Maria Barbati, Betty Avendano-Collante, and Eduardo Navarro-Jimenez. Artificial intelligence and discrete-event simulation for capacity management of intensive care units during the Covid-19 pandemic: A case study. *Journal of Business Research*, 160:113806, May 2023. doi:10.1016/j.jbusres.2023.113806.

[125] Pramod Kumar Voola, Aravind Ayyagiri, Aravindsundeep Musunuri, Anshika Aggarwal, and Shalu Jain. Leveraging GenAI for clinical data analysis: Applications and challenges in real-time patient monitoring. *Modern Dynamics: Mathematical Progressions*, 1(2):204–223, August 2024. doi:10.36676/mdmp.v1.i2.21.

[126] Dinesh Mendhe, Akriti Dogra, Prabha Shreeraj Nair, S Punitha, K S Preetha, and S. B G Tilak Babu. AI-enabled data-driven approaches for personalized medicine and healthcare analytics. In *2024 Ninth International Conference on Science Technology Engineering and Mathematics (ICONSTEM)*, pages 1–5. IEEE, April 2024. doi:10.1109/iconstem60960.2024.10568722.

[127] James Van Yperen, Eduard Campillo-Funollet, Rebecca Inkpen, Anjum Memon, and Anotida Madzvamuse. A hospital demand and capacity intervention approach for COVID-19. *PLOS ONE*, 18(5):e0283350, May 2023. doi:10.1371/journal.pone.0283350.

[128] Teo Susnjak and Paula Maddigan. Forecasting patient demand at urgent care clinics using explainable machine learning. *CAAI Transactions on Intelligence Technology*, 8(3):712–733, July 2023. doi:10.1049/cit2.12258.

[129] Mariann Békésy. Forecasting patient arrival trends to the emergency department based on weather: A scoping review. In *2023 IEEE 21st Jubilee International Symposium on Intelligent Systems and Informatics (SISY)*, volume 33, pages 555–558. IEEE, September 2023. doi:10.1109/sisy60376.2023.10417922.

[130] Jing Wang, Yanbing Xiong, Qi Cai, Ying Wang, Lijing Du, and Kevin Xiong. *A Review of Epidemic Prediction and Control from a POM Perspective*, pages 734–744. Springer Nature Switzerland, 2023. doi:10.1007/978-3-031-36115-9_65.

[131] Mahesh Babu Mariappan, Kanniga Devi, Yegnanarayanan Venkataraman, Ming K. Lim, and Panneerselvam Theivendren. Using AI and ML to predict shipment times of therapeutics, diagnostics and vaccines in e-pharmacy supply chains during covid-19 pandemic. *The International Journal of Logistics Management*, 34(2):390–416, January 2022. doi:10.1108/ijlm-05-2021-0300.

[132] Abdulqadir J Nashwan and Ahmad A Abujaber. Nursing in the artificial intelligence (AI) era: Optimizing staffing for tomorrow. *Cureus*, October 2023. doi:10.7759/cureus.47275.

[133] Angelina R. Wilton, Katharine Sheffield, Quantia Wilkes, Sherry Chesak, Joel Pacyna, Richard Sharp, Paul E. Croarkin, Mohit Chauhan, Liselotte N. Dyrbye,

William V. Bobo, and Arjun P. Athreya. The Burnout PRedictiOn Using Wearable aNd ArtIficial IntelligEnce (BROWNIE) study: a decentralized digital health protocol to predict burnout in registered nurses. *BMC Nursing*, 23(1), February 2024. doi:10.1186/s12912-024-01711-8.

[134] Markus Bertl, Peeter Ross, and Dirk Draheim. Systematic AI support for decision-making in the healthcare sector: Obstacles and success factors. *Health Policy and Technology*, 12(3):100748, September 2023. doi:10.1016/j.hlpt.2023.100748.

[135] Rohan Khera, Atul J. Butte, Michael Berkwits, Yulin Hswen, Annette Flanagin, Hannah Park, Gregory Curfman, and Kirsten Bibbins-Domingo. AI in medicine–JAMA's focus on clinical outcomes, patient-centered care, quality, and equity. *JAMA*, 330(9):818, September 2023. doi:10.1001/jama.2023.15481.

[136] Aurelia Sauerbrei, Angeliki Kerasidou, Federica Lucivero, and Nina Hallowell. The impact of artificial intelligence on the person-centred, doctor-patient relationship: some problems and solutions. *BMC Medical Informatics and Decision Making*, 23(1), April 2023. doi:10.1186/s12911-023-02162-y.

[137] Emilie Cauet, Gabrielle Schittecatte, Marc Van Den Bulcke, Valentina Albarani, El Maati Allaoui, Helene Antoine-Poirel, Sarah Baatout, Glenn Broeckx, Marcela Chavez, Emmanuel Coche, Romaric Croes, Sofie De Broe, Pieter Demetter, Chloe De Witte, Louis Delsupehe, Frederik Deman, Amelie Dendooven, Jennifer Dhont, Gokhan Ertaylan, Thierry Gevaert, Stefan Gijssels, Koen Hasaers, Karin Haustermans, Rudy Hovelinck, Roland Hustinx, Sebastien Jodogne, Lies Lahousse, Steven Lauwers, Stephane Lejeune, Arthur Leloup, Evi Lippens, Benoit Macq, Brigitte Maes, Carlos Meca, Ward Rommel, Roberto Salgado, Bart Schelfhout, Wim Schreurs, Gwen Sys, Lien Van De Voorde, Isabelle Van Den Bulck, Johan Van Lint, Wim Van Roose, Kristel Van Steen, Ad Vandermeulen, Pieter-Jan Volders, and Suresh Yogeswaran. Policy brief belgian ebcp mirror group artificial intelligence in cancer care. *Archives of Public Health*, 82(S1), August 2024. doi:10.1186/s13690-024-01367-5.

[138] Filippo Lorè, Pierpaolo Basile, Annalisa Appice, Marco de Gemmis, Donato Malerba, and Giovanni Semeraro. An ai framework to support decisions on GDPR compliance. *Journal of Intelligent Information Systems*, 61(2):541–568, March 2023. doi:10.1007/s10844-023-00782-4.

[139] Marco Guevara, Shan Chen, Spencer Thomas, Tafadzwa L. Chaunzwa, Idalid Franco, Benjamin H. Kann, Shalini Moningi, Jack M. Qian, Madeleine Goldstein, Susan Harper, Hugo J. W. L. Aerts, Paul J. Catalano, Guergana K. Savova, Raymond H. Mak, and Danielle S. Bitterman. Large language models to identify social determinants of health in electronic health records. *npj Digital Medicine*, 7(1), January 2024. doi:10.1038/s41746-023-00970-0.

[140] Justyna Stypinska and Annette Franke. AI revolution in healthcare and medicine and the (re-)emergence of inequalities and disadvantages for ageing population. *Frontiers in Sociology*, 7, January 2023. doi:10.3389/fsoc.2022.1038854.

[141] Jon Rueda, Janet Delgado Rodriguez, Iris Parra Jounou, Joaquín Hortal-Carmona, Txetxu Ausin, and David Rodriguez-Arias. "just" accuracy? procedural fairness demands explainability in ai-based medical resource allocations. *AI & SOCIETY*, 39(3):1411–1422, December 2022. doi:10.1007/s00146-022-01614-9.

[142] Petra Apell and Henrik Eriksson. Artificial intelligence (AI) healthcare technology innovations: the current state and challenges from a life science industry perspective. *Technology Analysis & Strategic Management*, 35(2):179–193, September 2021. doi:10.1080/09537325.2021.1971188.

[143] Maryam Ramezani, Amirhossein Takian, Ahad Bakhtiari, Hamid R. Rabiee, Sadegh Ghazanfari, and Hakimeh Mostafavi. The application of artificial intelligence in health policy: a scoping review. *BMC Health Services Research*, 23(1), December 2023. doi:10.1186/s12913-023-10462-2.

[144] David O. Shumway and Hayes J. Hartman. Medical malpractice liability in large language model artificial intelligence: legal review and policy recommendations. *Journal of Osteopathic Medicine*, 124(7):287–290, January 2024. doi:10.1515/jom-2023-0229.

[145] Elarbi Badidi. Edge AI for early detection of chronic diseases and the spread of infectious diseases: Opportunities, challenges, and future directions. *Future Internet*, 15(11):370, November 2023. doi:10.3390/fi15110370.

[146] Nigam H. Shah, John D. Halamka, Suchi Saria, Michael Pencina, Troy Tazbaz, Micky Tripathi, Alison Callahan, Hailey Hildahl, and Brian Anderson. A nationwide network of health AI assurance laboratories. *JAMA*, 331(3):245, January 2024. doi:10.1001/jama.2023.26930.

[147] Alfred Addy, Johnson Mensah Sukah Selorm, Francis Mawunyo Ahotoh, Abraham Gborfuh, and George Benneh Mensah. Analysis of ghana's public health act 2012 and ai's role in augmenting vaccine supply and distribution challenges in ghana. *Journal of Law, Policy and Globalization*, 139, January 2024. doi:10.7176/jlpg/139-03.

[148] Sayash Kapoor and Arvind Narayanan. Leakage and the reproducibility crisis in machine-learning-based science. *Patterns*, 4(9):100804, September 2023. doi:10.1016/j.patter.2023.100804.

[149] Richard D Riley, Lucinda Archer, Kym I E Snell, Joie Ensor, Paula Dhiman, Glen P Martin, Laura J Bonnett, and Gary S Collins. Evaluation of clinical prediction models (part 2): how to undertake an external validation study. *BMJ*, page e074820, January 2024. doi:10.1136/bmj-2023-074820.

[150] Molly Bekbolatova, Jonathan Mayer, Chi Wei Ong, and Milan Toma. Transformative potential of AI in healthcare: Definitions, applications, and navigating the ethical landscape and public perspectives. *Healthcare*, 12(2):125, January 2024. doi:10.3390/healthcare12020125.

[151] Steven M. Williamson and Victor Prybutok. Balancing privacy and progress: A review of privacy challenges, systemic oversight, and patient perceptions in ai-driven healthcare. *Applied Sciences*, 14(2):675, January 2024. doi:10.3390/app14020675.

[152] Rajiv Avacharmal. Explainable AI: Bridging the gap between machine learning models and human understanding. *Journal of Informatics Education and Research*, 4(2), September 2024. doi:10.52783/jier.v4i2.960.

[153] Upol Ehsan and Mark O. Riedl. Explainability pitfalls: Beyond dark patterns in explainable AI. *Patterns*, 5(6):100971, June 2024. doi:10.1016/j.patter.2024.100971.

[154] L.E. Murray and M. Barnes. Policy brief: Proposal for a US-EU AI code of conduct, 2023. Available from https://www.ced.org/pdf/CED_Policy_Brief_US-EU_AI_Code_of_Conduct_FINAL.pdf, accessed on: May 22, 2025.

[155] Andrea Berber and Sanja Sreckovic. When something goes wrong: Who is responsible for errors in ML decision-making? *AI & Society*, 39(4):1891–1903, February 2023. doi:10.1007/s00146-023-01640-1.

[156] Tom Lawton, Philip Morgan, Zoe Porter, Shireen Hickey, Alice Cunningham, Nathan Hughes, Ioanna Iacovides, Yan Jia, Vishal Sharma, and Ibrahim Habli. Clinicians risk becoming "liability sinks" for artificial intelligence. *Future Healthcare Journal*, 11(1):100007, March 2024. doi:10.1016/j.fhj.2024.100007.

[157] Phillip Morgan. Chapter 6: Tort law and artificial intelligence - vicarious liability. In Ernest Lim and Phillip Morgan, editors, *The Cambridge Handbook of Private Law and Artificial Intelligence*. Cambridge University Press, Cambridge, 2024.

[158] Ryan Abbott. *The Reasonable Robot: Artificial Intelligence and the Law*. Cambridge University Press, Cambridge, 2020.

[159] Milan Toma, Faiz Syed, Lise McCoy, Michael Nizich, and William Blazey. Engineering in medicine: Bridging the cognitive and emotional distance between medical and non-medical students. *International Journal of Education in Mathematics, Science and Technology*, 12(1):99–113, October 2023. doi:10.46328/ijemst.3089.

[160] Michael Haenlein and Andreas Kaplan. A brief history of artificial intelligence: On the past, present, and future of artificial intelligence. *California Management Review*, 61(4):5–14, 2019. doi:10.1177/0008125619864925.

[161] L. Li, N. N. Zheng, and F. Y. Wang. On the crossroad of artificial intelligence: A revisit to alan turing and norbert wiener. *IEEE Transactions on Cybernetics*, 49(9):3618–3626, 2019. doi:10.1109/TCYB.2019.2922807.

[162] D. Monett, C. W. P. Lewis, K. R. Thórisson, J. Bach, G. Baldassarre, G. Granato, I. S. N. Berkeley, F. Chollet, M. Crosby, H. Shevlin, et al. Special issue "on defining artificial intelligence"—commentaries and author's response. *Journal of Artificial General Intelligence*, 11(2):1–100, 2020. doi:10.2478/jagi-2020-0002.

[163] Andre Esteva, Brett Kuprel, Roberto A. Novoa, Justin Ko, Susan M. Swetter, Helen M. Blau, and Sebastian Thrun. Dermatologist-level classification of skin cancer with deep neural networks. *Nature*, 542(7639):115–118, January 2017. doi:10.1038/nature21056.

[164] Alessandro Gasparetto and Luca Scalera. From the unimate to the delta robot: The early decades of industrial robotics. In Marco Ceccarelli, editor, *Explorations in the History and Heritage of Machines and Mechanisms*, pages 284–295. Springer International Publishing, Berlin/Heidelberg, Germany, 2018. doi:10.1007/978-3-319-93435-4_27.

[165] Heung-Yeung Shum, Xiaodong He, and Di Li. From eliza to xiaoice: Challenges and opportunities with social chatbots. *Frontiers of Information Technology & Electronic Engineering*, 19(1):10–26, 2018. doi:10.1631/FITEE.1700826.

[166] Benjamin Kuipers, Edward A. Feigenbaum, Peter E. Hart, and Nils J. Nilsson. Shakey: From conception to history. *AI Magazine*, 38(4):88–103, 2017. doi:10.1609/aimag.v38i4.2737.

[167] Adam Bohr and Kaveh Memarzadeh. The rise of artificial intelligence in healthcare applications. In Adam Bohr and Kaveh Memarzadeh, editors, *Artificial Intelligence in Healthcare*, pages 25–60. Elsevier, Amsterdam, The Netherlands, 2020. doi: 10.1016/B978-0-12-818438-7.00002-2.

[168] Casimir A. Kulikowski and Steven M. Weiss. Representation of expert knowledge for consultation: The casnet and expert projects. In Peter Szolovits, editor, *Artificial Intelligence In Medicine*, pages 21–55. Routledge, London, UK, 1982.

[169] H. Alder, B. A. Michel, C. Marx, G. Tamborrini, T. Langenegger, P. Bruehlmann, J. Steurer, and L. M. Wildi. Computer-based diagnostic expert systems in rheumatology: Where do we stand in 2014? *International Journal of Rheumatology*, 2014:672714, 2014. doi:10.1155/2014/672714.

[170] Eric I. George, Thomas C. Brand, Andrew LaPorta, Jacques Marescaux, and Richard M. Satava. Origins of robotic surgery: From skepticism to standard of care. *JSLS: Journal of the Society of Laparoendoscopic Surgeons*, 22(4):e2018.00039, 2018. doi:10.4293/JSLS.2018.00039.

[171] Vivek Kaul, Samuel Enslin, and Sachin A. Gross. History of artificial intelligence in medicine. *Gastrointestinal Endoscopy*, 92:807–812, 2020. doi:10.1016/j.gie.2020.06.040.

[172] M. Toma and R. Concu. Computational biology: A new frontier in applied biology. *Biology*, 10:374, 2021. doi:10.3390/biology10050374.

[173] M. Toma, S.K. Guru, W. Wu, M. Ali, and C.W. Ong. Addressing discrepancies between experimental and computational procedures. *Biology*, 10:536, 2021. doi:10.3390/biology10060536.

[174] A. Ramesh, C. Kambhampati, J. Monson, and P. Drew. Artificial intelligence in medicine. *Annals of the Royal College of Surgeons of England*, 86:334–338, 2004. doi:10.1308/147870804290.

[175] S. Roy, T. Meena, and S.J. Lim. Demystifying supervised learning in healthcare 4.0: A new reality of transforming diagnostic medicine. *Diagnostics*, 12:2549, 2022. doi:10.3390/diagnostics12102549.

[176] C. Anitescu, E. Atroshchenko, N. Alajlan, and T. Rabczuk. Artificial neural network methods for the solution of second order boundary value problems. *Computational Materials Continuum*, 59:345–359, 2019. doi:10.32604/cmc.2019.05861.

[177] J. Gu, Z. Wang, J. Kuen, L. Ma, A. Shahroudy, B. Shuai, T. Liu, X. Wang, G. Wang, J. Cai, et al. Recent advances in convolutional neural networks. *Pattern Recognition*, 77:354–377, 2018. doi:10.1016/j.patcog.2017.10.013.

[178] P. Ongsulee. Artificial intelligence, machine learning and deep learning. In *2017 15th International Conference on ICT and Knowledge Engineering (ICT & KE)*, pages 1–6, 2017. doi:10.1109/ICTKE.2017.8259629.

[179] D. Wang, Y. Zhang, K. Zhang, and L. Wang. Focalmix: Semi-supervised learning for 3d medical image detection. In *2020 IEEE/CVF Conference on Computer Vision and Pattern Recognition (CVPR)*, pages 3951–3960, 2020. doi:10.1109/CVPR42600.2020.00399.

[180] M. Lowe, R. Qin, and X. Mao. A review on machine learning, artificial intelligence, and smart technology in water treatment and monitoring. *Water*, 14(9):1384, 2022. doi:10.3390/w14091384.

[181] G. Yang, Q. Ye, and J. Xia. Unbox the black-box for the medical explainable ai via multi-modal and multi-centre data fusion: A mini-review, two showcases and beyond. *Information Fusion*, 77:29–52, 2022. doi:10.1016/j.inffus.2021.06.008.

[182] Y.K. Kim, J.H. Koo, S.J. Lee, H.S. Song, and M. Lee. Explainable artificial intelligence warning model using an ensemble approach for in-hospital cardiac arrest prediction: Retrospective cohort study. *Journal of Medical Internet Research*, 25:e48244, 2023. doi:10.2196/48244.

[183] F. Mohsen, B. Al-Saadi, N. Abdi, S. Khan, and Z. Shah. Artificial intelligence-based methods for precision cardiovascular medicine. *Journal of Personalized Medicine*, 13(8):1268, 2023. doi:10.3390/jpm13081268.

[184] N.C.d. Silva, M.K. Albertini, A.R. Backes, and G.d.G. Pena. Machine learning for hospital readmission prediction in pediatric population. *Computer Methods and Programs in Biomedicine*, 244:107980, 2024. doi:10.1016/j.cmpb.2023.107980.

[185] J.D. Fuhrman, N. Gorre, Q. Hu, H. Li, I.E. Naqa, and M.L. Giger. A review of explainable and interpretable ai with applications in covid-19 imaging. *Med. Phys.*, 49:1–14, 2021. doi:10.1002/mp.15253.

[186] M. Toma and O.C. Wei. Predictive modeling in medicine. *Encyclopedia*, 3:590–601, 2023. doi:10.3390/encyclopedia3020040.

[187] H. Nosrati and M. Nosrati. Artificial intelligence in regenerative medicine: Applications and implications. *Biomimetics*, 8:442, 2023. doi:10.3390/biomimetics8080442.

[188] D. Roosan, P. Padua, R. Khan, H. Khan, C. Verzosa, and Y. Wu. Effectiveness of chatgpt in clinical pharmacy and the role of artificial intelligence in medication therapy management. *J. Am. Pharm. Assoc.*, 2023. in press. doi:10.1016/j.japh.2023.06.012.

[189] S. Dayarathna, K.T. Islam, S. Uribe, G. Yang, M. Hayat, and Z. Chen. Deep learning based synthesis of mri, ct and pet: Review and analysis. *Med. Image Anal.*, 92:103046, 2024. doi:10.1016/j.media.2024.103046.

[190] C. Weng and J.R. Rogers. Ai uses patient data to optimize selection of eligibility criteria for clinical trials. *Nature*, 592:512–513, 2021. doi:10.1038/d41586-021-00999-2.

[191] C. Barbieri, L. Neri, S. Stuard, F. Mari, and J.D. Martín-Guerrero. From electronic health records to clinical management systems: How the digital transformation can support healthcare services. *Clin. Kidney J.*, 16:1878–1884, 2023. doi:10.1093/ckj/sfad181.

[192] B. Fuchs, G. Studer, B. Bode-Lesniewska, and P. Heesen. The next frontier in sarcoma care: Digital health, ai, and the quest for precision medicine. *J. Pers. Med.*, 13:1530, 2023. doi:10.3390/jpm13091530.

[193] Baptiste Vasey, Myura Nagendran, Bruce Campbell, David A Clifton, Gary S Collins, Spiros Denaxas, Alastair K Denniston, Livia Faes, Bart Geerts, Mudathir

Ibrahim, Xiaoxuan Liu, Bilal A Mateen, Piyush Mathur, Melissa D McCradden, Lauren Morgan, Johan Ordish, Campbell Rogers, Suchi Saria, Daniel S W Ting, Peter Watkinson, Wim Weber, Peter Wheatstone, and Peter McCulloch. Reporting guideline for the early stage clinical evaluation of decision support systems driven by artificial intelligence: Decide-ai. *BMJ*, page e070904, May 2022. URL: http://dx.doi.org/10.1136/bmj-2022-070904, doi:10.1136/bmj-2022-070904.

[194] M. Stasevych and V. Zvarych. Innovative robotic technologies and artificial intelligence in pharmacy and medicine: Paving the way for the future of health care—a review. *Big Data Cogn. Comput.*, 7:147, 2023. doi:10.3390/bdcc7040147.

[195] A. Philip, B. Samuel, S. Bhatia, S. Khalifa, and H. El-Seedi. Artificial intelligence and precision medicine: A new frontier for the treatment of brain tumors. *Life*, 13:24, 2022. doi:10.3390/life13010024.

[196] A. Shirazibeheshti, A. Ettefaghian, F. Khanizadeh, G. Wilson, T. Radwan, and C. Luca. Automated detection of patients at high risk of polypharmacy including anticholinergic and sedative medications. *Int. J. Environ. Res. Public Health*, 20:6178, 2023. doi:10.3390/ijerph20126178.

[197] L.L. Văduva, A.-M. Nedelcu, D. Stancu, C. Bălan, I.-M. Purcărea, M. Gurău, and D.A. Cristian. Digital technologies for public health services after the covid-19 pandemic: A risk management analysis. *Sustainability*, 15:3146, 2023. doi:10.3390/su15043146.

[198] B.I. Ciubotaru, G.V. Sasu, N. Goga, A. Vasilateanu, I. Marin, M. Goga, R. Popovici, and G. Datta. Prototype results of an internet of things system using wearables and artificial intelligence for the detection of frailty in elderly people. *Appl. Sci.*, 13:8702, 2023. doi:10.3390/app13148702.

[199] S. Sharma, R. Rawal, and D. Shah. Addressing the challenges of ai-based telemedicine: Best practices and lessons learned. *J. Educ. Health Promot.*, 12:338, 2023. doi:10.4103/jehp.jehp_1677_22.

[200] A. Amjad, P. Kordel, and G. Fernandes. A review on innovation in healthcare sector (telehealth) through artificial intelligence. *Sustainability*, 15:6655, 2023. doi:10.3390/su15086655.

[201] S. Singh, R. Kumar, S. Payra, and S.K. Singh. Artificial intelligence and machine learning in pharmacological research: Bridging the gap between data and drug discovery. *Cureus*, 15:e44359, 2023. doi:10.7759/cureus.44359.

[202] D.G. Poalelungi, C.L. Musat, A. Fulga, M. Neagu, A.I. Neagu, A.I. Piraianu, and I. Fulga. Advancing patient care: How artificial intelligence is transforming healthcare. *J. Pers. Med.*, 13:1214, 2023. doi:10.3390/jpm13071214.

[203] F. Aydin, O.T. Yildirim, A.H. Aydin, B. Murat, and C.H. Basaran. Comparison of artificial intelligence-assisted informed consent obtained before coronary angiography with the conventional method: Medical competence and ethical assessment. *Digital Health*, 9:20552076231218141, 2023. doi:10.1177/20552076231218141.

[204] W.H. Shrank, T.L. Rogstad, and N. Parekh. Waste in the us health care system. *JAMA*, 322:1501, 2019. doi:10.1001/jama.2019.13978.

[205] S.M. Erickson, B. Rockwern, M. Koltov, and R.M. McLean. Putting patients first by reducing administrative tasks in health care: A position paper of the

american college of physicians. *Annals of Internal Medicine*, 166:659, 2017 `doi:`
`10.7326/M16-2687`.

[206] T. Davenport and R. Kalakota. The potential for artificial intelligence in healthcare.
Future Healthcare Journal, 6:94–98, 2019. `doi:10.7861/futurehosp.6-2-94`.

[207] Y. Kaneda, M. Takita, T. Hamaki, A. Ozaki, and T. Tanimoto. Chatgpt's potential
in enhancing physician efficiency: A japanese case study. *Cureus*, 15:e48235, 2023.
`doi:10.7759/cureus.48235`.

[208] S.P. TerKonda, A.A. TerKonda, J.M. Sacks, B.M. Kinney, G.C. Gurtner, J.M.
Nachbar, S.K. Reddy, and L.L. Jeffers. Artificial intelligence: Singularity approaches.
Plastic and Reconstructive Surgery, 2023. publish ahead of print. `doi:10.1097/`
`PRS.0000000000010376`.

[209] A.S. Alzahrani, V. Gay, R. Alturki, and M.J. AlGhamdi. Towards understanding
the usability attributes of ai-enabled ehealth mobile applications. *Journal of
Healthcare Engineering*, 2021:5313027, 2021. `doi:10.1155/2021/5313027`.

[210] S.M. Tăranu, R. Ştefăniu, T. Ştefan Rotaru, A.M. Turcu, A.I. Pîslaru, I.A. Sandu,
A.M. Herghelegiu, G.I. Prada, I.D. Alexa, and A.C. Ilie. Factors associated
with burnout in medical staff: A look back at the role of the covid-19 pandemic.
Healthcare, 11:2533, 2023. `doi:10.3390/healthcare11182533`.

[211] C.P. West, L.N. Dyrbye, and T.D. Shanafelt. Physician burnout: Contributors,
consequences and solutions. *Journal of Internal Medicine*, 283:516–529, 2018.
`doi:10.1111/joim.12752`.

[212] T. Tajirian, V. Stergiopoulos, G. Strudwick, L. Sequeira, M. Sanches, J. Kemp,
K. Ramamoorthi, T. Zhang, and D. Jankowicz. The influence of electronic health
record use on physician burnout: Cross-sectional survey. *Journal of Medical
Internet Research*, 22(7):e19274, 2020. `doi:10.2196/19274`.

[213] P. Yu, H. Xu, X. Hu, and C. Deng. Leveraging generative ai and large language
models: A comprehensive roadmap for healthcare integration. *Healthcare*, 11:2776,
2023. `doi:10.3390/healthcare11192776`.

[214] P. Suryanarayanan, E.A. Epstein, A. Malvankar, B.L. Lewis, L. DeGenaro, J.J.
Liang, C.H. Tsou, and D. Pathak. Timely and efficient ai insights on ehr: Sys-
tem design. In *AMIA Annual Symposium Proceedings*, pages 1180–1189, 2020.
[PubMed].

[215] J.-a. Sim, X. Huang, M.R. Horan, C.M. Stewart, L.L. Robison, M.M. Hudson,
J.N. Baker, and I.-C. Huang. Natural language processing with machine learning
methods to analyze unstructured patient-reported outcomes derived from electronic
health records: A systematic review. *Artificial Intelligence in Medicine*, 146:102701,
2023. `doi:10.1016/j.artmed.2023.102701`.

[216] F. Yasmin, S.M.I. Shah, A. Naeem, S.M. Shujauddin, A. Jabeen, S. Kazmi, S.A.
Siddiqui, P. Kumar, S. Salman, S.A. Hassan, and et al. Artificial intelligence in the
diagnosis and detection of heart failure: The past, present, and future. *Reviews in
Cardiovascular Medicine*, 22:1095, 2021. `doi:10.31083/j.rcm2204105`.

[217] M. Toma, S. Singh-Gryzbon, E. Frankini, Z.A. Wei, and A.P. Yoganathan. Clinical
impact of computational heart valve models. *Materials*, 15:3302, 2022. `doi:`
`10.3390/ma15093302`.

[218] T.G. Myers, P.N. Ramkumar, B.F. Ricciardi, K.L. Urish, J. Kipper, and C. Ketonis. Artificial intelligence and orthopaedics. *Journal of Bone and Joint Surgery*, 102:830–840, 2020. doi:10.2106/JBJS.19.01205.

[219] V. Bagaria and A. Tiwari. Augmented intelligence in joint replacement surgery: How can artificial intelligence (ai) bridge the gap between the man and the machine? *Arthroplasty*, 4:4, 2022. doi:10.1186/s42836-022-00132-2.

[220] M. Cellina, M. Cè, N. Khenkina, P. Sinichich, M. Cervelli, V. Poggi, S. Boemi, A.M. Ierardi, and G. Carrafiello. Artificial intelligence in the era of precision oncological imaging. *Technology in Cancer Research & Treatment*, 21:153303382211417, 2022. doi:10.1177/15330338221141713.

[221] C. Frascarelli, G. Bonizzi, C.R. Musico, E. Mane, C. Cassi, E. Guerini Rocco, A. Farina, A. Scarpa, R. Lawlor, L. Reggiani Bonetti, and et al. Revolutionizing cancer research: The impact of artificial intelligence in digital biobanking. *Journal of Personalized Medicine*, 13:1390, 2023. doi:10.3390/jpm13081390.

[222] S. Huang, J. Yang, S. Fong, and Q. Zhao. Artificial intelligence in cancer diagnosis and prognosis: Opportunities and challenges. *Cancer Letters*, 471:61–71, 2020. doi:10.1016/j.canlet.2019.12.007.

[223] A. Fron, A. Semianiuk, U. Lazuk, K. Ptaszkowski, A. Siennicka, A. Lemiński, W. Krajewski, T. Szydełko, and B. Małkiewicz. Artificial intelligence in urooncology: What we have and what we expect. *Cancers*, 15:4282, 2023. doi:10.3390/cancers15174282.

[224] B. Bhinder, C. Gilvary, N.S. Madhukar, and O. Elemento. Artificial intelligence in cancer research and precision medicine. *Cancer Discovery*, 11:900–915, 2021. doi:10.1158/2159-8290.CD-20-1530.

[225] A. Grzybowski, P. Brona, G. Lim, P. Ruamviboonsuk, G.S.W. Tan, M. Abramoff, and D.S.W. Ting. Artificial intelligence for diabetic retinopathy screening: A review. *Eye*, 34:451–460, 2019. doi:10.1038/s41433-019-0547-y.

[226] D.S.W. Ting, L.R. Pasquale, L. Peng, J.P. Campbell, A.Y. Lee, R. Raman, G.S.W. Tan, L. Schmetterer, P.A. Keane, and T.Y. Wong. Artificial intelligence and deep learning in ophthalmology. *British Journal of Ophthalmology*, 103:167–175, 2018. doi:10.1136/bjophthalmol-2018-313173.

[227] J. Sumner, H.W. Lim, L.S. Chong, A. Bundele, A. Mukhopadhyay, and G. Kayambu. Artificial intelligence in physical rehabilitation: A systematic review. *Artificial Intelligence in Medicine*, 146:102693, 2023. doi:10.1016/j.artmed.2023.102693.

[228] R.A. Vulpoi, M. Luca, A. Ciobanu, A. Olteanu, O. Bărboi, D.E. Iov, L. Nichita, I. Ciortescu, C. Cijevschi Prelipcean, G. S, tefaňescu, and et al. The potential use of artificial intelligence in irritable bowel syndrome management. *Diagnostics*, 13:3336, 2023. doi:10.3390/diagnostics13183336.

[229] H.J. Kim, E.J. Gong, and C.S. Bang. Application of machine learning based on structured medical data in gastroenterology. *Biomimetics*, 8:512, 2023. doi:10.3390/biomimetics8080512.

[230] D. Gala and A.N. Makaryus. The utility of language models in cardiology: A narrative review of the benefits and concerns of chatgpt-4. *International Journal of Environmental Research and Public Health*, 20:6438, 2023. doi:10.3390/ijerph20156438.

[231] A. Salinari, M. Machì, Y. Armas Diaz, D. Cianciosi, Z. Qi, B. Yang, M.S. Ferreiro Cotorruelo, S.G. Vilar, L.A. Dzul Lopez, M. Battino, and et al. The application of digital technologies and artificial intelligence in healthcare: An overview on nutrition assessment. *Diseases*, 11:97, 2023. doi:10.3390/diseases11040097.

[232] K. Minamimura, K. Hara, S. Matsumoto, T. Yasuda, H. Arai, D. Kakinuma, Y. Ohshiro, Y. Kawano, M. Watanabe, H. Suzuki, and et al. Current status of robotic gastrointestinal surgery. *J. Nippon Med. Sch.*, 90:308–315, 2023. doi:10.1272/jnms.JNMS.2023_90-308.

[233] S.I. Ahmed, G. Javed, B. Mubeen, S.B. Bareeqa, H. Rasheed, A. Rehman, M.M. Phulpoto, S.S. Samar, and K. Aziz. Robotics in neurosurgery: A literature review. *J. Pak. Med. Assoc.*, 68:258–263, 2018.

[234] J.D. Opfermann, S. Leonard, R.S. Decker, N.A. Uebele, C.E. Bayne, A.S. Joshi, and A. Krieger. Semi-autonomous electrosurgery for tumor resection using a multi-degree of freedom electrosurgical tool and visual servoing. In *Proceedings of the 2017 IEEE/RSJ International Conference on Intelligent Robots and Systems (IROS)*, pages 2371–2378, Vancouver, BC, Canada, 2017. doi:10.1109/IROS.2017.8206062.

[235] A. Shademan, R.S. Decker, J.D. Opfermann, S. Leonard, A. Krieger, and P.C.W. Kim. Supervised autonomous robotic soft tissue surgery. *Sci. Transl. Med.*, 8:337ra64, 2016. doi:10.1126/scitranslmed.aad9398.

[236] M. Kam, H. Saeidi, S. Wei, J.D. Opfermann, S. Leonard, M.H. Hsieh, J.U. Kang, and A. Krieger. Semi-autonomous robotic anastomoses of vaginal cuffs using marker enhanced 3d imaging and path planning. In *Lecture Notes in Computer Science*, pages 65–73. Springer International Publishing, Berlin/Heidelberg, Germany, 2019. doi:10.1007/978-3-030-32254-0_8.

[237] M. Salman, T. Bell, J. Martin, K. Bhuva, R. Grim, and V. Ahuja. Use, cost, complications, and mortality of robotic versus nonrobotic general surgery procedures based on a nationwide database. *Am. Surg.*, 79:553–560, 2013. doi:10.1177/000313481307900606.

[238] H. Saeidi, J.D. Opfermann, M. Kam, S. Raghunathan, S. Leonard, and A. Krieger. A confidence-based shared control strategy for the smart tissue autonomous robot (star). In *Proceedings of the 2018 IEEE/RSJ International Conference on Intelligent Robots and Systems (IROS)*, pages 1–6, Madrid, Spain, 2018. doi:10.1109/IROS.2018.8594442.

[239] A.A. Gumbs, S. Ferretta, B. d'Allemagne, and E. Chouillard. What is artificial intelligence surgery? *Artif. Intell. Surg.*, 1:1–10, 2021. doi:10.1016/j.aisurg.2021.03.001.

[240] T. Tragaris, I.S. Benetos, J. Vlamis, and S. Pneumaticos. Machine learning applications in spine surgery. *Cureus*, 15:e48078, 2023. doi:10.7759/cureus.48078.

[241] W.G. Bradley. History of medical imaging. *Proc. Am. Philos. Soc.*, 152:349–361, 2008.

[242] M.L. Giger. Machine learning in medical imaging. *J. Am. Coll. Radiol.*, 15:512–520, 2018. doi:10.1016/j.jacr.2017.12.035.

[243] G.M. Currie. Intelligent imaging: Artificial intelligence augmented nuclear medicine. *J. Nucl. Med. Technol.*, 47:217–222, 2019. doi:10.2967/jnmt.119.227603.

[244] X. Tang. The role of artificial intelligence in medical imaging research. *BJR—Open*, 2:20190031, 2020. `doi:10.1259/bjro.20190031`.

[245] C. Liew. The future of radiology augmented with artificial intelligence: A strategy for success. *Eur. J. Radiol.*, 102:152–156, 2018. `doi:10.1016/j.ejrad.2018.03. 019`.

[246] S. Huang, J. Yang, S. Fong, and Q. Zhao. Artificial intelligence in the diagnosis of covid-19: Challenges and perspectives. *Int. J. Biol. Sci.*, 17:1581–1587, 2021. `doi:10.7150/ijbs.58830`.

[247] A. Shukla, U. Ramdasani, G. Vinzuda, M.S. Obaidat, S. Tanwar, and N. Kumar. Bcovx: Blockchain-based covid diagnosis scheme using chest x-ray for isolated location. In *Proceedings of the ICC 2021—IEEE International Conference on Communications*, pages 1–6, Montreal, QC, Canada, 2021. `doi:10.1109/ICC42927. 2021.9500747`.

[248] R. Najjar. Redefining radiology: A review of artificial intelligence integration in medical imaging. *Diagnostics*, 13:2760, 2023. `doi:10.3390/diagnostics13152760`.

[249] S.N. Qayyum. A comprehensive review of applications of artificial intelligence in echocardiography. *Curr. Probl. Cardiol.*, 49:102250, 2023. `doi:10.1016/j. cpcardiol.2023.102250`.

[250] L. Ledzinski and G. Grzesk. Artificial intelligence technologies in cardiology. *J. Cardiovasc. Dev. Dis.*, 10:202, 2023. `doi:10.3390/jcdd10040202`.

[251] J. Huang, X. Fan, and W. Liu. Applications and prospects of artificial intelligence-assisted endoscopic ultrasound in digestive system diseases. *Diagnostics*, 13:2815, 2023. `doi:10.3390/diagnostics13162815`.

[252] S. M. and V.K. Chattu. A review of artificial intelligence, big data, and blockchain technology applications in medicine and global health. *Big Data Cogn. Comput.*, 5:41, 2021. `doi:10.3390/bdcc5040041`.

[253] C. Lauri, F. Shimpo, and M.M. Sokołowski. Artificial intelligence and robotics on the frontlines of the pandemic response: The regulatory models for technology adoption and the development of resilient organisations in smart cities. *J. Ambient. Intell. Humaniz. Comput.*, 2023:1–12, 2023. `doi:10.1007/s12652-023-04567-2`.

[254] F.W. Pun, I.V. Ozerov, and A. Zhavoronkov. Ai-powered therapeutic target discovery. *Trends Pharmacol. Sci.*, 44:561–572, 2023. `doi:10.1016/j.tips.2023. 04.002`.

[255] E. Fountzilas, A.M. Tsimberidou, H.H. Vo, and R. Kurzrock. Clinical trial design in the era of precision medicine. *Genome Med.*, 14:101, 2022. `doi:10.1186/s13073-022-01109-2`.

[256] S. Shakibfar, F. Nyberg, H. Li, J. Zhao, H.M.E. Nordeng, G.K.F. Sandve, M. Pavlovic, M. Hajiebrahimi, M. Andersen, and M. Sessa. Artificial intelligence-driven prediction of covid-19-related hospitalization and death: A systematic review. *Front. Public Health*, 11:1183725, 2023. `doi:10.3389/fpubh.2023.1183725`.

[257] T.F. Tan, A.J. Thirunavukarasu, L. Jin, J. Lim, S. Poh, Z.L. Teo, M. Ang, R.V.P. Chan, J. Ong, A. Turner, and et al. Artificial intelligence and digital health in global eye health: Opportunities and challenges. *Lancet Glob. Health*, 11:e1432–e1443, 2023. `doi:10.1016/S2214-109X(23)00309-2`.

[258] D. Datta, S.G. Dalmida, L. Martinez, D. Newman, J. Hashemi, T.M. Khoshgoftaar, C. Shorten, C. Sareli, and P. Eckardt. Using machine learning to identify patient characteristics to predict mortality of in-patients with covid-19 in south florida. *Front. Digit. Health*, 5:1193467, 2023. `doi:10.3389/fdgth.2023.1193467`.

[259] L. Lösch, T. Zuiderent-Jerak, F. Kunneman, E. Syurina, M. Bongers, M.L. Stein, M. Chan, W. Willems, and A. Timen. Capturing emerging experiential knowledge for vaccination guidelines through natural language processing: A proof-of-concept study (preprint). *J. Med. Internet Res.*, 25:e44461, 2022. `doi:10.2196/44461`.

[260] P. Zhang and M.N. Kamel Boulos. Generative ai in medicine and healthcare: Promises, opportunities and challenges. *Future Internet*, 15:286, 2023. `doi:10.3390/fi15080286`.

[261] S.J. Hong and H. Cho. The role of uncertainty and affect in decision-making on the adoption of ai-based contact-tracing technology during the covid-19 pandemic. *Digit. Health*, 9:205520762311698, 2023. `doi:10.1177/20552076231169818`.

[262] D.K. Pasquale, W. Welsh, A. Olson, M. Yacoub, J. Moody, B.A.B. Gomez, K.L. Bentley-Edwards, J. McCall, M.L. Solis-Guzman, J.P. Dunn, and et al. Scalable strategies to increase efficiency and augment public health activities during epidemic peaks. *J. Public Health Manag. Pract.*, 2023. publish ahead of print. `doi:10.1097/PHH.0000000000001772`.

[263] M.H. Maras, M.D. Miranda, and A.S. Wandt. The use of covid-19 contact tracing app data as evidence of a crime. *Sci. Justice*, 63:158–163, 2023. `doi:10.1016/j.scijus.2023.01.003`.

[264] S. Barth, D. Ionita, and P. Hartel. Understanding online privacy—a systematic review of privacy visualizations and privacy by design guidelines. *ACM Comput. Surv.*, 55:1–37, 2022. `doi:10.1145/3491143`.

[265] G. Charkoftaki, R. Aalizadeh, A. Santos-Neto, W.Y. Tan, E.A. Davidson, V. Nikolopoulou, Y. Wang, B. Thompson, T. Furnary, Y. Chen, and et al. An ai-powered patient triage platform for future viral outbreaks using covid-19 as a disease model. *Hum. Genom.*, 17:80, 2023. `doi:10.1186/s40246-023-00541-2`.

[266] B. Hao, Y. Hu, S. Sotudian, Z. Zad, W.G. Adams, S.A. Assoumou, H. Hsu, R.G. Mishuris, and I.C. Paschalidis. Development and validation of predictive models for covid-19 outcomes in a safety-net hospital population. *J. Am. Med. Inform. Assoc.*, 29:1253–1262, 2022. `doi:10.1093/jamia/ocac089`.

[267] S.A. Wartman and C.D. Combs. Reimagining medical education in the age of ai. *AMA J. Ethics*, 21:146–152, 2019. `doi:10.1001/amajethics.2019.146`.

[268] E.R. Han, S. Yeo, M.J. Kim, Y.H. Lee, K.H. Park, and H. Roh. Medical education trends for future physicians in the era of advanced technology and artificial intelligence: An integrative review. *BMC Med. Educ.*, 19:460, 2019. `doi:10.1186/s12909-019-1891-5`.

[269] A.J. Buabbas, B Miskin, A.A. Alnaqi, A.K. Ayed, A.A. Shehab, S. Syed-Abdul, and M. Uddin. Investigating students' perceptions towards artificial intelligence in medical education. *Healthcare*, 11:1298, 2023. `doi:10.3390/healthcare11091298`.

[270] B.C. Dobey. Educating medical providers in the era of artificial intelligence. *J. Physician Assist. Educ.*, 34:168–170, 2023. `doi:10.1097/JPA.0000000000000487`.

[271] K.S. Chan and N. Zary. Applications and challenges of implementing artificial intelligence in medical education: Integrative review. *JMIR Med. Educ.*, 5:e13930, 2019. doi:10.2196/13930.

[272] Z.C. Lum. Can artificial intelligence pass the american board of orthopaedic surgery examination? orthopaedic residents versus chatgpt. *Clin. Orthop. Relat. Res.*, 481:1623–1630, 2023. doi:10.1097/CORR.0000000000002672.

[273] D. Qi, A. Ryason, N. Milef, S. Alfred, M.R. Abu-Nuwar, M. Kappus, S. De, and D.B. Jones. Virtual reality operating room with ai guidance: Design and validation of a fire scenario. *Surg. Endosc.*, 35:779–786, 2020. doi:10.1007/s00464-020-07913-2.

[274] I. Mese. The impact of artificial intelligence on radiology education in the wake of coronavirus disease 2019. *Korean J. Radiol.*, 24:478, 2023. doi:10.3348/kjr.2022.0792.

[275] J. Krive, M. Isola, L. Chang, T. Patel, M. Anderson, and R. Sreedhar. Grounded in reality: Artificial intelligence in medical education. *JAMIA Open*, 6:ooad037, 2023. doi:10.1093/jamiaopen/ooad037.

[276] E.A. Wood, B.L. Ange, and D.D. Miller. Are we ready to integrate artificial intelligence literacy into medical school curriculum: Students and faculty survey. *J. Med. Educ. Curric. Dev.*, 8:238212052110240, 2021. doi:10.1177/23821205211024043.

[277] B.S. Aylward, H. Abbas, S. Taraman, C. Salomon, D. Gal-Szabo, C. Kraft, L. Ehwerhemuepha, A. Chang, and D.P. Wall. An introduction to artificial intelligence in developmental and behavioral pediatrics. *J. Dev. Behav. Pediatr.*, 44:e126–e134, 2022. doi:10.1097/DBP.0000000000001172.

[278] F. Tustumi, N.A. Andreollo, and J.E. de Aguilar-Nascimento. Future of the language models in healthcare: The role of chatgpt. *ABCD. Arquivos Brasileiros de Cirurgia Digestiva (São Paulo)*, 36:e1727, 2023. doi:10.1590/0102-672020230002e1727.

[279] N. Naik, B.M.Z. Hameed, D.K. Shetty, D. Swain, M. Shah, R. Paul, K. Aggarwal, S. Ibrahim, V. Patil, K. Smriti, and et al. Legal and ethical consideration in artificial intelligence in healthcare: Who takes responsibility? *Front. Surg.*, 9:266, 2022. doi:10.3389/fsurg.2022.862322.

[280] D. Rao. The urgent need for healthcare workforce upskilling and ethical considerations in the era of ai-assisted medicine. *Indian J. Otolaryngol. Head Neck Surg.*, 75:2638–2639, 2023. doi:10.1007/s12070-023-03744-2.

[281] S. Reddy, S. Allan, S. Coghlan, and P. Cooper. A governance model for the application of ai in healthcare. *J. Am. Med. Inform. Assoc.*, 27:491–497, 2019. doi:10.1093/jamia/ocz192.

[282] D. Oniani, J. Hilsman, Y. Peng, R.K. Poropatich, J.C. Pamplin, G.L. Legault, and Y. Wang. Adopting and expanding ethical principles for generative artificial intelligence from military to healthcare. *Npj Digit. Med.*, 6:225, 2023. doi:10.1038/s41746-023-00961-2.

[283] W. Wang, L. Chen, M. Xiong, and Y. Wang. Accelerating ai adoption with responsible ai signals and employee engagement mechanisms in health care. *Inf. Syst. Front.*, 2021. doi:10.1007/s10796-021-10182-2.

[284] U. Sivarajah, Y. Wang, H. Olya, and S. Mathew. Responsible artificial intelligence (ai) for digital health and medical analytics. *Inf. Syst. Front.*, 25:2117–2122, 2023. doi:10.1007/s10796-023-10461-6.

[285] T. Siriborvornratanakul. Advanced artificial intelligence methods for medical applications. In *Digital Human Modeling and Applications in Health, Safety, Ergonomics and Risk Management*, pages 329–340. Springer Nature, Cham, Switzerland, 2023. doi:10.1007/978-3-031-35762-5_25.

[286] American Medical Association. Principles for augmented intelligence development, deployment, and use. Technical report, American Medical Association, Chicago, IL, USA, 2023.

[287] Z. Obermeyer, B. Powers, C. Vogeli, and S. Mullainathan. Dissecting racial bias in an algorithm used to manage the health of populations. *Science*, 366:447–453, 2019. doi:10.1126/science.aax2342.

[288] A.J. Larrazabal, N. Nieto, V. Peterson, D.H. Milone, and E. Ferrante. Gender imbalance in medical imaging datasets produces biased classifiers for computer-aided diagnosis. *Proc. Natl. Acad. Sci. USA*, 117:12592–12594, 2020. doi:10.1073/pnas.1919012117.

[289] Y.J. Juhn, E. Ryu, C.I. Wi, K.S. King, M. Malik, S. Romero-Brufau, C. Weng, S. Sohn, R.R. Sharp, and J.D. Halamka. Assessing socioeconomic bias in machine learning algorithms in health care: A case study of the houses index. *J. Am. Med. Inform. Assoc.*, 29:1142–1151, 2022. doi:10.1093/jamia/ocac073.

[290] A. De, A. Sarda, S. Gupta, and S. Das. Use of artificial intelligence in dermatology. *Indian J. Dermatol.*, 65:352, 2020. doi:10.4103/ijd.IJD_528_19.

[291] A. Kawsar, K. Hussain, D. Kalsi, P. Kemos, H. Marsden, and L. Thomas. Patient perspectives of artificial intelligence as a medical device in a skin cancer pathway. *Front. Med.*, 10:1259595, 2023. doi:10.3389/fmed.2023.1259595.

[292] R. Daneshjou, M.P. Smith, M.D. Sun, V. Rotemberg, and J. Zou. Lack of transparency and potential bias in artificial intelligence data sets and algorithms. *JAMA Dermatol.*, 157:1362, 2021. doi:10.1001/jamadermatol.2021.3129.

[293] H. Ejaz, H. McGrath, B.L. Wong, A. Guise, T. Vercauteren, and J. Shapey. Artificial intelligence and medical education: A global mixed-methods study of medical students' perspectives. *Digit. Health*, 8:205520762210890, 2022. doi:10.1177/20552076221089041.

[294] J. Bernal and C. Mazo. Transparency of artificial intelligence in healthcare: Insights from professionals in computing and healthcare worldwide. *Appl. Sci.*, 12:10228, 2022. doi:10.3390/app122010228.

[295] S. Larsson and F. Heintz. Transparency in artificial intelligence. *Internet Policy Rev.*, 9, 2020. doi:10.14763/2020.4.1510.

[296] L. Coventry and D. Branley. Cybersecurity in healthcare: A narrative review of trends, threats and ways forward. *Maturitas*, 113:48–52, 2018. doi:10.1016/j.maturitas.2018.04.008.

[297] B. Dash, M.F. Ansari, P. Sharma, and A. Ali. Threats and opportunities with ai-based cybersecurity intrusion detection: A review. *Int. J. Softw. Eng. Appl.*, 13:13–21, 2022. doi:10.21742/ijsea.2022.13.2.02.

[298] W. Ricciardi, P.P. Barros, A. Bourek, W. Brouwer, T. Kelsey, L. Lehtonen, C. Anastasy, P. Barros, M. Barry, A. Bourek, and et al. How to govern the digital transformation of health services. *Eur. J. Public Health*, 29:7–12, 2019. doi:10.1093/eurpub/ckz165.

[299] E. Biasin and E. Kamenjaševic. Cybersecurity of medical devices: New challenges arising from the ai act and nis 2 directive proposals. *Int. Cybersecur. Law Rev.*, 3:163–180, 2022. doi:10.1365/s43439-022-00061-2.

[300] J. Rickert. On patient safety: The lure of artificial intelligence—are we jeopardizing our patients' privacy? *Clin. Orthop. Relat. Res.*, 478:712–714, 2020. doi:10.1097/CORR.0000000000001178.

[301] M. Kayaalp. Patient privacy in the era of big data. *Balk. Med. J.*, 35:8–17, 2018. doi:10.4274/balkanmedj.2018.0023.

[302] S. Gao, L. He, Y. Chen, D. Li, and K. Lai. Public perception of artificial intelligence in medical care: Content analysis of social media. *J. Med. Internet Res.*, 22:e16649, 2020. doi:10.2196/16649.

[303] A. Tyson, G. Pasquini, A. Spencer, and C. Funk. 60% of americans would be uncomfortable with provider relying on ai in their own health care. Technical report, Pew Research Center, Washington, DC, USA, 2023.

[304] A. Spencer and C. Funk. Public trust in artificial intelligence varies by education and experience. *Pew Research Center*, 2023.

[305] C. Funk, A. Tyson, A. Spencer, and G. Pasquini. Americans' views on ai in health care: Concerns and opportunities. *Pew Research Center*, 2023.

[306] J. Wang, V. Ravi, and A. Alwan. Non-uniform speaker disentanglement for depression detection from raw speech signals. In *Proceedings of the INTERSPEECH 2023, Dublin, Ireland, 20–24 August 2023*, pages 2343–2347, 2023. doi:10.21437/Interspeech.2023-1462.

[307] A. Abd-alrazaq, R. AlSaad, M. Harfouche, S. Aziz, A. Ahmed, R. Damseh, and J. Sheikh. Wearable artificial intelligence for detecting anxiety: Systematic review and meta-analysis. *J. Med. Internet Res.*, 25:e48754, 2023. doi:10.2196/48754.

[308] V. Vo, G. Chen, Y.S.J. Aquino, S.M. Carter, Q.N. Do, and M.E. Woode. Multi-stakeholder preferences for the use of artificial intelligence in healthcare: A systematic review and thematic analysis. *Soc. Sci. Med.*, 338:116357, 2023. doi:10.1016/j.socscimed.2023.116357.

[309] O.E. Karpov, E.N. Pitsik, S.A. Kurkin, V.A. Maksimenko, A.V. Gusev, N.N. Shusharina, and A.E. Hramov. Analysis of publication activity and research trends in the field of ai medical applications: Network approach. *International Journal of Environmental Research and Public Health*, 20:5335, 2023. doi:10.3390/ijerph20075335.

[310] Ethan Goh, Robert Gallo, Jason Hom, Eric Strong, Yingjie Weng, Hannah Kerman, Joséphine A. Cool, Zahir Kanjee, Andrew S. Parsons, Neera Ahuja, Eric Horvitz, Daniel Yang, Arnold Milstein, Andrew P. J. Olson, Adam Rodman, and Jonathan H. Chen. Large language model influence on diagnostic reasoning: A randomized clinical trial. *JAMA Network Open*, 7(10):e2440969, October 2024. doi:10.1001/jamanetworkopen.2024.40969.

[311] Rohith Ravindranath, Joshua D. Stein, Tina Hernandez-Boussard, A. Caroline Fisher, Sophia Y. Wang, Sejal Amin, Paul A. Edwards, Divya Srikumaran, Fasika Woreta, Jeffrey S. Schultz, Anurag Shrivastava, Baseer Ahmad, Paul Bryar, Dustin French, Brian L. Vanderbeek, Suzann Pershing, Anne M. Lynch, Jennifer L. Patnaik, Saleha Munir, Wuqaas Munir, Joshua Stein, Lindsey DeLott, Brian C. Stagg, Barbara Wirostko, Brian McMillian, Arsham Sheybani, Soshian Sarrapour, Kristen Nwanyanwu, Michael Deiner, Catherine Sun, Houston: Robert Feldman, and Rajeev Ramachandran. The impact of race, ethnicity, and sex on fairness in artificial intelligence for glaucoma prediction models. *Ophthalmology Science*, 5(1):100596, January 2025. doi:10.1016/j.xops.2024.100596.

[312] U.S. Food and Drug Administration (FDA). Considerations for the use of artificial intelligence to support regulatory decision-making for drug and biological products. Technical report, U.S. Department of Health and Human Services, Food and Drug Administration, January 2025. Available from https://www.fda.gov/media/184830/download, accessed on: May 22, 2025.

[313] Qi An, Saifur Rahman, Jingwen Zhou, and James Jin Kang. A comprehensive review on machine learning in healthcare industry: Classification, restrictions, opportunities and challenges. *Sensors*, 23(9):4178, April 2023. doi:10.3390/s23094178.

[314] Antoine Decoux, Loic Duron, Paul Habert, Victoire Roblot, Emina Arsovic, Guillaume Chassagnon, Armelle Arnoux, and Laure Fournier. Comparative performances of machine learning algorithms in radiomics and impacting factors. *Scientific Reports*, 13(1), August 2023. doi:10.1038/s41598-023-39738-7.

[315] Yinan Huang, Jieni Li, Mai Li, and Rajender R. Aparasu. Application of machine learning in predicting survival outcomes involving real-world data: a scoping review. *BMC Medical Research Methodology*, 23(1), November 2023. doi:10.1186/s12874-023-02078-1.

[316] Md. Siraj-Ud Doulah and Md. Nazmul Islam. Performance evaluation of machine learning algorithm in various datasets. *Journal of Artificial Intelligence, Machine Learning and Neural Network*, 3(2):14–32, February 2023. doi:10.55529/jaimlnn.32.14.32.

[317] F. Pasa, V. Golkov, F. Pfeiffer, D. Cremers, and D. Pfeiffer. Efficient deep network architectures for fast chest x-ray tuberculosis screening and visualization. *Scientific Reports*, 9(1), April 2019. doi:10.1038/s41598-019-42557-4.

[318] Nguyen Van Thieu. Permetrics: A framework of performance metrics for machine learning models. *Journal of Open Source Software*, 9(95):6143, March 2024. doi:10.21105/joss.06143.

[319] Ross Upton, Angela Mumith, Arian Beqiri, Andrew Parker, William Hawkes, Shan Gao, Mihaela Porumb, Rizwan Sarwar, Patricia Marques, Deborah Markham, Jake Kenworthy, Jamie M. O'Driscoll, Neelam Hassanali, Kate Groves, Cameron Dockerill, William Woodward, Maryam Alsharqi, Annabelle McCourt, Edmund H. Wilkes, Stephen B. Heitner, Mrinal Yadava, David Stojanovski, Pablo Lamata, Gary Woodward, and Paul Leeson. Automated echocardiographic detection of severe coronary artery disease using artificial intelligence. *JACC: Cardiovascular Imaging*, 15(5):715–727, May 2022. doi:10.1016/j.jcmg.2021.10.013.

[320] Ying Guo, Chenxi Xia, You Zhong, Yiliang Wei, Huolan Zhu, Jianqiang Ma, Guang Li, Xuyang Meng, Chenguang Yang, Xiang Wang, and Fang Wang. Machine learning-enhanced echocardiography for screening coronary artery disease. *BioMedical Engineering OnLine*, 22(1), May 2023. doi:10.1186/s12938-023-01106-x.

[321] Manish Motwani, Damini Dey, Daniel S. Berman, Guido Germano, Stephan Achenbach, Mouaz H. Al-Mallah, Daniele Andreini, Matthew J. Budoff, Filippo Cademartiri, Tracy Q. Callister, Hyuk-Jae Chang, Kavitha Chinnaiyan, Benjamin J.W. Chow, Ricardo C. Cury, Augustin Delago, Millie Gomez, Heidi Gransar, Martin Hadamitzky, Joerg Hausleiter, Niree Hindoyan, Gudrun Feuchtner, Philipp A. Kaufmann, Yong-Jin Kim, Jonathon Leipsic, Fay Y. Lin, Erica Maffei, Hugo Marques, Gianluca Pontone, Gilbert Raff, Ronen Rubinshtein, Leslee J. Shaw, Julia Stehli, Todd C. Villines, Allison Dunning, James K. Min, and Piotr J. Slomka. Machine learning for prediction of all-cause mortality in patients with suspected coronary artery disease: a 5-year multicentre prospective registry analysis. *European Heart Journal*, page ehw188, June 2016. doi:10.1093/eurheartj/ehw188.

[322] Dongwoo Kang, Damini Dey, Piotr J. Slomka, Reza Arsanjani, Ryo Nakazato, Hyunsuk Ko, Daniel S. Berman, Debiao Li, and C.-C. Jay Kuo. Structured learning algorithm for detection of nonobstructive and obstructive coronary plaque lesions from computed tomography angiography. *Journal of Medical Imaging*, 2(1):014003, March 2015. doi:10.1117/1.jmi.2.1.014003.

[323] Kanako K Kumamaru, Shinichiro Fujimoto, Yujiro Otsuka, Tomohiro Kawasaki, Yuko Kawaguchi, Etsuro Kato, Kazuhisa Takamura, Chihiro Aoshima, Yuki Kamo, Yosuke Kogure, Hidekazu Inage, Hiroyuki Daida, and Shigeki Aoki. Diagnostic accuracy of 3d deep-learning-based fully automated estimation of patient-level minimum fractional flow reserve from coronary computed tomography angiography. *European Heart Journal - Cardiovascular Imaging*, June 2019. doi:10.1093/ehjci/jez160.

[324] Chad Hunter, Eric Moulton, Aun Yeong Chong, Rob Beanlands, and Robert deKemp. Deep learning improves diagnosis of obstructive cad using rb-82 pet imaging of myocardial blood flow. *Journal of Nuclear Medicine*, 65(supplement 2):241721, June 2024.

[325] Mei Zhou, Yongjian Deng, Yi Liu, Xiaolin Su, and Xiaocong Zeng. Echocardiography-based machine learning algorithm for distinguishing ischemic cardiomyopathy from dilated cardiomyopathy. *BMC Cardiovascular Disorders*, 23(1), September 2023. doi:10.1186/s12872-023-03520-4.

[326] Vanathi Gopalakrishnan, Prahlad G Menon, and Shobhit Madan. cmri-bed: A novel informatics framework for cardiac mri biomarker extraction and discovery applied to pediatric cardiomyopathy classification. *BioMedical Engineering OnLine*, 14(Suppl 2):S7, 2015. doi:10.1186/1475-925x-14-s2-s7.

[327] Caiwei Zhang, Junhao Qu, Weicheng Li, and Lehan Zheng. Predicting cardiovascular events by machine learning. *Journal of Physics: Conference Series*, 1693(1):012093, December 2020. doi:10.1088/1742-6596/1693/1/012093.

[328] Sourya Sengupta and Mark A. Anastasio. A test statistic estimation-based approach for establishing self-interpretable cnn-based binary classifiers. *IEEE Transactions on Medical Imaging*, 43(5):1753–1765, May 2024. doi:10.1109/tmi.2023.3348699.

[329] Ali Madani, Ramy Arnaout, Mohammad Mofrad, and Rima Arnaout. Fast and accurate view classification of echocardiograms using deep learning. *npj Digital Medicine*, 1(1), March 2018. doi:10.1038/s41746-017-0013-1.

[330] Akhil Narang, Richard Bae, Ha Hong, Yngvil Thomas, Samuel Surette, Charles Cadieu, Ali Chaudhry, Randolph P. Martin, Patrick M. McCarthy, David S. Rubenson, Steven Goldstein, Stephen H. Little, Roberto M. Lang, Neil J. Weissman, and James D. Thomas. Utility of a deep-learning algorithm to guide novices to acquire echocardiograms for limited diagnostic use. *JAMA Cardiology*, 6(6):624, June 2021. doi:10.1001/jamacardio.2021.0185.

[331] Ambarish Pandey, Nobuyuki Kagiyama, Naveena Yanamala, Matthew W. Segar, Jung S. Cho, Marton Tokodi, and Partho P. Sengupta. Deep-learning models for the echocardiographic assessment of diastolic dysfunction. *JACC: Cardiovascular Imaging*, 14(10):1887–1900, October 2021. doi:10.1016/j.jcmg.2021.04.010.

[332] Ahmed S. Fahmy, Ulf Neisius, Raymond H. Chan, Ethan J. Rowin, Warren J. Manning, Martin S. Maron, and Reza Nezafat. Three-dimensional deep convolutional neural networks for automated myocardial scar quantification in hypertrophic cardiomyopathy: A multicenter multivendor study. *Radiology*, 294(1):52–60, January 2020. doi:10.1148/radiol.2019190737.

[333] Iulian Emil Tampu, Anders Eklund, and Neda Haj-Hosseini. Inflation of test accuracy due to data leakage in deep learning-based classification of oct images. *Scientific Data*, 9(1), September 2022. doi:10.1038/s41597-022-01618-6.

[334] Jeffery T. Leek and Roger D. Peng. What is the question? *Science*, 347(6228):1314–1315, March 2015. doi:10.1126/science.aaa6146.

[335] Sharen Lee, Jiandong Zhou, Cheuk To Chung, Rebecca On Yu Lee, George Bazoukis, Konstantinos P Letsas, Wing Tak Wong, Ian Chi Kei Wong, Ngai Shing Mok, Tong Liu, Qingpeng Zhang, and Gary Tse. Comparing the performance of published risk scores in brugada syndrome: A multi-center cohort study. *Current Problems in Cardiology*, 47(12):101381, December 2022. doi:10.1016/j.cpcardiol.2022.101381.

[336] Bharath Ambale-Venkatesh, Xiaoying Yang, Colin O. Wu, Kiang Liu, W. Gregory Hundley, Robyn McClelland, Antoinette S. Gomes, Aaron R. Folsom, Steven Shea, Eliseo Guallar, David A. Bluemke, and Joao A.C. Lima. Cardiovascular event prediction by machine learning: The multi-ethnic study of atherosclerosis. *Circulation Research*, 121(9):1092–1101, October 2017. doi:10.1161/circresaha.117.311312.

[337] Haomin Chen, Catalina Gomez, Chien-Ming Huang, and Mathias Unberath. Explainable medical imaging ai needs human-centered design: guidelines and evidence from a systematic review. *npj Digital Medicine*, 5:156, October 2022. doi:10.1038/s41746-022-00699-2.

[338] Bobak J. Mortazavi, Emily M. Bucholz, Nihar R. Desai, Chenxi Huang, Jeptha P. Curtis, Frederick A. Masoudi, Richard E. Shaw, Sahand N. Negahban, and Harlan M. Krumholz. Comparison of machine learning methods with national cardiovascular data registry models for prediction of risk of bleeding after percutaneous coronary intervention. *JAMA Network Open*, 2(7):e196835, July 2019. doi:10.1001/jamanetworkopen.2019.6835.

[339] Anders Holt, Gunnar H Gislason, Morten Schou, Bochra Zareini, Tor Biering-Sørensen, Matthew Phelps, Kristian Kragholm, Charlotte Andersson, Emil L Fosbøl, Morten Lock Hansen, Thomas A Gerds, Lars Køber, Christian Torp-Pedersen, and Morten Lamberts. New-onset atrial fibrillation: incidence, characteristics, and related events following a national covid-19 lockdown of 5.6 million people. *European Heart Journal*, 41(32):3072–3079, June 2020. doi:10.1093/eurheartj/ehaa494.

[340] C H Hsu, Y L Chen, C H Hsieh, Y J Liang, S H Liu, and D Pei. Hemogram-based decision tree for predicting the metabolic syndrome and cardiovascular diseases in the elderly. *QJM: An International Journal of Medicine*, 114(6):363–373, June 2020. doi:10.1093/qjmed/hcaa205.

[341] June-Goo Lee, Jiyuon Ko, Hyeonyong Hae, Soo-Jin Kang, Do-Yoon Kang, Pil Hyung Lee, Jung-Min Ahn, Duk-Woo Park, Seung-Whan Lee, Young-Hak Kim, Cheol Whan Lee, Seong-Wook Park, and Seung-Jung Park. Intravascular ultrasound-based machine learning for predicting fractional flow reserve in intermediate coronary artery lesions. *Atherosclerosis*, 292:171–177, January 2020. doi:10.1016/j.atherosclerosis.2019.10.022.

[342] Yin-Hao Lee, Tsung-Hsien Tsai, Jun-Hong Chen, Chi-Jung Huang, Chern-En Chiang, Chen-Huan Chen, and Hao-Min Cheng. Machine learning of treadmill exercise test to improve selection for testing for coronary artery disease. *Atherosclerosis*, 340:23–27, January 2022. doi:10.1016/j.atherosclerosis.2021.11.028.

[343] Xiaobing Cheng, Weixing Han, Youfeng Liang, Xianhe Lin, Juanjuan Luo, Wansheng Zhong, and Dong Chen. Risk prediction of coronary artery stenosis in patients with coronary heart disease based on logistic regression and artificial neural network. *Computational and Mathematical Methods in Medicine*, 2022:1–8, March 2022. doi:10.1155/2022/3684700.

[344] Jin-Yu Sun, Yue Qiu, Hong-Cheng Guo, Yang Hua, Bo Shao, Yu-Cong Qiao, Jin Guo, Han-Lin Ding, Zhen-Ye Zhang, Ling-Feng Miao, Ning Wang, Yu-Min Zhang, Yan Chen, Juan Lu, Min Dai, Chang-Ying Zhang, and Ru-Xing Wang. A method to screen left ventricular dysfunction through ecg based on convolutional neural network. *Journal of Cardiovascular Electrophysiology*, 32(4):1095–1102, February 2021. doi:10.1111/jce.14936.

[345] Mohammad Mahbubur Rahman Khan Mamun and Tarek Elfouly. Detection of cardiovascular disease from clinical parameters using a one-dimensional convolutional neural network. *Bioengineering*, 10(7):796, July 2023. doi:10.3390/bioengineering10070796.

[346] Fariba Asadi, Reza Homayounfar, Yaser Mehrali, Chiara Masci, Samaneh Talebi, and Farid Zayeri. Detection of cardiovascular disease cases using advanced tree-based machine learning algorithms. *Scientific Reports*, 14(1), September 2024. doi:10.1038/s41598-024-72819-9.

[347] Andreas J. Morguet, Steffen Behrens, Olaf Kosch, Christine Lange, Markus Zabel, Daniela Selbig, Dieter L. Munz, Heinz-Peter Schultheiss, and Hans Koch. Myocardial viability evaluation using magnetocardiography in patients with coronary artery disease. *Coronary Artery Disease*, 15(3):155–162, May 2004. doi:10.1097/00019501-200405000-00004.

[348] Edward J. Ciaccio, Angelo B. Biviano, and Hasan Garan. The dominant morphology of fractionated atrial electrograms has greater temporal stability in persistent as compared with paroxysmal atrial fibrillation. *Computers in Biology and Medicine*, 43(12):2127–2135, December 2013. doi:10.1016/j.compbiomed.2013.08.027.

[349] Eka Miranda, Edy Irwansyah, Alowisius Y. Amelga, Marco M. Maribondang, and Mulyadi Salim. Detection of cardiovascular disease risk's level for adults using naive bayes classifier. *Healthcare Informatics Research*, 22(3):196, 2016. doi:10.4258/hir.2016.22.3.196.

[350] Zeyang Zhu, Wenyan Liu, Yang Yao, Xuewei Chen, Yingxian Sun, and Lisheng XU. Adaboost based ecg signal quality evaluation. In *2019 Computing in Cardiology Conference (CinC)*, CinC2019. Computing in Cardiology, December 2019. doi:10.22489/cinc.2019.151.

[351] Xiangkun Xie, Mingwei Yang, Shan Xie, Xiaoying Wu, Yuan Jiang, Zhaoyu Liu, Huiying Zhao, Yangxin Chen, Yuling Zhang, and Jingfeng Wang. Early prediction of left ventricular reverse remodeling in first-diagnosed idiopathic dilated cardiomyopathy: A comparison of linear model, random forest, and extreme gradient boosting. *Frontiers in Cardiovascular Medicine*, 8, August 2021. doi:10.3389/fcvm.2021.684004.

[352] Adindra Vickar Ega, Gigin Ginanjar, and Muhammad Azzumar. Monitoring and data acquisition of automated non-invasive blood pressure reading with esp32-cam and yolo algorithm. In *Proceedings of the 10th International Conference on Sustainable Energy Engineering and Application 2022 (ICSEEA2022)*, volume 3069, page 020114. AIP Publishing, 2024. doi:10.1063/5.0206265.

[353] W. H. Wolberg, W. N. Street, and O. L. Mangasarian. Image analysis and machine learning applied to breast cancer diagnosis and prognosis. *Analytical and Quantitative Cytology and Histology*, 17(2):77–87, 1995.

[354] J. W. Agar and G. I. Webb. Application of machine learning to a renal biopsy database. *Nephrology, Dialysis, Transplantation: Official Publication of the European Dialysis and Transplant Association - European Renal Association*, 7(6):472–478, 1992.

[355] W.Z. Liu, A.P. White, M.T. Hallissey, and J.W.L. Fielding. Machine learning techniques in early screening for gastric and oesophageal cancer. *Artificial Intelligence in Medicine*, 8(4):327–341, 1996. doi:10.1016/0933-3657(95)00039-9.

[356] Matjaz Kukar, Igor Kononenko, and Toma Silvester. Machine learning in prognosis of the femoral neck fracture recovery. *Artificial Intelligence in Medicine*, 8(5):431–451, 1996. doi:10.1016/s0933-3657(96)00351-x.

[357] Jorma Laurikkala and Martti Juhola. A genetic-based machine learning system to discover the diagnostic rules for female urinary incontinence. *Computer Methods and Programs in Biomedicine*, 55(3):217–228, 1998. doi:10.1016/s0169-2607(97)00067-9.

[358] W. R. Shankle, S. Mania, M. B. Dick, and M. J. Pazzani. Simple models for estimating dementia severity using machine learning. *Studies in Health Technology and Informatics*, 52(Pt 1):472–476, 1998.

[359] Hulin Kuang, Yahui Wang, Xianzhen Tan, Jialin Yang, Jiarui Sun, Jin Liu, Wu Qiu, Jingyang Zhang, Jiulou Zhang, Chunfeng Yang, Jianxin Wang, and Yang Chen. Lw-ctrans: A lightweight hybrid network of cnn and transformer for 3d medical image segmentation. *Medical Image Analysis*, 102:103545, 2025. doi:10.1016/j.media.2025.103545.

[360] Lin Zhang, Xinyu Guo, Hongkun Sun, Weigang Wang, and Liwei Yao. Alternate encoder and dual decoder cnn-transformer networks for medical image segmentation. *Scientific Reports*, 15(1), 2025. doi:10.1038/s41598-025-93353-2.

[361] Sanuwani Dayarathna, Kh Tohidul Islam, Sergio Uribe, Guang Yang, Munawar Hayat, and Zhaolin Chen. Deep learning based synthesis of mri, ct and pet: Review and analysis. *Medical Image Analysis*, 92:103046, 2024. doi:10.1016/j.media.2023.103046.

[362] Xuxin Chen, Ximin Wang, Ke Zhang, Kar-Ming Fung, Theresa C. Thai, Kathleen Moore, Robert S. Mannel, Hong Liu, Bin Zheng, and Yuchen Qiu. Recent advances and clinical applications of deep learning in medical image analysis. *Medical Image Analysis*, 79:102444, 2022. doi:10.1016/j.media.2022.102444.

[363] Marleen de Bruijne. Machine learning approaches in medical image analysis: From detection to diagnosis. *Medical Image Analysis*, 33:94–97, 2016. doi:10.1016/j.media.2016.06.032.

[364] Aaishwarya Sanjay Bajaj and Usha Chouhan. A review of various machine learning techniques for brain tumor detection from mri images. *Current Medical Imaging Formerly Current Medical Imaging Reviews*, 16(8):937–945, 2020. doi:10.2174/1573405615666190903144419.

[365] Adam Fauzi, Yuyun Yueniwati, Agus Naba, and Rachmi Fauziah Rahayu. Performance of deep learning in classifying malignant primary and metastatic brain tumors using different mri sequences: A medical analysis study. *Journal of X-Ray Science and Technology*, 31(5):893–914, 2023. doi:10.3233/xst-230046.

[366] Liwen Song, Chuanpu Li, Lilian Tan, Menghong Wang, Xiaqing Chen, Qiang Ye, Shisi Li, Rui Zhang, Qinghai Zeng, Zhuoyao Xie, Wei Yang, and Yinghua Zhao. A deep learning model to enhance the classification of primary bone tumors based on incomplete multimodal images in x-ray, ct, and mri. *Cancer Imaging*, 24(1), 2024. doi:10.1186/s40644-024-00784-7.

[367] JoonNyung Heo, Jihoon G. Yoon, Hyungjong Park, Young Dae Kim, Hyo Suk Nam, and Ji Hoe Heo. Machine learning–based model for prediction of outcomes in acute stroke. *Stroke*, 50(5):1263–1265, 2019. doi:10.1161/strokeaha.118.024293.

[368] Junzi Dong, Ting Feng, Binod Thapa-Chhetry, Byung Gu Cho, Tunu Shum, David P. Inwald, Christopher J. L. Newth, and Vinay U. Vaidya. Machine learning model for early prediction of acute kidney injury (aki) in pediatric critical care. *Critical Care*, 25(1), 2021. doi:10.1186/s13054-021-03724-0.

[369] Chip M. Lynch, Behnaz Abdollahi, Joshua D. Fuqua, Alexandra R. de Carlo, James A. Bartholomai, Rayeanne N. Balgemann, Victor H. van Berkel, and Hermann B. Frieboes. Prediction of lung cancer patient survival via supervised machine learning classification techniques. *International Journal of Medical Informatics*, 108:1–8, 2017. doi:10.1016/j.ijmedinf.2017.09.013.

[370] Abbas M. Hassan, Andrea Biaggi-Ondina, Aashish Rajesh, Malke Asaad, Jonas A. Nelson, J. Henk Coert, Babak J. Mehrara, and Charles E. Butler. Predicting patient-reported outcomes following surgery using machine learning. *The American Surgeon*, 89(1):31–35, 2022. doi:10.1177/00031348221109478.

[371] Timothy Zhang, Anton Nikouline, David Lightfoot, and Brodie Nolan. Machine learning in the prediction of trauma outcomes: A systematic review. *Annals of Emergency Medicine*, 80(5):440–455, 2022. doi:10.1016/j.annemergmed.2022.05.011.

[372] Samson J. Mataraso, Camilo A. Espinosa, David Seong, S. Momsen Reincke, Eloise Berson, Jonathan D. Reiss, Yeasul Kim, Marc Ghanem, Chi-Hung Shu, Tomin James, Yuqi Tan, Sayane Shome, Ina A. Stelzer, Dorien Feyaerts, Ronald J. Wong, Gary M. Shaw, Martin S. Angst, Brice Gaudilliere, David K. Stevenson, and Nima Aghaeepour. A machine learning approach to leveraging electronic health records for enhanced omics analysis. *Nature Machine Intelligence*, 7(2):293–306, 2025. doi:10.1038/s42256-024-00974-9.

[373] William Lotter, Abdul Rahman Diab, Bryan Haslam, Jiye G. Kim, Giorgia Grisot, Eric Wu, Kevin Wu, Jorge Onieva Onieva, Yun Boyer, Jerrold L. Boxerman, Meiyun Wang, Mack Bandler, Gopal R. Vijayaraghavan, and A. Gregory Sorensen. Robust breast cancer detection in mammography and digital breast tomosynthesis using an annotation-efficient deep learning approach. *Nature Medicine*, 27(2):244–249, 2021. doi:10.1038/s41591-020-01174-9.

[374] Nikos Tsiknakis, Dimitris Theodoropoulos, Georgios Manikis, Emmanouil Ktistakis, Ourania Boutsora, Alexa Berto, Fabio Scarpa, Alberto Scarpa, Dimitrios I. Fotiadis, and Kostas Marias. Deep learning for diabetic retinopathy detection and classification based on fundus images: A review. *Computers in Biology and Medicine*, 135:104599, 2021. doi:10.1016/j.compbiomed.2021.104599.

[375] Katharina Wenderott, Jim Krups, Fiona Zaruchas, and Matthias Weigl. Effects of artificial intelligence implementation on efficiency in medical imaging—a systematic literature review and meta-analysis. *npj Digital Medicine*, 7(1), 2024. doi:10.1038/s41746-024-01248-9.

[376] Luigi M Preti, Vittoria Ardito, Amelia Compagni, Francesco Petracca, and Giulia Cappellaro. Implementation of machine learning applications in health care organizations: Systematic review of empirical studies. *Journal of Medical Internet Research*, 26:e55897, 2024. doi:10.2196/55897.

[377] Isabelle Boutron, Matthew J Page, Julian PT Higgins, Douglas G Altman, Andreas Lundh, and Asbjørn Hrobjartsson. Considering bias and conflicts of interest among the included studies, 2019. doi:10.1002/9781119536604.ch7.

[378] Michał Paweł Wierzbicki, Barbara Anna Jantos, and Michał Tomaszewski. A review of approaches to standardizing medical descriptions for clinical entity recognition: Implications for artificial intelligence implementation. *Applied Sciences*, 14(21):9903, 2024. doi:10.3390/app14219903.

[379] Anmol Arora, Joseph E. Alderman, Joanne Palmer, Shaswath Ganapathi, Elinor Laws, Melissa D. McCradden, Lauren Oakden-Rayner, Stephen R. Pfohl, Marzyeh Ghassemi, Francis McKay, Darren Treanor, Negar Rostamzadeh, Bilal Mateen, Jacqui Gath, Adewole O. Adebajo, Stephanie Kuku, Rubeta Matin, Katherine

Heller, Elizabeth Sapey, Neil J. Sebire, Heather Cole-Lewis, Melanie Calvert, Alastair Denniston, and Xiaoxuan Liu. The value of standards for health datasets in artificial intelligence-based applications. *Nature Medicine*, 29(11):2929–2938, 2023. doi:10.1038/s41591-023-02608-w.

[380] Tai-Won Um, Jinsul Kim, Sunhwan Lim, and Gyu Myoung Lee. Trust management for artificial intelligence: A standardization perspective. *Applied Sciences*, 12(12):6022, 2022. doi:10.3390/app12126022.

[381] Daniel M. Goldenholz, Haoqi Sun, Wolfgang Ganglberger, and M. Brandon Westover. Sample size analysis for machine learning clinical validation studies. *Biomedicines*, 11(3):685, 2023. doi:10.3390/biomedicines11030685.

[382] Gazi Husain, Daniel Nasef, Rejath Jose, Jonathan Mayer, Molly Bekbolatova, Timothy Devine, and Milan Toma. Smote vs. smoteenn: A study on the performance of resampling algorithms for addressing class imbalance in regression models. *Algorithms*, 18(1):37, 2025. doi:10.3390/a18010037.

[383] International Council for Harmonisation of Technical Requirements for Pharmaceuticals for Human Use (ICH). Q13 continuous manufacturing of drug substances and drug products: Guidance for industry. Technical report, U.S. Department of Health and Human Services, Food and Drug Administration, Center for Drug Evaluation and Research (CDER), Center for Biologics Evaluation and Research (CBER), March 2023. Available from https://www.fda.gov/media/165775/download, accessed on: May 22, 2025.

[384] U.S. Food and Drug Administration (FDA), Center for Drug Evaluation and Research (CDER). Artificial intelligence in drug manufacturing: Discussion paper. Technical report, U.S. Department of Health and Human Services, Food and Drug Administration, Center for Drug Evaluation and Research, February 2023. Available from https://www.fda.gov/media/165743/download, accessed on: May 22, 2025.

[385] European Parliament and Council of the European Union. Regulation (eu) 2017/745 of the european parliament and of the council of 5 april 2017 on medical devices, amending directive 2001/83/ec, regulation (ec) no 178/2002 and regulation (ec) no 1223/2009 and repealing council directives 90/385/eec and 93/42/eec (text with eea relevance). Technical report, European Union, April 2017. Available from https://eur-lex.europa.eu/legal-content/EN/TXT/PDF/?uri=CELEX:32017R0745, accessed on: May 22, 2025.

[386] European Parliament and Council of the European Union. Regulation (eu) 2024/1689 of the european parliament and of the council of 13 june 2024 laying down harmonised rules on artificial intelligence and amending regulations (ec) no 300/2008, (eu) no 167/2013, (eu) no 168/2013, (eu) 2018/858, (eu) 2018/1139 and (eu) 2019/2144 and directives 2014/90/eu, (eu) 2016/797 and (eu) 2020/1828 (artificial intelligence act). Technical report, European Union, July 2024. Available from https://eur-lex.europa.eu/legal-content/EN/TXT/PDF/?uri=OJ:L_202401689, accessed on: May 22, 2025.

[387] World Health Organization (WHO). Ethics and governance of artificial intelligence for health: Who guidance. Technical report, World Health Organization, June 2021. Available from https://apps.who.int/iris/handle/10665/341996, accessed on: May 19, 2025.

[388] U.S. Food and Drug Administration (FDA), Health Canada, and Medicines and Healthcare products Regulatory Agency (MHRA). Good machine learning practice for medical device development: Guiding principles. Technical report, U.S. Food and Drug Administration (FDA), Health Canada, and MHRA, October 2021. Available from https://www.fda.gov/medical-devices/software-medical-device-samd/good-machine-learning-practice-medical-device-development-guiding-principles, accessed on: May 22, 2025.

[389] Beau Norgeot, Giorgio Quer, Brett K. Beaulieu-Jones, Ali Torkamani, Raquel Dias, Milena Gianfrancesco, Rima Arnaout, Isaac S. Kohane, Suchi Saria, Eric Topol, Ziad Obermeyer, Bin Yu, and Atul J. Butte. Minimum information about clinical artificial intelligence modeling: the mi-claim checklist. *Nature Medicine*, 26(9):1320–1324, 2020. doi:10.1038/s41591-020-1041-y.

[390] Xiaoxuan Liu, Samantha Cruz Rivera, David Moher, Melanie J. Calvert, Alastair K. Denniston, An-Wen Chan, Ara Darzi, Christopher Holmes, Christopher Yau, Hutan Ashrafian, Jonathan J. Deeks, Lavinia Ferrante di Ruffano, Livia Faes, Pearse A. Keane, Sebastian J. Vollmer, Aaron Y. Lee, Adrian Jonas, Andre Esteva, Andrew L. Beam, An-Wen Chan, Maria Beatrice Panico, Cecilia S. Lee, Charlotte Haug, Christopher J. Kelly, Christopher Yau, Cynthia Mulrow, Cyrus Espinoza, John Fletcher, Dina Paltoo, Elaine Manna, Gary Price, Gary S. Collins, Hugh Harvey, James Matcham, Joao Monteiro, M. Khair ElZarrad, Lavinia Ferrante di Ruffano, Luke Oakden-Rayner, Melissa McCradden, Pearse A. Keane, Richard Savage, Robert Golub, Rupa Sarkar, and Samuel Rowley. Reporting guidelines for clinical trial reports for interventions involving artificial intelligence: the consort-ai extension. *Nature Medicine*, 26(9):1364–1374, 2020. doi:10.1038/s41591-020-1034-x.

[391] Minh Long Hoang, Guido Matrella, and Paolo Ciampolini. Comparison of machine learning algorithms for heartbeat detection based on accelerometric signals produced by a smart bed. *Sensors*, 24(6):1900, 2024. doi:10.3390/s24061900.

[392] Daniel Nasef, Demarcus Nasef, Michael Sher, and Milan Toma. A standardized validation framework for clinically actionable healthcare machine learning with knee osteoarthritis grading as a case study. *Algorithms*, 18(6):343, 2025. doi:10.3390/a18060343.

[393] Panagiotis Tziachris, Melpomeni Nikou, Vassilis Aschonitis, Andreas Kallioras, Katerina Sachsamanoglou, Maria Dolores Fidelibus, and Evangelos Tziritis. Spatial or random cross-validation? the effect of resampling methods in predicting groundwater salinity with machine learning in mediterranean region. *Water*, 15(12):2278, 2023. doi:10.3390/w15122278.

[394] Kwok Sun Cheng, Pei-Chi Huang, Tae-Hyuk Ahn, and Myoungkyu Song. Tool support for improving software quality in machine learning programs. *Information*, 14(1):53, 2023. doi:10.3390/info14010053.

[395] Daniel Nasef, Demarcus Nasef, Viola Sawiris, Peter Girgis, and Milan Toma. Deep learning for automated kellgren–lawrence grading in knee osteoarthritis severity assessment. *Surgeries*, 6(1):3, 2024. doi:10.3390/surgeries6010003.

[396] Hafiz Nouman Ahmad. Annotated dataset for knee arthritis detection, 2023. Avaliable from https://www.kaggle.com/datasets/hafiznouman786/annotated-dataset-for-knee-arthritis-detection/, accessed on May 22, 2025.

[397] Pingjun Chen. Knee osteoarthritis severity grading dataset, 2018. Avaliable from `https://data.mendeley.com/datasets/56rmx5bjcr/1`, accessed on May 22, 2025. `doi:10.17632/56RMX5BJCR.1.`

[398] Lionel Chong, Gazi Husain, Daniel Nasef, Prince Vathappallil, Mihir Matalia, and Milan Toma. Machine learning strategies for improved cardiovascular disease detection. *Medical Research Archives*, 13(1), 2025. `doi:10.18103/mra.v13i1.6245.`

[399] David Remyes, Daniel Nasef, Sarah Remyes, Joseph Tawfellos, Michael Sher, Demarcus Nasef, and Milan Toma. Clinical applicability and cross-dataset validation of machine learning models for binary glaucoma detection. *Information*, 16(6):432, 2025. `doi:10.3390/info16060432.`

[400] Rejath Jose, Nicholas Lewis, Zain Satti, Robert Steinberg, Alec Toufexis, Daniel Nasef, and Milan Toma. Machine-learning-based diagnosis and progression analysis of knee osteoarthritis. *Discover Data*, 3(1), 2025. `doi:10.1007/s44248-025-00026-6.`

[401] Xing Xing, Yining Wang, Jianan Zhu, Ziyuan Shen, Flavia Cicuttini, Graeme Jones, Dawn Aitken, and Guoqi Cai. Predictive validity of consensus-based mri definition of osteoarthritis plus radiographic osteoarthritis for the progression of knee osteoarthritis: A longitudinal cohort study. *Osteoarthritis and Cartilage Open*, 7(2):100582, 2025. `doi:10.1016/j.ocarto.2025.100582.`

[402] Milad Yousefi, Matin Akhbari, Zhina Mohamadi, Shaghayegh Karami, Hediyeh Dasoomi, Alireza Atabi, Seyed Amirali Sarkeshikian, Mahdi Abdoullahi Dehaki, Hesam Bayati, Negin Mashayekhi, Shirin Varmazyar, Zahra Rahimian, Mahsa Asadi Anar, Daniel Shafiei, and Alireza Mohebbi. Machine learning based algorithms for virtual early detection and screening of neurodegenerative and neurocognitive disorders: a systematic-review. *Frontiers in Neurology*, 15, 2024. `doi:10.3389/fneur.2024.1413071.`

[403] Jordi Martorell-Marugán, Marco Chierici, Sara Bandres-Ciga, Giuseppe Jurman, and Pedro Carmona-Sáez. Machine learning applications in the study of parkinson's disease: A systematic review. *Current Bioinformatics*, 18(7):576–586, 2023. `doi:10.2174/1574893618666230406085947.`

[404] Hajar Rabie and Moulay A. Akhloufi. A review of machine learning and deep learning for parkinson's disease detection. *Discover Artificial Intelligence*, 5(1), 2025. `doi:10.1007/s44163-025-00241-9.`

[405] Thasina Tabashum, Robert Cooper Snyder, Megan K O'Brien, and Mark V Albert. Machine learning models for parkinson disease: Systematic review. *JMIR Medical Informatics*, 12:e50117–e50117, 2024. `doi:10.2196/50117.`

[406] Hwayoung Park, Changhong Youm, Sang-Myung Cheon, Bohyun Kim, Hyejin Choi, Juseon Hwang, and Minsoo Kim. Using machine learning to identify parkinson's disease severity subtypes with multimodal data. *Journal of NeuroEngineering and Rehabilitation*, 22(1), 2025. `doi:10.1186/s12984-025-01648-2.`

[407] Farhad Maleki, Katie Ovens, Rajiv Gupta, Caroline Reinhold, Alan Spatz, and Reza Forghani. Generalizability of machine learning models: Quantitative evaluation of three methodological pitfalls. *Radiology: Artificial Intelligence*, 5(1), 2023. `doi:10.1148/ryai.220028.`

[408] Ekin Yagis, Selamawet Workalemahu Atnafu, Alba García Seco de Herrera, Chiara Marzi, Riccardo Scheda, Marco Giannelli, Carlo Tessa, Luca Citi, and Stefano Diciotti. Effect of data leakage in brain mri classification using 2d convolutional neural networks. *Scientific Reports*, 11(1), 2021. doi:10.1038/s41598-021-01681-w.

[409] Matthew Rosenblatt, Link Tejavibulya, Rongtao Jiang, Stephanie Noble, and Dustin Scheinost. Data leakage inflates prediction performance in connectome-based machine learning models. *Nature Communications*, 15(1), 2024. doi:10.1038/s41467-024-46150-w.

[410] Jie Mei, Christian Desrosiers, and Johannes Frasnelli. Machine learning for the diagnosis of parkinson's disease: A review of literature. *Frontiers in Aging Neuroscience*, 13, 2021. doi:10.3389/fnagi.2021.633752.

[411] Charalampos Sotirakis, Zi Su, Maksymilian A. Brzezicki, Niall Conway, Lionel Tarassenko, James J. FitzGerald, and Chrystalina A. Antoniades. Identification of motor progression in parkinson's disease using wearable sensors and machine learning. *npj Parkinson's Disease*, 9(1), 2023. doi:10.1038/s41531-023-00581-2.

[412] Hong Lai, Xu-Ying Li, Fanxi Xu, Junge Zhu, Xian Li, Yang Song, Xianlin Wang, Zhanjun Wang, and Chaodong Wang. Applications of machine learning to diagnosis of parkinson's disease. *Brain Sciences*, 13(11):1546, 2023. doi:10.3390/brainsci13111546.

[413] Ibrahim Serag, Ahmed Y. Azzam, Amr K. Hassan, Rehab Adel Diab, Mohamed Diab, Mahmoud Tarek Hefnawy, Mohamed Ahmed Ali, and Ahmed Negida. Multimodal diagnostic tools and advanced data models for detection of prodromal parkinson's disease: a scoping review. *BMC Medical Imaging*, 25(1), 2025. doi:10.1186/s12880-025-01620-5.

[414] Mabrouka Salmi, Dalia Atif, Diego Oliva, Ajith Abraham, and Sebastian Ventura. Handling imbalanced medical datasets: review of a decade of research. *Artificial Intelligence Review*, 57(10), 2024. doi:10.1007/s10462-024-10884-2.

[415] Marc Ghanem, Abdul Karim Ghaith, Victor Gabriel El-Hajj, Archis Bhandarkar, Andrea de Giorgio, Adrian Elmi-Terander, and Mohamad Bydon. Limitations in evaluating machine learning models for imbalanced binary outcome classification in spine surgery: A systematic review. *Brain Sciences*, 13(12):1723, 2023. doi:10.3390/brainsci13121723.

[416] Jonathan Starcke, James Spadafora, Jonathan Spadafora, Phillip Spadafora, and Milan Toma. The effect of data leakage and feature selection on machine learning performance for early parkinson's disease detection. *Bioengineering*, 12(8):845, August 2025. doi:10.3390/bioengineering12080845.

[417] Rabie El Kharoua. Parkinson's disease dataset analysis, 2024. Accessed on: May 22, 2025. doi:10.34740/KAGGLE/DSV/8668551.

[418] Yibrah Gebreyesus, Damian Dalton, Sebastian Nixon, Davide De Chiara, and Marta Chinnici. Machine learning for data center optimizations: Feature selection using shapley additive explanation (shap). *Future Internet*, 15(3):88, 2023. doi:10.3390/fi15030088.

[419] Abdullah Marish Ali, Farsana Salim, and Faisal Saeed. Parkinson's disease detection using filter feature selection and a genetic algorithm with ensemble learning. *Diagnostics*, 13(17):2816, 2023. doi:10.3390/diagnostics13172816.

[420] Zeinab Noroozi, Azam Orooji, and Leila Erfannia. Analyzing the impact of feature selection methods on machine learning algorithms for heart disease prediction. *Scientific Reports*, 13(1), 2023. doi:10.1038/s41598-023-49962-w.

[421] Sheng-Chieh Lu, Christine L. Swisher, Caroline Chung, David Jaffray, and Chris Sidey-Gibbons. On the importance of interpretable machine learning predictions to inform clinical decision making in oncology. *Frontiers in Oncology*, 13, 2023. doi:10.3389/fonc.2023.1129380.

[422] David Nickson, Henrik Singmann, Caroline Meyer, Carla Toro, and Lukasz Walasek. Replicability and reproducibility of predictive models for diagnosis of depression among young adults using electronic health records. *Diagnostic and Prognostic Research*, 7(1), 2023. doi:10.1186/s41512-023-00160-2.

[423] Milad Mirbabaie, Stefan Stieglitz, and Nicholas R. J. Frick. Artificial intelligence in disease diagnostics: A critical review and classification on the current state of research guiding future direction. *Health and Technology*, 11(4):693–731, 2021. doi:10.1007/s12553-021-00555-5.

[424] Myura Nagendran, Yang Chen, Christopher A Lovejoy, Anthony C Gordon, Matthieu Komorowski, Hugh Harvey, Eric J Topol, John P A Ioannidis, Gary S Collins, and Mahiben Maruthappu. Artificial intelligence versus clinicians: systematic review of design, reporting standards, and claims of deep learning studies. *BMJ*, page m689, 2020. doi:10.1136/bmj.m689.

[425] Burak Kocak. Key concepts, common pitfalls, and best practices in artificial intelligence and machine learning: focus on radiomics. *Diagnostic and Interventional Radiology*, 28(5):450–462, 2022. doi:10.5152/dir.2022.211297.

[426] Alexandre Chiavegatto Filho, André Filipe De Moraes Batista, and Hellen Geremias dos Santos. Data leakage in health outcomes prediction with machine learning. comment on "prediction of incident hypertension within the next year: Prospective study using statewide electronic health records and machine learning". *Journal of Medical Internet Research*, 23(2):e10969, 2021. doi:10.2196/10969.

[427] Tom Viering and Marco Loog. The shape of learning curves: A review. *IEEE Transactions on Pattern Analysis and Machine Intelligence*, 45(6):7799–7819, 2023. doi:10.1109/tpami.2022.3220744.

[428] Juseon Hwang, Changhong Youm, Hwayoung Park, Bohyun Kim, Hyejin Choi, and Sang-Myung Cheon. Machine learning for early detection and severity classification in people with parkinson's disease. *Scientific Reports*, 15(1), 2025. doi:10.1038/s41598-024-83975-3.

[429] Rajib Kumar Halder, Mohammed Nasir Uddin, Md. Ashraf Uddin, Sunil Aryal, and Ansam Khraisat. Enhancing k-nearest neighbor algorithm: a comprehensive review and performance analysis of modifications. *Journal of Big Data*, 11(1), 2024. doi:10.1186/s40537-024-00973-y.

[430] Pedro Domingos. A few useful things to know about machine learning. *Communications of the ACM*, 55(10):78–87, 2012. doi:10.1145/2347736.2347755.

[431] Yanru Jiang and Rick Dale. Mapping the learning curves of deep learning networks. *PLOS Computational Biology*, 21(2):e1012286, 2025. doi:10.1371/journal.pcbi.1012286.

[432] Mohamed Aly Bouke and Azizol Abdullah. An empirical study of pattern leakage impact during data preprocessing on machine learning-based intrusion detection models reliability. *Expert Systems with Applications*, 230:120715, 2023. doi:10.1016/j.eswa.2023.120715.

[433] John R. Zech, Marcus A. Badgeley, Manway Liu, Anthony B. Costa, Joseph J. Titano, and Eric Karl Oermann. Variable generalization performance of a deep learning model to detect pneumonia in chest radiographs: A cross-sectional study. *PLOS Medicine*, 15(11):e1002683, 2018. doi:10.1371/journal.pmed.1002683.

[434] Adara Nogueira, Artur Ferreira, and Mario Figueiredo. A machine learning pipeline for cancer detection on microarray data: The role of feature discretization and feature selection. *BioMedInformatics*, 3(3):585–604, 2023. doi:10.3390/biomedinformatics3030040.

[435] Wei Zeng, Zhangbo Peng, Yang Chen, and Shaoyi Du. Multi-scale temporal analysis with a dual-branch attention network for interpretable gait-based classification of neurodegenerative diseases. *IEEE Journal of Biomedical and Health Informatics*, page 1–19, 2025. doi:10.1109/jbhi.2025.3580944.

[436] Ling-Chun Sun, Chun-Wei Tseng, Ke-Feng Lin, and Ping-Nan Chen. Hybrid preprocessing and ensemble classification for enhanced detection of parkinson's disease using multiple speech signal databases. *Digital Health*, 11, 2025. doi:10.1177/20552076251352941.

[437] Zhiheng Xu, Liwen Li, Xining Liu, Xiaoniu Liang, Mindi Yang, Yi Chen, Xixi Han, Jian Wang, Yilin Tang, Menghan Zhang, and Jianjun Wu. Evaluating the clinical utility of a machine learning model for diagnosing parkinson's disease using acoustic parameters. *Journal of Voice*, 2025. doi:10.1016/j.jvoice.2025.05.024.

[438] Milosz Dudek, Daria Hemmerling, Marta Kaczmarska, Joanna Stepien, Mateusz Daniol, Marek Wodzinski, and Magdalena Wojcik-Pedziwiatr. Analysis of voice, speech, and language biomarkers of parkinson's disease collected in a mixed reality setting. *Sensors*, 25(8):2405, 2025. doi:10.3390/s25082405.

[439] Giuseppe Marano, Sara Rossi, Ester Maria Marzo, Alice Ronsisvalle, Laura Artuso, Gianandrea Traversi, Antonio Pallotti, Francesco Bove, Carla Piano, Anna Rita Bentivoglio, Gabriele Sani, and Marianna Mazza. Writing the future: Artificial intelligence, handwriting, and early biomarkers for parkinson's disease diagnosis and monitoring. *Biomedicines*, 13(7):1764, 2025. doi:10.3390/biomedicines13071764.

[440] Francesco Asci, Gaetano Saurio, Giulia Pinola, Marco Falletti, Alessandro Zampogna, Martina Patera, Francesco Fattapposta, Simone Scardapane, and Antonio Suppa. Micrographia in parkinson's disease: Automatic recognition through artificial intelligence. *Movement Disorders Clinical Practice*, 2025. doi:10.1002/mdc3.70208.

[441] Ali Mohd Ali, Mohammad R. Hassan, Faisal Aburub, Mohammad Alauthman, Amjad Aldweesh, Ahmad Al-Qerem, Issam Jebreen, and Ahmad Nabot. Explainable machine learning approach for hepatitis c diagnosis using sfs feature selection. *Machines*, 11(3):391, 2023. doi:10.3390/machines11030391.

[442] Daniel Nasef, Demarcus Nasef, Viola Sawiris, Brett Weinstein, Jodan Garcia, and Milan Toma. Integrating artificial intelligence in clinical practice, hospital management, and health policy: literature review. *Journal of Hospital Management and Health Policy*, 9:20–20, 2025. `doi:10.21037/jhmhp-24-138`.

[443] Muhammad Farooq Siddique, Faisal Saleem, Muhammad Umar, Cheol Hong Kim, and Jong-Myon Kim. A hybrid deep learning approach for bearing fault diagnosis using continuous wavelet transform and attention-enhanced spatiotemporal feature extraction. *Sensors*, 25(9):2712, 2025. `doi:10.3390/s25092712`.

[444] Wasim Zaman, Muhammad Farooq Siddique, Shafi Ullah Khan, and Jong-Myon Kim. A new dual-input cnn for multimodal fault classification using acoustic emission and vibration signals. *Engineering Failure Analysis*, 179:109787, 2025. `doi:10.1016/j.engfailanal.2025.109787`.

[445] Gary S Collins, Karel G M Moons, Paula Dhiman, Richard D Riley, Andrew L Beam, Ben Van Calster, Marzyeh Ghassemi, Xiaoxuan Liu, Johannes B Reitsma, Maarten van Smeden, Anne-Laure Boulesteix, Jennifer Catherine Camaradou, Leo Anthony Celi, Spiros Denaxas, Alastair K Denniston, Ben Glocker, Robert M Golub, Hugh Harvey, Georg Heinze, Michael M Hoffman, André Pascal Kengne, Emily Lam, Naomi Lee, Elizabeth W Loder, Lena Maier-Hein, Bilal A Mateen, Melissa D McCradden, Lauren Oakden-Rayner, Johan Ordish, Richard Parnell, Sherri Rose, Karandeep Singh, Laure Wynants, and Patricia Logullo. Tripod+ai statement: updated guidance for reporting clinical prediction models that use regression or machine learning methods. *BMJ*, page e078378, April 2024. URL: `http://dx.doi.org/10.1136/bmj-2023-078378`, `doi:10.1136/bmj-2023-078378`.

Dawning Research Press

Founded in 20_9, Dawning Research Press is dedicated to publishing scholarly works that bridge academic rigor with public understanding. Our mission is to illuminate complex issues at the intersection of science, society, and human experience.

Contact Information

Email: admin@dawningresearch.org
Website: www.dawningresearch.org

For information about permissions, bulk purchases, educational discounts, or media inquiries, please contact us at the email address above.

Committed to evidence-based scholarship and accessible science communication.

www.ingramcontent.com/pod-product-compliance
Lightning Source LLC
Chambersburg PA
CBHW071848270326
41929CB00013B/2139